Mental Health Policy
for Older Americans

Mental Health Policy for Older Americans: Protecting Minds at Risk

Edited by

Barry S. Fogel, M.D.
*Associate Professor of Psychiatry and Human Behavior
and Associate Director, Center for Gerontology and
Health Care Research, Brown University*

Antonio Furino, Ph.D.
*Professor of Economics and Director,
Center for Studies in Health Economics,
The University of Texas Health Science Center at San Antonio*

Gary L. Gottlieb, M.D., M.B.A.
*Associate Professor of Psychiatry;
Director, Section of Geriatric Psychiatry,
University of Pennsylvania; and Senior Fellow,
Leonard Davis Institute for Health Economics*

American Psychiatric Press, Inc.

Washington, D.C.
London, England

Copyright © 1990 American Psychiatric Press, Inc.
ALL RIGHTS RESERVED
Manufactured in the United States of America
90 91 92 93 94 5 4 3 2 1

American Psychiatric Press, Inc.
1400 K Street, N.W.
Washington, DC 20005

The paper used in this publication meets the minimum requirements of American National Standard for Information Sciences—Permanence of Paper for Printed Library Materials, ANSI Z39.48-1984.

Library of Congress Cataloging-in-Publication Data

Mental health policy for older Americans : protecting minds at risk / edited by Barry S. Fogel, Antonio Furino, Gary L. Gottlieb.
    p.   cm.
    Includes bibliographical references.
    ISBN 0-88048-320-2 (alk. paper)
    1. Mental health policy—United States. 2. Aged—Mental health services—United States. I. Fogel, Barry S. II. Furino, Antonio. III. Gottlieb, Gary L.
    [DNLM: 1. Health Policy—United States. 2. Mental Disorders—in old age. 3. Mental Health Services—economics—United States. 4. Mental Health Services—in old age—United States.   WT 150 M5495]
  RA790.6.M443 1990
  362.2′0973—dc20
  DNLM/DLC
  for Library of Congress   90-86
                                                CIP

British Cataloguing in Publication Data

A CIP record is available from the British Library

Contents

Contributors . . . . *vii*

Acknowledgments . . . . *ix*

Preface . . . . *xi*

DIMENSIONS OF THE PROBLEM

1 Minds at Risk 1
   Barry S. Fogel, M.D.
   Gary L. Gottlieb, M.D., M.B.A.
   Antonio Furino, Ph.D.

2 The Economic Perspective 23
   Antonio Furino, Ph.D.
   Barry S. Fogel, M.D.

3 The Nature and Efficacy of Interventions for
   Depression and Dementia 37
   Barbara Kamholz, M.D.
   Gary L. Gottlieb, M.D., M.B.A.

4 Mental Health Services in General Medical
   Care and in Nursing Homes 63
   Barbara J. Burns, Ph.D.
   Carl A. Taube, Ph.D.

PAYING THE BILL

5 Division of Responsibility Among Payers . . . 85
   Howard H. Goldman, M.D., Ph.D.
   Richard G. Frank, Ph.D.

6 Payment for Services: A Provider's
   Perspective 97
   Steven S. Sharfstein, M.D.

7 Physician Payment Reform 109
   Barry S. Fogel, M.D.

8 The Cost-Offset Effect 125
   Judith R. Lave, Ph.D.

PROVIDING SERVICES

9 Market Segmentation 135
   Gary L. Gottlieb, M.D., M.B.A.

10 The Psychiatric Component of Long-Term
   Care Models 157
   Gail K. Robinson, Ph.D.

11 Testing New Models of Service Delivery . . . 179
   Robert L. Kane, M.D.

MANAGING CARE

12 The Relevance of Case Management 201
   Rosalie A. Kane, Ph.D.

13 Managed Care 221
   Terrie Wetle, Ph.D.
   Hal Mark, Ph.D.

14 Chronic Mental Illness 239
   Linda H. Aiken, Ph.D.

ASSESSING THE PRESENT AND SHAPING THE FUTURE

15 Present and Future Solutions 257
   Barry S. Fogel, M.D.
   Gary L. Gottlieb, M.D., M.B.A.
   Antonio Furino, Ph.D.

APPENDICES

I.   A Window on the Debate: Dialogues from the
     National Conference 279

II. The Organization of the Psychiatric Inpatient
     Services System 305

III. Glossary 323

IV. Conference Participants 345

     Index 349

Contributors

Linda H. Aiken, Ph.D.
Trustee Professor of Nursing and Sociology, University of Pennsylvania; and Associate Director, Leonard Davis Institute for Health Economics

Barbara J. Burns, Ph.D.
Professor of Medical Psychology, Department of Psychiatry, Duke University Medical Center

Barry S. Fogel, M.D.
Associate Professor of Psychiatry and Human Behavior and Associate Director, Center for Gerontology and Health Care Research, Brown University

Richard G. Frank, Ph.D.
Associate Professor, Health Services Research and Development Center, Department of Health Policy and Management, School of Hygiene and Public Health, The Johns Hopkins University

Antonio Furino, Ph.D.
Professor of Economics and Director, Center for Studies in Health Economics, The University of Texas Health Science Center at San Antonio

Howard H. Goldman, M.D., Ph.D.
Professor of Psychiatry, School of Medicine; and Director, Mental Health Policy Studies, University of Maryland

Gary L. Gottlieb, M.D., M.B.A.
Associate Professor of Psychiatry; Director, Section of Geriatric Psychiatry, University of Pennsylvania; and Senior Fellow, Leonard Davis Institute for Health Economics

Barbara Kamholz, M.D.
Clinical Assistant Professor, Hospital of the University of Pennsylvania; and Staff, Institute of Pennsylvania Hospital

Robert L. Kane, M.D.
Dean, School of Public Health, University of Minnesota

Rosalie A. Kane, Ph.D.
Professor, School of Social Work, and School of Public Health; and Director, University of Minnesota National Long-Term Care Decisions Resource Center, Division of Health Services Research and Policy, University of Minnesota

Judith R. Lave, Ph.D.
Professor of Health Economics, Graduate School of Public Health, University of Pittsburgh

Hal Mark, Ph.D.
Assistant Professor, Department of Community Medicine and Health Care, School of Medicine, University of Connecticut; and Director of Managed Care Research, Institute of Living

Gail K. Robinson, Ph.D.
Associate Director, Mental Health Policy Resource Center, Washington, D.C.

Steven S. Sharfstein, M.D.
Executive Vice President and Medical Director, Sheppard and Enoch Pratt Hospital; and Clinical Professor of Psychiatry, University of Maryland

Carl A. Taube, Ph.D.[*]
Professor, Mental Hygiene Department, School of Hygiene and Public Health, The Johns Hopkins University

Terrie Wetle, Ph.D.
Director of Research, Braceland Center for Mental Health and Aging, Institute of Living; Associate Professor of Community Medicine and Health Care, School of Medicine, University of Connecticut; and Lecturer on Medicine, Harvard Medical School

*Deceased.

Acknowledgments

This book was written in connection with the National Conference on Access and Financing for Neuropsychiatric Care for the Elderly, held at Brown University in October 1988. Financial support for the Conference, and for the preparation of the manuscript for this book, was provided by The RGK Foundation, the Upjohn Company, Brown University, the Rhode Island Department of Health, the National Institute of Mental Health, the Voluntary Hospitals of America, and the American Association of Retired Persons. We are indebted for intellectual contributions to all of the participants in the National Conference, and especially to all those who contributed manuscripts, recorded conference sessions, and critiqued manuscripts. A complete list of conference participants and their institutional affiliations is found in the final appendix to this book. Ms. Christine Ferguson of Senator John Chafee's office, Ms. Lauren Gross of Senator Claiborne Pell's office, and Ms. Lori Gibson of Representative Claudine Schneider's office, were extraordinarily helpful in introducing us to legislative staff people, and in educating us about some of the intricacies of legislative process.

We thank Ms. Janice Miller and Ms. Rita St. Pierre of Brown University for administrative support for the conference and post-conference activities, and all of our secretaries for their assistance in the typing and retyping of manuscripts.

Our families, of course, deserve credit for their support and forbearance during this time-consuming endeavor.

Finally, special thanks are due to Dr. George Kozmetsky, who inspired thousands of hours of human effort by a few provocative questions over the breakfast table.

Preface

Informed discussion of policy issues concerning the mental health of older Americans requires the integration of epidemiologic and clinical perspectives with historical, political, and pragmatic viewpoints on the organization and financing of mental health care. This interdisciplinary volume comprises efforts toward that end. It is written for policymakers and advocates, for entrepreneurs and intrapreneurs in the business of providing health and mental health services to the elderly, and for clinicians treating the elderly who wish to know more about the context in which they provide care.

The book is divided into five main sections, addressing: overall dimensions of the problem, financing care, providing services, managing care, and assessing present and future directions for policy development. The main text is followed by four appendices.

In Chapter 1, the editors describe seven major risks to the mental health of older people, estimate their prevalence, and indicate when effective treatment is known to exist. We also describe general features of neuropsychiatric assessment and treatment.

In Chapter 2, Antonio Furino and Barry S. Fogel discuss the economic implications of neuropsychiatric disorders in an aging American population. They emphasize not only familiar concerns about health care and long-term care costs, but also the relevance of mental health issues to the economic productivity of the elderly.

In Chapter 3, Barbara Kamholz and Gary L. Gottlieb review the nature and efficacy of therapeutic interventions for depression and dementia. Readers seeking a summary of specific biologic and psychotherapeutic treatments will find it here; those concerned more narrowly with policy implications, or lacking in a clinical background, might skip the middle sections and read the introductory and concluding sections that address the generalities of treatment and their implications for service delivery.

In Chapter 4, Barbara Burns and Carl Taube, drawing upon recent national epidemiologic studies, estimate the need for mental health services in primary medical care settings and in nursing homes. They establish a substantial unmet need for services in primary care, and a profound deficit in services for nursing home residents. Options for change, both in policy and in provider behavior, are identified.

In Chapter 5, Howard Goldman and Richard Frank explore the historical roots and current status of the division of responsibility between the states and the Federal government in paying for mental health care. They discuss the relative advantages and disadvantages of direct governmental responsibility for service provision as opposed to contractual relationships with non-governmental providers. For interested readers, further detail of the current elaborate division of responsibility for payment for inpatient psychiatric services is provided in Appendix II, which reprints an outstanding recent review article by Dr. Goldman and his colleagues Carl Taube and Stephen Jencks.

In Chapter 6, Steven Sharfstein, the medical director of a large private psychiatric hospital, addresses issues of third-party payment from a provider's perspective. The critical insurance concepts of adverse selection, moral hazard, and cost-sharing are defined and discussed. While supporting the concept of more favorable reimbursement for "medical management" of psychiatric disorders, he points out the risks of developing incentives for a narrowly biomedical approach to late-life mental illness.

In Chapter 7, the senior editor offers a detailed analysis of the recent Harvard Resource-Based Relative Value Scale (RBRVS) study. It is argued that a relative value scale based only on primary diagnosis, and not taking into account multiple diagnoses including neuropsychiatric disorders, is unlikely to provide physicians with proper incentives for addressing their elderly patients' complex problems in a holistic and comprehensive fashion. The chapter offers a "microscopic" analysis of how the Harvard study approached evaluation of psychiatric services for the elderly, and presents reasons why geriatric psychiatric care often is time-consuming and effortful.

In Chapter 8, Judith Lave defines and analyzes the potential for mental health services to reduce, or "offset," the costs of other medical and supportive care. She identifies several major areas where cost-offset effects may exist, and where future clinical and economic investigation is warranted. However, she emphasizes that improved access for the elderly to mental health services is already warranted by the evidence for their *clinical* efficacy.

In Chapter 9, Gary L. Gottlieb defines and differentiates the many classes of providers that render mental health services, and estimates their degree of involvement in the care of the elderly. He advocates the development of an empirical basis for assigning specific roles for particular provider groups. Division of the mental health services market into rational "market segments" could lead to more efficient care than is currently provided under conditions of unrestricted competition, often political as well as economic, among provider groups.

In Chapter 10, Gail Robinson examines the psychiatric aspects of four current models for comprehensive long-term care services for older adults. She observes that existing long-term care models insufficiently address the mental health needs of their clients, but that they do offer a promising structure for coordinating care. Potentially, models could then offer improved access to mental health services at a containable and acceptable cost. She also notes that problems of stigma and of limited human resources have limited mental health services even in plans where they are adequately funded.

In Chapter 11, Robert Kane establishes a framework for evaluating new models of service delivery. Drawing on his extensive experience in geriatric assessment research, he recommends desirable features of new service delivery models, and offers specific guidelines for program evaluation. Crucial issues addressed include the choice of goals and measures, legal and administrative constraints on innovation, and the need to choose an appropriate timeframe for evaluation. He makes a strong plea for evaluation to be designed prospectively and integrated with program planning.

In Chapter 12, Rosalie Kane defines "case management," placing the often-used concept into historical and disciplinary context. Arguing from empirical studies (or their lack), she establishes that case management is no panacea for managing frail or mentally ill elderly, but that it may have a valuable role in coordinating services for the chronically mentally ill, and in helping older people obtain needed services from overlapping and fragmented sources of care.

In Chapter 13, Terrie Wetle and Hal Mark explore the potential of comprehensive managed care systems, particularly exclusive provider organizations (EPOs), to facilitate access to mental health care by making the service provider at risk for the adverse medical and social consequences of undertreated mental illness. They advocate demonstration projects that focus on groups at high risk for service use. Such projects could shed light on the difficult technical questions that must be resolved if managed care plans are to take on the challenge of improving mental health services for their clients.

In Chapter 14, Linda Aiken focuses attention on the elderly with severe and chronic mental illnesses—especially those with long-standing mental illnesses who have grown old. She emphasizes that state mental health systems must continue to play a major role in the care of this group of elderly mentally ill, as other providers are neither organized nor funded to assume that function. Medicaid reform, however, could improve incentives for the development of innovative programs that would provide a broader range of community-based treatment alternatives for the chronically mentally ill elderly.

In the concluding chapter, the editors recapitulate the policy recommendations of the preceding chapters. Following this summary, we present a personal view of the present Federal policy environment, as it is expressed in recent legislation. We conclude by offering three guiding themes for future policy development.

The main text is followed by four appendices. The first offers vignettes and brief summaries of actual dialogues among policymakers, advocates, researchers, and service providers, derived from transcripts of the 1988 National Conference on Access and Financing for Neuropsychiatric Care of the Elderly. The vignettes offer interested readers a feel for the shared assumptions and qualitative differences in viewpoint among various actors in the policy debate.

The second appendix, reprinted with permission from *Medical Care,* offers a detailed description of the organization and financing of inpatient psychiatric services. As inpatient care is the most costly, best-reimbursed, and most highly regulated part of the mental health service system, a grasp of its structure would be particularly helpful to those concerned with coverage policy.

The third appendix is a glossary of terms frequently encountered in discussions of mental health policy. While primarily intended to assist readers with the interpretation of jargon, it occasionally offers comments on the context and connotations of the terminology.

A final appendix lists the participants in the National Conference on Access and Financing for Neuropsychiatric Care of the Elderly, and their institutional affiliations.

The broad scope of this book implies that not all of its content will be relevant for all of its readers. The glossary, and the cross-references within chapters, are designed to permit selective reading. However, we strongly encourage all readers to begin with Chapter 1, and to consider the summary recommendations, current issues, and future options presented in the concluding chapter. Readers primarily concerned with professional issues might focus on Chapters 2, 3, 6, 7, 8, and 9. Public mental health program directors and administrators might find Chapters 4, 5, 10, 11, 12, 13, and 14 specifically relevant. Elderly advocates might focus on Chapters 2, 3, 4, 6, 10, 11, and 14.

1

Minds at Risk

Barry S. Fogel, M.D.
Gary L. Gottlieb, M.D., M.B.A.
Antonio Furino, Ph.D.

Risks to the mind, including Alzheimer's disease, depression, confusional states, and the emotional consequences of brain disease and physical disability loom large among the concerns of elderly people and their families. Not uncommonly, older people express a preference for death over loss of their mental faculties. In addition, family caretakers cope better with the physical care of a disabled relative than they cope with agitation, uncooperativeness, or personality changes that make a positive personal relationship difficult. While public awareness of the mental disorders of late life has grown substantially, medical practice, medical education, and health care financing are still a long way from fully incorporating a sophisticated understanding of mental and behavioral issues into the health care of the elderly. In the hope of contributing to the eventual integration of physical and mental health care for the elderly, this book will describe various aspects of the problem, and indicate some promising directions for policy development and for research.

Seven major risks to elderly minds, hereafter referred to as neuropsychiatric disorders, are: 1) dementia (Alzheimer's disease and related disorders); 2) depression; 3) schizophrenia and other chronic mental illnesses; 4) behavioral and emotional consequences, other than dementia, of brain disease or dysfunction; 5) prescription drug psychotoxicity; 6) alcoholism and prescription drug abuse; and 7) maladaptive emotional reactions to predictable crises of later life, including bereavement, retirement, and acute medical illness.

Each of these problems has different implications for health service delivery. For example, patients with chronic schizophrenia

1

are highly likely to become clients of public sector mental health systems. When these people grow old, they may continue to look to these systems for access to care and for coordination of services. By contrast, individuals with complicated bereavement and no prior history of mental illness are highly unlikely to avail themselves of public sector mental health systems, because these systems are unfamiliar, stigmatized, and not geared to address that type of problem. Older adults with depression are most likely to seek relief from their primary care physicians; specialty mental health services of any kind are unlikely to be used unless the primary physician initiates or supports an appropriate referral.

Financial responsibility also differs among the different neuropsychiatric disorders. Traditionally, through community mental health centers (CMHCs) and state hospitals, the states have had the primary financial burden of caring for people with chronic schizophrenia. On the other hand, the acute treatment of depression or confusional states is funded by Medicare. Long-term care in nursing homes is primarily the responsibility of Medicaid. Even though the problems of aged schizophrenics may overlap substantially with the problems of individuals with dementia, recent federal legislation has focused on attempting to exclude chronic schizophrenics from receiving Medicaid-funded nursing home treatment, largely on the grounds that this has traditionally been a state responsibility.

Because the problem of minds at risk is segmented, advocates and policy-makers are frequently in peril of advancing the interests of one group of patients or providers at the expense of another. Consciousness of the different segments of the problem is a first step toward preventing destructive competition of diverse and equally legitimate interests.

A Note on Nomenclature

In discussing the issue of risks to elderly minds, an immediate problem presents regarding nomenclature. Traditionally, the term *mental illness* has been associated with severe disturbances of thought or behavior, such as those produced by schizophrenia. Some people even associate mental illness mainly with disturbed people who are violent. The term *mental health* is somewhat better. It implies a concern with the emotional problems of ordinary people, and suggests the possibility of prevention. Unfortunately, *mental health facilities* are still the places where *mentally ill* people go, and so they are associated with stigma. Furthermore, mental health has no necessary connection with the medical profession, or with the assumption of a medical orientation in evaluating and treating disturbances of behavior and mood. *Psychiatric* and *psychological* may be slightly less stigmatized terms, but they too have drawbacks. They are associated with specific provider disciplines. Also, psychiatry is equated in some circles with psychotherapy, and in others with a rather narrow medication-oriented approach. Psychologists, depending on their community, may be seen primarily as people who administer psychological tests, or perhaps as behavior therapists. *Emotional problems* does not capture the issue either, as many of the problems of the elderly involve disturbances of intellect, perception, and other brain functions that are not primarily emotional. For these reasons, the editors have chosen the term *neuropsychiatric* as a relatively unfamiliar and hopefully less stigmatized term that captures the relevance of both mind and brain, cognition and emotion, to the behavioral problems of late life. In its narrow usage, neuropsychiatry refers to the diagnosis and treatment of psychiatric complications of brain disease and dysfunction, and to an approach to mental illness that emphasizes brain dysfunction. If the term is used this narrowly, it too is perhaps unsatisfactory, but still may have fewer negatives than the alternatives. Throughout this book, the terms *neuropsychiatry* and *neuropsychiatric* will be the preferred terms to describe that field of health care that addresses the cognitive, emotional, and behavioral dimensions of patients' problems, with special attention to the role of brain disease and dysfunction in causing or aggravating those problems. The term will not be used to imply primacy of any particular provider group, as many medical specialties, nonmedical health providers, providers of social services, and paraprofessionals have a role to play in addressing various aspects of neuropsychiatric disorders. On occasion, contributors to this volume will use the terms *mental health* and *mental illness;* it should be clear from context whether these terms are intended as synonyms for *neuropsychiatric* or whether a different meaning is intended.

The Common Neuropsychiatric Disorders

Each of the common neuropsychiatric disorders is now discussed with attention to epidemiology, complications, and health services implications. The reader primarily interested in health services can abbreviate this section by reading the first paragraph of each subsection, and then skipping to the concluding paragraph or two of the subsection. These concluding paragraphs are marked with bullets in the left margin.

Dementia

Approximately 5% of the population over age 65 suffer from severe cognitive impairment (Cummings and Benson 1983). The most common cause is senile dementia of the Alzheimer type, or Alzheimer's disease. At age 80, 15%–20% of the population have significant cognitive impairment (Thompson 1987; Jarvik 1980; Campbell et al. 1983); about half of those have Alzheimer's disease (Katzman and Terry 1983; Katzman et al. 1988). For every patient with a definite dementia, there are two to three more with mild to moderate symptoms of cognitive impairment sufficient to impair some area of everyday function (Kral 1978; Mortimer 1980). About two-thirds of nursing home residents suffer from dementia (Schneck 1982; Chandler and Chandler 1988). For each demented patient in a nursing home, there are two to three more in the community with an equal level of impairment who are cared for by some combination of family, friends, and paid caretakers (Katzman and Terry 1983; U.S. Department of Health and Human Services 1982).

Ten percent to 25% of patients with dementia have causative neurological, psychiatric, or medical disorders that can be either arrested or completely reversed (Thompson 1987; Cummings and Benson 1983). Thus, while most patients with dementia have an irreversible disorder, the proportion with specific, treatable causative or aggravating factors is large enough to warrant a search for these factors in virtually all cases severe enough to impair everyday function (Katzman et al. 1988). (Exhaustive evaluation of the early, pre symptomatic stages of dementia is controversial. Robert Kane addresses this issue in Chapter 11.)

Coexisting depression or psychosis affects at least one-third of patients with Alzheimer's disease (Thompson 1987; Reifler 1986; Rubin et al. 1988; Wragg and Jeste 1989); depression occurs in approximately one-half of patients with multi-infarct dementia, the second most common dementing disorder (Lechner et al. 1988). These psychiatric complications of dementia aggravate functional impairment and substantially increase the burden of care, whether the patient is at home or in a nursing facility.

Family caretakers of patients with Alzheimer's disease are highly vulnerable to depression and to stress-related physical and emotional complaints. Some studies have suggested that more than half of family caretakers of demented patients may suffer from a diagnosable depression at some time during the course of care (Cohen and Eisdorfer 1988).

• The initial object of the medical assessment of patients with suspected dementia is the confirmation of the diagnosis and a diligent search for remediable factors that are causal or contributory. Subsequent medical intervention focuses on management of comorbid medical problems and on treating specific behavioral complications, such as depression, psychosis, or sleep-wake disturbances that may contribute excess disability. In the longer term, care focuses on educating and supporting family caretakers to preserve the patient in the community for as long as possible. Ultimately, if a patient becomes so severely impaired that the need for care goes beyond what the family can provide, the patient is placed in a nursing facility. Acute medical services for demented patients generally are covered by Medicare as well as by private insurance. However, outpatient psychiatric services, apart from initial evaluation and medical management, are subject to a 50% copayment. Outpatient therapeutic services by psychologists and social workers have been covered only since the recent passage of OBRA 1989 and are also subject to the 50% copayment. Medicare reimbursement for therapeutic services by clinical social workers does not apply to services rendered in hospitals or nursing homes. Patients and families must rely on private resources for the support of home help and nursing home care, until they become so impoverished that they are eligible for Medicaid support of these services.

Ideal care for dementia also addresses the needs of caretaking families before, during, and after the placement process. These needs include education, concrete services, respite, and assistance with emotional reactions to the patient's changed behavior (Szwabo 1988). These services when available may be partially funded by various state, local, and nonprofit voluntary agencies. Treatment for caretaker emotional problems is not funded by Medicare unless the caretaker herself is a Medicare beneficiary.

Depression

Approximately 15% of elderly living in the community have a clinically significant degree of dysphoria—that is, they feel bad persistently to an extent that impairs their function and/or ability to enjoy life. About 4% have a major depression not associated with a medical illness, another 6.5% have depression associated with medical illness, and 4.5% have a dysphoric mood that does not reach major depressive proportions (Blazer and Williams 1980). In ambulatory medical care settings the proportions are higher: 30% to 50%

of the elderly have significant depressive symptoms, often reaching the full syndrome of major depression. In institutional long-term care facilities such as nursing homes, about 25% of the best functioning residents have major depression (Katz et al. 1988). Depressive symptoms and signs may be even more prevalent among patients with worse function, but with sufficient cognitive capacity to perceive their situation.

Depression is associated with increased mortality, both from suicide and from cardiovascular and cerebrovascular disease. The age-specific suicide rate is highest for the elderly, and the majority of elderly suicide victims are depressed prior to committing suicide (Katz et al. 1988).

Patients with physical illness and disability who are also depressed are less likely to regain function than similarly disabled patients who are not depressed (Harris et al. 1988; Gurland et al. 1986). Depression has been associated with worse functional outcomes from a physical condition (e.g., stroke), and its treatment has been associated with improved function (Reding et al. 1986).

• Acute treatment of depression in late life usually begins with a primary care physician. More severe cases, particularly if accompanied by psychotic features or suicidal behavior, usually find their way to psychiatrists or mental health facilities; however, depressions in which major symptoms are physical rather than mental may escape the mental health system, and receive less-than-adequate treatment in the general health sector (Fogel and Fretwell 1985; see Chapter 4).

Medicare is the usual funding for the acute treatment of late-life depression. There are substantial copayments for outpatient treatment and lifetime limits on inpatient treatment in psychiatric hospitals. Therapeutic services by psychologists and clinical social workers, covered only since the passage of OBRA 1989, are also subject to substantial copayments. Therefore, individuals with chronic, treatment-resistant, or frequently recurring depressions may ultimately exhaust their Medicare inpatient psychiatric benefits and/or private resources and come to depend, like many demented patients, upon Medicaid.

Schizophrenia and Paranoia

Chronic *schizophrenia* afflicts 0.3% to 1.0% of community-dwelling elderly persons. One-third of chronically institutionalized elderly, in state hospitals and in nursing homes, are also afflicted (Katz et al. 1988; Babigian and Lehman 1987; Siegel and Goodman

1987). In late life, some chronic schizophrenics may show less dramatic psychopathology, such as hallucinations and overtly bizarre behavior, than do younger schizophrenics. In many cases, these patients' behavioral syndromes overlap with those displayed by individuals with dementia, with the prominent findings being impaired abstract reasoning, impaired memory, and diminished ability to cope with life, in association with unusual or idiosyncratic ideas (Harrow et al. 1987; Heaton and Drexler 1987; Craig and Bregman 1988).

The vast majority of patients with chronic schizophrenia have an onset of illness prior to middle age. They are most likely to receive treatment in the public sector, either from a state hospital, a community mental health center, or a Veterans Administration hospital. Patients with the late-onset form of schizophrenia, called *paraphrenia,* may enter treatment through the general health system. Since paraphrenics usually present with florid delusions (Roth 1987), referral from the general health sector to the specialty mental health sector usually occurs rapidly after presentation.

- For the most part, care of patients with chronic schizophrenia takes place in state mental health systems, and is funded by state and local governments with support from Federal block grants. However, when elderly schizophrenics are placed in nursing homes, Medicaid may become the primary payer.

Persecutory ideation, or *paranoia,* is present in 4% of elderly people living in the community. Half of these individuals are cognitively intact, the other half cognitively impaired (Christenson and Blazer 1984). Unlike patients with the full syndrome of schizophrenia, individuals with persecutory ideation are not necessarily impaired in their ability to cope with everyday life. However, paranoia becomes highly problematic when individuals must be hospitalized, -must move, or must be treated for acute medical illness. In these situations, ideas of persecution may become major barriers to cooperation with care or adaptation to new surroundings.

- Since the adaptational problems of patients with persecutory ideation are acute though their disorder is chronic, treatment is usually by general physicians, and is paid for by Medicare.

Behavioral and Emotional Consequences of Brain Disease and Dysfunction, Other Than Dementia

This heterogeneous group of disorders, which includes delirium, or the acute confusional state, is highly prevalent among elderly people, and constitutes the core of neuropsychiatry in the narrow sense. While these conditions are studied by neurologists, psychiatrists, geriatricians, and neuropsychologists, they are most often encountered in the practice of primary care medicine with the elderly. Most are treatable, if not completely reversible. The greatest risks of these disorders lie in misdiagnosis, or lack of diagnosis, where, in the worst case, delay leads to a reversible condition becoming irreversible. Several of the most common are detailed below.

Delirium. Delirium, or the acute confusional state, affects at least 20% of elderly patients admitted to general hospitals with acute medical or surgical illness, and at least 10% of elderly patients admitted to mental hospitals with behavioral symptoms (Lipowski 1984; Beresin 1988). Patients with specific acute medical conditions, like hip fracture or recent open heart surgery, have an especially high prevalence of delirium (Levitan and Kornfeld 1981; Smith and Dimsdale 1989; Gustafson et al. 1988). Delirium often is associated with specific disturbances of blood chemistry or metabolism, or with drug intoxication or withdrawal. However, particularly in frail elderly patients, it may be produced by the stress of physical illness, trauma, or even environmental change, in the absence of readily measurable changes in blood chemistry.

While in its most florid forms delirium is unmistakable, milder forms may be overlooked by physicians completely, or thought to represent disorders of purely emotional origin (Sullivan and Fogel 1986).

Compared with nondelirious patients with the same medical diagnoses, delirious patients have a significantly higher mortality rate, as great as double in some studies (Wise 1987; Guze and Daengsurisri 1967). In one prospective controlled study, early recognition and intervention in post-hip fracture delirium reduced hospital length of stay and the proportion of nursing home placements following discharge (Levitan and Kornfeld 1981).

• Treatment of delirium comprises making a diagnosis, correcting remediable causes, and managing the patient's disturbed behavior until the confusion resolves. Diagnosis and management of the medical dimension is the task of the primary care physician, often assisted by other medical subspecialty consultants. Behavioral management will tend to involve psychiatrists if the patient is violent, dangerous to self, or psychotic. In this situation, the patient usually remains on a medical inpatient service, with the psychiatrist offering ongoing consultation or occasionally concurrent care. The primary physician's medical care is covered by Medicare; the psychiatric interventions are incompletely reimbursed because of Medicare limits on follow-up consultations. Treatment of delirium frequently necessitates counseling family members, who can be frightened and perplexed by the patient's abrupt change in behavior and mentation. This counseling, which is neither psychotherapy nor a direct medical service to the patient, tends to be poorly reimbursed by Medicare, and is not covered at all if the counseling is provided in the hospital or nursing home by a clinical social worker or nurse clinician.

Parkinson's disease. This condition affects almost 2% of the population at age 70, and an even larger proportion at older ages (Evans and Caird 1982). The disorder is complicated by significant depression in approximately 40% of cases (Mayeux 1984; Santamaria et al. 1986), and by cognitive impairment in approximately 50% of cases (Portin and Rinne 1986; Growdon and Corkin 1986). Both the depression and the cognitive impairment are direct consequences of the brain degeneration, rather than separate and concurrent problems, or merely emotional reactions to disability (Mayeux et al. 1986). Biologic treatment of the depressive symptomatology usually is effective, and may improve functional status. Many of the drugs used to treat Parkinson's disease, including L-dopa, Sinemet, and amantadine, may produce confusional states or psychosis (Lishman 1987b). Adjustment of drug therapy to balance physical and mental considerations can be quite subtle.

- Treatment of the psychiatric complications usually is carried out by the neurologist treating the Parkinson's disease, and is covered by Medicare. Psychiatrists and other mental health specialists usually are not involved unless the symptomatology is remarkably florid, with psychotic or suicidal behavior, or is refractory to the neurologist's efforts at treatment.

Stroke. The prevalence of stroke is at least 5% of the population over age 65, with a higher prevalence among blacks and people of lower socioeconomic status (Wolf et al. 1984). Approximately 50% of strokes are complicated by depression. Post-stroke depression appears to be a direct consequence of the brain damage, rather than emotional reaction to disability, as the severity and symptomatology of depression correlates well with the precise location of the brain injury, rather than with the degree of disability (Robinson and Forrester 1987). In addition to depression, more unusual behavioral syndromes specific to particular stroke locations are described in the literature of behavioral neurology (Lishman

1987c). Post-stroke depression has been shown to respond to anti-depressant drug therapy in a placebo-controlled trial (Lipsey et al. 1984), and in one study physical and cognitive function improved with antidepressants (Reding et al. 1986).

- Treatment of post-stroke depression, when it is undertaken, usually is carried out by neurologists, primary care physicians, or rehabilitation specialists; referrals to psychiatrists are relatively infrequent and generally are reserved for patients with unusually severe or refractory symptoms. As with other organically caused mood states, under-diagnosis and under-treatment are the rule. Under-diagnosis has been attributed to erroneous attribution of depressed mood as a transient emotional reaction, and to diffi-culties in assessing mood in the presence of brain damage. Under-treatment is explained in part by a reluctance to prescribe adequate doses of antidepressant drugs in the face of significant physical illness. Nonetheless, many stroke patients can tolerate therapeutic doses of antidepressant medication (Robinson and Forrester 1987).

Epilepsy. Epilepsy affects at least 2% of the population over age 60 (Evans and Caird 1982). Approximately one-third of epileptic patients suffer from clinically significant depression. The adminis-tration of drug treatment to epileptic patients is complicated by drug interactions between antidepressant drugs and anticonvulsant drugs; on occasion antidepressant drugs may aggravate the patients' seizures (McNamara 1987; Fogel 1988).

- Treatment usually is undertaken by neurologists, although more difficult cases are referred to psychiatrists and other specialty mental health providers.

Hypothyroidism. Deficiency of thyroid hormone occurs in 3% to 4% of community elderly (Hurley 1983; Sawin et al. 1985) and up to 9% of hospitalized elderly (Livingston et al. 1987). Depression, cognitive impairment, and other mental status changes are among the most common early symptoms, and they may precede the development of overt physical signs such as reduced body temperature or abnormal reflexes (Lishman 1987a). The diagnosis is easily made through a blood test, the thyroid-stimulating hor-mone (TSH) level, and treatment by replacement of thyroid hor-mone is 100% effective. However, if a patient has severe hypothy-roidism and has gone untreated for a prolonged period, some changes in cognition and behavior may be permanent.

- Since synthetic thyroid hormone is cheap and readily available, treatment is trivial once the diagnosis is made. The diagnosis requires the administration of a suitably sensitive test of thyroid function to patients at risk. Despite the ease of making the diagnosis, it remains among the most common previously unsuspected medical diagnoses encountered by inpatient geropsychiatric units (Felicetta 1988).

Vitamin B$_{12}$ deficiency. This disorder, which can occur spontaneously or as a complication of gastrointestinal surgery or general malnutrition, may be a causal or contributory factor to psychiatric illness in as many as 12% of elderly people with severe mental symptoms (Shulman 1967). In a general population without risk factors, the prevalence rate is no less than 1% (Lishman 1987d). B$_{12}$ deficiency may present with confusion and memory loss, with depression, or with personality change. Mental symptoms can occur alone or in combination with anemia or disturbance in gait. Routine laboratory tests may be normal, the diagnosis may not be made unless it is considered and a level of vitamin B$_{12}$ checked.

- Treatment with vitamin B$_{12}$ injections is always effective in arresting the progression of symptoms, and will usually reverse symptoms if the disease has not been too long-standing. As with hypothyroidism, treatment is trivial as long as the diagnosis is not excessively delayed (Adams and Victor 1981).

Psychotoxicity of Prescription Drugs

The precise incidence of psychotoxicity of prescription drugs is difficult to ascertain, because the majority of psychotoxic reactions go either undetected or unreported. However, it is well known that the incidence of adverse reactions to prescription drugs increases with age, and is estimated to be three to seven times greater in the elderly than in young people (Caird and Scott 1986). Particularly problematic drugs include cardiac drugs such as digitalis, beta-blockers, calcium-channel blockers, and anti-arrhythmics; anti-inflammatory drugs including both steroids and nonsteroidal agents, and most of the common psychotropic drugs, including antidepressants and sedatives (Besdine 1988). Depression, anxiety, memory loss, insomnia, apathy, and confusional states are all common presentations and may occur at usual therapeutic doses of these drugs in vulnerable patients. These conditions are aggravated by the prescription of multiple drugs to the same patient, a common occurrence. Over-the-counter drugs purchased by patients for problems such as insomnia, cold symptoms, and minor aches and pains may contain active ingredients with psychotoxic effects. Often, patients are treated by multiple physicians, leading to a drug list that is not completely known by anyone. Systematic elimination of psychotoxic drugs and rationalization of drug regimens may improve function and reduce mental and behavioral symptoms.

- The evaluation of patients for potential drug toxicity generally is performed by primary care physicians, although pharmacists are increasingly taking a role in this activity, since they often are the only professionals with complete lists of all the drugs patients are taking. Specialists in geriatrics, psychiatry, or clinical pharmacology sometimes are involved when the diagnosis of drug toxicity is obscure, or when patients appear to have unusual drug sensitivities or interactions.

Alcoholism and Prescription Drug Abuse

Alcoholism, which is frequently associated with the misuse of prescription drugs, is present in 5% to 10% of community elderly, and in more than 10% of elderly patients seeking medical care (Beresford et al. 1988). In particular populations such as V.A. hospitals and inner city public hospitals, more than 20% of patients may suffer from alcoholism (Blazer and Pennybacker 1984; Curtis et al. 1989).

Alcoholism in the elderly is associated with cognitive impairment, mood disorder, and a wide variety of physical complications, including increased risk of liver disease, blood disorders, cancer, and respiratory infection (Gambert et al. 1984). A particular type of dementia is associated with chronic alcoholism, although its precise neurological etiology is not known (Meyer et al. 1984).

- Treatment of elderly patients with alcoholism involves the same elements as treatment of younger patients with alcoholism, including confrontation of the patient and family by the physician, insistence on total abstinence as a goal, and the use of group support, including Alcoholics Anonymous. There is some evidence that elderly patients do best in homogeneous groups of elderly alcoholics, rather than mixed-age groups. Despite the evidence that alcohol treatment in the elderly can be effective, both diagnosis and referral for treatment are less likely to occur in elderly medical patients with alcoholism than with their younger counterparts (Curtis et al. 1989).

Treatment for alcoholism is funded by Medicare, with 50% copayments for outpatient services by covered specialty providers.

Inpatient care is subject to prospective payment by a single diagnostic-related group (DRG), so that elderly alcoholics who were medically complicated or slow to regain function might be money-losers for an inpatient alcohol facility. The provision of supervision and social services for demented or chronically deteriorated alcoholics falls upon state mental health systems, or Medicaid. Private insurance coverages vary.

Prescription drug abuse in the absence of alcoholism often is associated with long-standing personality problems. Its precise prevalence is not known, although it is not uncommon in general medical settings (Busse and Blazer 1980). Successful management of the problem requires some coordination of care among the various physicians, clinics, and pharmacists with whom the patient does business.

Maladaptive Emotional Reactions to Predictable Crises of Later Life, Including Bereavement, Retirement, and Acute Medical Illness

Stressful life events, particularly losses, are ubiquitous in late life. For the most part, older persons cope with them without any need for professional help, relying on their inner resources and upon the social support provided by family, friends, community, and religion. However, certain stresses, such as life-threatening illness or the loss of a lifelong companion, are of such magnitude that they may combine with the physiologic vulnerabilities of an older person to produce a clinically significant depression or anxiety state. These problems may aggravate the person's chronic medical problems or cognitive impairments, or may lead to bad judgments such as impulsive decisions to retire, change residence, go to a nursing home, or move in with children.

The prevalence of a clinically significant depression following the loss of a spouse in late life is more than 30% one month later and at least 16% after one year (Stroebe and Stroebe 1987). The prevalence of depression in conjunction with major medical illness is likewise at least 30% (Katz et al. 1988). The epidemiology of maladaptive anxiety is less well established but it is known that generalized anxiety, panic attacks, and phobias affect at least 6% of the general population, and that these disorders tend to be aggravated by major life stresses, especially losses (Faravelli and Pallanti 1989).

Risk factors for the development of clinically significant anxiety or depression include a personal or family history of depression or anxiety, preexisting medical conditions associated with mood disturbance, and consumption of psychotoxic prescription. Untreated, these depression and anxiety states may lead to more severe or chronic neuropsychiatric problems. The greatest risks are of medical or social consequences from impulsive decisions or maladaptive health behaviors carried out during the period of the crisis.

Patients who experience these disorders often seek no treatment, even if they are experiencing considerable distress, because they expect themselves to cope with the problem, or to rely upon informal social support. Those who do seek treatment tend to obtain it from their primary care physician, whose usual response is medication, most often an anti-anxiety drug (see Chapter 4). More effective treatment, to be described below, would probably include psychotherapeutic and medical interventions (Marmar et al. 1988). Most acute mental problems occurring in the context of life crises respond to relatively short-term treatment, which is covered by Medicare if rendered by a psychiatrist or, since the passage of OBRA 1989, by a psychologist or clinical social worker. A 50% copayment applies. Most private insurance plans also have significant copayments or apply annual caps to total reimbursement for mental health treatment.

General Features of Neuropsychiatric Assessment and Treatment

Neuropsychiatric assessment and treatment of the elderly differs from generic psychiatric or "mental health" treatment, because the relative role of organic factors, concurrent medical illness, and functional disability is much larger in the elderly than in most other populations that seek psychiatric treatment (Jenike 1988).

Regardless of the presenting problem, there are several features common to comprehensive neuropsychiatric evaluation of the elderly. These are discussed here, and are listed in Table 1-1.

The elderly patient with a probable neuropsychiatric disorder requires the collection of a history of present illness, family background, and personal development, as do all patients with significant behavioral complaints. In addition, the history must include an exhaustive exploration of past and present medical problems, and the treatments for those problems. The majority of elderly people with mental complaints have one or more active medical illnesses, and may have a history of prior illness, trauma, or surgery that may have late effects relevant to brain function, for example a past stroke or a history of gastrectomy predisposing to vitamin B_{12} deficiency.

Elicitation of the medical history and establishment of a drug history may require the use of collateral sources, particularly if memory impairment or confusion is part of the identified problem. This may involve review of outside medical records, conversations with other care providers, or having the patient or family bring in a paper bag filled with the entire contents of the medicine cabinet.

Once a medical history is fully established, a formal mental status examination must be performed. This examination must pay special attention to disturbances in memory, cognition, and perception. Given the high prevalence of delirium and dementia in elderly patients, the presence or absence of these disorders must be established. Knowledge of the patient's cognitive capacities and memory also are necessary to establish the patient's ability to follow advice or prescriptions, or to profit from psychotherapeutic interventions.

A physical examination must be performed, not only to establish whether there are untreated or inadequately treated active medical problems, but also to establish the status of vision, hearing, and neurologic functions including gait and coordination. Impairment of vision affects almost half of elderly people by age 85 (Wright and Henkind 1983), and hearing impairment affects half of elderly by age 80 (Ruben and Kruger 1983). These sensory impairments not only affect an elderly person's general quality of life, but also are relevant to their ability to communicate, to understand medical instructions, to read prescriptions, and to carry on a meaningful dialogue with family members or care providers.

A neurological examination may detect the earliest evidence of a primary brain disease such as Parkinson's disease or a small stroke, which not only may be causative of the patient's neuropsychiatric problem, but may also require further assessment or treatment in its own right.

Laboratory data, particularly concerning metabolic status, drug levels, and brain function must be reviewed. This will include review of CT scans, magnetic resonance images, and EEG, if they are performed. In many cases, these tests must be completed before a firm diagnosis can be made.

A final component of assessment is an evaluation of the patient's ability to function in everyday life. This includes assessment both of physical functions such as bathing, dressing, toileting, transfers, and continence, and also the so-called instrumental activities of daily living, including the ability to shop, use public transportation, and handle one's own finances (Katz and Stroud 1989). Evaluation of function is necessary to determine what supportive services an individual may require, and to set realistic functional goals for treatment.

Table 1–1.   Components of comprehensive neuropsychiatric
evaluation

- History of present illness
- Medical history
- Family history
- Personal developmental history
- Information from collateral sources
- Complete drug review
- Physical examination
- Neurological examination, including gait
  assessment
- Hearing and vision screening
- Mental status examination
- Review of laboratory data
- Neurodiagnostic tests
- Functional assessment

Treatment

Once assessment is complete, treatment must begin with remediation of whatever untreated or under-treated medical problems the patient has, as well as removal or substitution whenever possible of drugs and substances with psychotoxic effects (Larson et al. 1985; Fogel and Kroessler 1987). This is accompanied or followed by more specific psychosocial and psychopharmacologic interventions directed at the patient's specific problem. Psychotherapy generally is reserved for patients whose neuropsychiatric problem is linked to a clear-cut emotional conflict, personal crisis, or disturbance of personality. Major mood disturbances and psychotic thinking are virtually always treated with appropriate medications or with electroconvulsive therapy (ECT). Finally, environmental interventions, including family therapy, institutional placement, or various community support services are mobilized for individuals who need supervision, ongoing emotional support, or concrete services.

In the selection of drug therapy for those who require it, great attention must be given to the patient's medical illnesses and medical drug regimen, to avoid toxicity and dangerous drug interactions. Drug therapy often involves careful and repeated monitoring of drug effects or drug levels to protect the patient from these adverse consequences (Stoudemire and Fogel 1987).

Thus, generic neuropsychiatric care for the elderly is remarkable for the intensity of medical involvement, the close integration of medical and psychiatric services, the emphasis on functional assessment, and the frequent involvement of family or formal social services to render support.

References

Adams RD, Victor M: The neurologic manifestations of vitamin B_{12} deficiency, in Principles of Neurology, 2nd ed. Adams RD, Victor M. New York, McGraw-Hill, 1981

Babigian HM, Lehman AF: Functional psychoses in later life: epidemiological patterns from the Monroe County Psychiatric Register, in Schizophrenia and Aging. Edited by Miller NE, Cohen GD. New York, Guilford Press, 1987

Beresford TP, Blow FC, Bower KJ, et al: Alcoholism and aging in the general hospital. Psychosomatics 29:61-72, 1988

Beresin EV: Delirium in the elderly. Journal of Geriatric Psychiatry and Neurology 1:127-143, 1988

Besdine RW: Dementia and Delirium in Geriatric Medicine, 2nd ed. Edited by Rowe JW, Besdine RW. Boston, Little Brown, 1988

Blazer DG, Pennybacker MR: Epidemiology of alcoholism in the elderly, in Alcoholism in the Elderly. Edited by Hartford JT, Samorjski T. New York, Raven Press, 1984

Blazer D, Williams CD: Epidemiology of dysphoria and depression in an elderly population. American Journal of Psychiatry 139:439-444, 1980

Busse EW, Blazer DG: Disorders related to biological functioning, in Handbook of Geriatric Psychiatry. Edited by Busse EW, Blazer DG. New York, Van Nostrand Reinhold, 1980

Caird FI, Scott PJW: Drug-Induced Diseases in the Elderly. Amsterdam, Elsevier, 1986

Campbell A, McCosh L, Reinken J, et al: Dementia in old age and the need for services. Age and Ageing 12:11-16, 1983

Chandler JD, Chandler JE: The prevalence of neuropsychiatric disorders in the nursing home population. Journal of Geriatric Psychiatry and Neurology 1:71-76, 1988

Christenson R, Blazer D: Epidemiology of persecutory ideation in an elderly population in the community. Am J Psychiatry 141:1088-1091, 1984

Cohen D, Eisdorfer C: Depression in family members caring for a relative with Alzheimer's disease. Journal of the American Geriatrics Society 36:885-889, 1988

Craig TJ, Bregman Z: Late-onset schizophrenia-like illness. Journal of the American Geriatrics Society 36:104-107, 1988

Cummings JL, Benson DF: Dementia: a clinical approach. Boston, Butterworth, 1983

Curtis JR, Geller G, Stokes EJ, et al: Characteristics, diagnosis, and treatment of alcoholism in elderly patients. Journal of the American Geriatrics Society 37:310-316, 1989

Evans JG, Caird FI: Epidemiology of neurological disorders in old age, in Neurological Disorders in the Elderly. Edited by Caird FI. Bristol, Wright-PSG, 1982

Faravelli C, Pallanti: Recent life events and panic disorder. American Journal of Psychiatry 146:622-626, 1989

Felicetta JV: The thyroid and aging, in The Endocrinology of Aging. Edited by Sowers JR, Felicetta JV. New York, Raven Press, 1988

Fogel B: Combining anticonvulsants with conventional psychotropic drugs, in Use of Anticonvulsants in Psychiatry: Recent Advances. Edited by McElroy S, Pope HG. Clifton, NJ, Oxford Health Care, 1988

Fogel B, Fretwell M: Reclassification of depression in the medically ill elderly. Journal of the American Geriatrics Society 33:446-448, 1985

Fogel BS, Kroessler D: Treating late-life depression on a medical psychiatric unit. Hospital and Community Psychiatry 38:829-831, 1987

Gambert SR, Newton M, Duthie EH: Medical issues in alcoholism, in the Elderly in Alcoholism in the Elderly. Edited by Hartford JT, Samorjski T. New York, Raven Press, 1984

Growdon JH, Corkin S: Cognitive impairments in Parkinson's disease. Advances in Neurology 45:383-392, 1986

Gurland BJ, Golden R, Lantigua R, et al: The overlap between physical conditions and depression in the elderly: a key to improvement in service delivery, in The Patient and Those Who Care: The Mental Health Aspect of Long-Term Physical Illness. Edited by Nayer D. Nantucket, MA, Watson Publishers International, 1986

Gustafson Y, Berggreen D, Bramnstrom B, et al: Acute confusional states in elderly patients treated for a femoral neck fracture. Journal of the American Geriatrics Society 36:525-530, 1988

Guze SB, Daengsurisri S: Organic brain syndromes: prognostic significance in general medical patients. Archives of General Psychiatry 17:365-366, 1967

Harris RE, Mion LC, Patterson MB, et al: Severe illness in older patients: the association between depressive disorders and functional dependency during the recovery phase. Journal of the American Geriatrics Society 36:890-896, 1988

Harrow M, Marengo J, Pogue-Geile M, et al: Schizophrenic deficits in intelligence and abstract thinking: influence of aging and long-term care institutionalization, in Schizophrenia and Aging. Edited by Miller NE, Cohen GD. New York, Guilford Press, 1987

Heaton RK, Drexler M: Clinical neuropsychological findings, in Schizophrenia and Aging. Edited by Miller NE, Cohen GD. New York, Guilford Press, 1987

Hurley JR: Thyroid disease in the elderly. Medical Clinics of North American 67:497, 1983

Jarvik L: Diagnosis of dementia in the elderly: A 1980 perspective, in Annual Review of Gerontology and Geriatrics, Vol 1. Edited by Eisdorfer C. New York, Springer, 1980

Jenike MA: Assessment and treatment of affective illness in the elderly. Journal of Geriatric Psychiatry and Neurology 1:89-107, 1988

Katz IR, Curlik S, Nemetz P: Functional psychiatric disorders in the elderly, in Essentials of Geriatric Psychiatry. Edited by Lazarus LW. New York, Springer, 1988

Katz S, Stroud MW: Functional assessment in geriatrics: a review of progress and directions. Journal of the American Geriatrics Society 37:267-271, 1989

Katzman R, Terry R: The Neurology of Aging. Philadelphia, F. A. Davis, 1983

Katzman R, Lasker B, Bernstein N: Advance in the diagnosis of dementia: accuracy of diagnosis and consequences of misdiagnosis of disorders causing dementia, in Aging and the Brain. Edited by Terry RD. New York, Raven Press, 1988

Kral VA: Benign senescent forgetfulness, in Aging, Vol 7. Edited by Katzman R, Terry RD, Bick KL. New York, Raven Press, 1978

Lechner H, Bertha G, Ott E: Results of a five-year prospective study of 94 patients with vascular and multi-infarct dementia, in Vascular and Multi-Infarct Dementia. Edited by Meyer JS, Lechner H, Marshall J, Toole JF. Mt. Kisco, NY, Futura Publishing Company, 1988

Levitan SJ, Kornfeld DS: Clinical and cost benefits of liaison psychiatry. American Journal of Psychiatry 138:790-793, 1981

Larson EB, Featherstone HJ, Reifler BV, et al: Medical aspects of care of elderly patients with cognitive impairment. Developmental Neuropsychology 1:145-171, 1985

Lipowski ZJ: Acute confusional states (delirium) in the elderly, in Clinical Neurology of Aging. Edited by Albert ML. New York, Oxford University Press, 1984

Lipsey JR, Robinson RG, Pearlson GD, et al: Nortriptyline treatment of post-stroke depression: a double-blind treatment trial. Lancet 1:297-300, 1984

Lishman WA: Hypothyroidism (myxoedema), in Organic Psychiatry. Edited by Lishman WA. Oxford, Blackwell, 1987a

Lishman WA: Parkinson's disease in the parkinsonian syndrome, in Organic Psychiatry. Edited by Lishman WA. Oxford, Blackwell, 1987b

Lishman WA: Symptoms and syndromes with regional affiliations, in Organic Psychiatry. Edited by Lishman WA. Oxford, Blackwell, 1987c

Lishman WA: Vitamin B_{12} Deficiency in Organic Psychiatry. Edited by Lishman WA. Oxford, Blackwell, 1987d

Livingston EH, Hershman JM, Sawin CT, et al: Prevalence of thyroid disease and abnormal thyroid tests in older hospitalized and ambulatory persons. Journal of the American Geriatrics Society 35:109-114, 1987

Marmar CR, Horowitz MJ, Weiss DS, et al: A controlled trial of brief psychotherapy and mutual-help group treatment of conjugal bereavement. American Journal of Psychiatry 145:203-209, 1988

Mayeux R, Williams JBW, Stern Y, et al: Depression in Parkinson's disease. Advances in Neurology 40:241-250, 1984

Mayeux R, Stern Y, Williams JBW, et al: Depression in Parkinson's disease. Advances in Neurology 45:451-455, 1986

McNamara ME: Neurology, in Principles of Medical Psychiatry. Edited by Stoudemire A, Fogel B. Orlando, Grune and Stratton, 1987

Meyer JS, Largen JW, Shaw T: Interactions of normal aging, senile dementia, multi-infarct dementia, and alcoholism in the elderly, in Alcoholism in the Elderly. Edited by Hartford JT, Samorjski T. New York, Raven Press, 1984

Mortimer JA: Epidemiologic aspects of Alzheimer's disease, in Advances in Neurogerontology, Vol 1: The Aging Nervous System. Edited by Maletta GJ, Perrozzolo FJ. New York, Praeger, 1980

Portin R, Rinne UK: Predictive factors for cognitive deterioration and dementia in Parkinson's disease. Advances in Neurology 45:413-416, 1986

Reding MJ, Orto LA, Winter SW, et al: Antidepressant therapy after stroke: a double-blind trial. Archives of Neurology 43:763-765, 1986

Reifler BV: Mixed cognitive-affective disturbances in the elderly: a new classification. Journal of Clinical Psychiatry 47:354-356, 1986

Robinson RG, Forrester AW: Neuropsychiatric aspects of cerebrovascular disease, in The American Psychiatric Press Textbook of Neuropsychiatry. Edited by Hales RE, Yudofsky SC. Washington, DC, American Psychiatric Press, 1987

Roth M: Late paraphrenia: phenomenology and etiological factors and their bearing upon the schizophrenic families of disorders, in Schizophrenia and Aging. Edited by Miller NE, Cohen GD. New York, Guilford Press, 1987

Ruben RJ, Kruger B: Hearing loss in the elderly, in The Neurology of Aging. Edited by Katzman R, Terry R. Philadelphia, F. A. Davis, 1983

Rubin EH, Drevets WC, Burke WJ: The Nature of psychotic symptoms in senile dementia of the Alzheimer type. Journal of Geriatric Psychiatry and Neurology 1:16-20, 1988

Santamaria J, Tolosa ES, Valles A, et al: Mental depression in untreated Parkinson's disease of recent onset. Advances in Neurology 45:443-446, 1986

Sawin CT, Castelli WP, Hershman JM, et al: The aging thyroid: thyroid deficiency in the Framingham study. Archives of Internal Medicine 145:1386-1388, 1985

Schneck SA: Aging of the nervous system and dementia, in Clinical Internal Medicine in the Aged. Edited by Schrier RW. Philadelphia, W. B. Saunders, 1982

Shulman R: A survey of vitamin B_{12} deficiency in an elderly psychiatric population. British Journal of Psychiatry 113:241-251, 1967

Siegel CE, Goodman AB: Mental illness among the elderly in a large state psychiatric facility: a comparison with other age groups, in Schizophrenia and Aging. Edited by Miller NE, Cohen GD. New York, Guilford Press, 1987

Smith LW, Dimsdale JE: Post-cardiotomy delirium: conclusions after 25 years. American Journal of Psychiatry 146:452-458, 1989

Stoudemire A, Fogel BS: Psychopharmacology in the medically ill, in Principles of Medical Psychiatry. Edited by Stoudemire A, Fogel BS. Orlando, Grune & Stratton, 1987

Stroebe W, Stroebe MS: Bereavement and Health. Cambridge, Cambridge University Press, 1987

Sullivan N, Fogel B: Could this be delirium? American Journal of Nursing 86:1359-1363, 1986

Szwabo PA: The family as an integral part of the management of central nervous system disorders, in Central Nervous System Disorders of Aging: Clinical Intervention and Research. Edited by Strong R, Wood WG, Burke WJ. New York, Raven Press, 1988

Thompson TL: Dementia, in The American Psychiatric Press Textbook of Neuropsychiatry. Edited by Hales RE, Yudofsky SC. Washington, DC, American Psychiatric Press, 1987

U.S. Department of Health and Human Services: White House Conference on Aging (1982). Bethesda, MD, U.S. Department of Health and Human Services, 1982

Wise MG: Delirium, in The American Psychiatric Press Textbook of Neuropsychiatry. Edited by Hales RE, Yudofsky SC. Washington, DC, American Psychiatric Press, 1987

Wolf PA, Kannel WB, Verter J: Cerebrovascular diseases in the elderly: epidemiology, in Clinical Neurology of Aging. Edited by Albert ML. New York, Oxford University Press, 1984

Wragg RE, Jeste DV: Overview of depression and psychosis in Alzheimer's disease. American Journal of Psychiatry 146:577-587, 1989

Wright BE, Henkind P: Aggravating changes in the eye, in The Neurology of Aging. Edited by Katzman R, Terry R. Philadelphia, F. A. Davis, 1983

2

The Economic Perspective

Antonio Furino, Ph.D.
Barry S. Fogel, M.D.

Lack of attention to the disorders of mood, cognition, and behavior, often accompanying physical illness in later life, may aggravate disability and functional impairments and worsen medical prognosis (Millard 1983; Cutler and Fine 1985; see Chapter 1). Yet, traditionally, primary care providers are not routinely trained to adequately evaluate and manage geriatric neuropsychiatric problems (Waxman and Carner 1984). And, older adults use specialty mental health services rarely (Walman et al. 1984; see Chapter 4).

Individuals and society may gain from timely treatment of neuropsychiatric disorders not only because it is likely to improve the overall outcome of medical care, but, under certain circumstances, it may reduce its cost (see Chapter 8).

Those aging Americans who are employed often must cope with decline in work efficiency due to neuropsychiatric disorders. Diminished productivity at work or increased absenteeism may be the consequence of subclinical physical illness, substance abuse, anxiety, depression, or mild cognitive impairment (Harwood et al. 1984; Lavizzo-Hourey et al. 1988; Luce et al. 1978; Gottlieb 1988). Workers experiencing diminished well-being because of undiagnosed neuropsychiatric disorders, particularly depression, may retire early, misattributing their withdrawal from the work force to age or to situation. Yet, as the age structure of the population changes, the contributions of older workers will be essential to the national economy (Soldo and Agree 1988). Promoting the health and productivity of older workers is one of the key outcomes of preventive gerontology as it goes beyond concern with survival and attempts to increase the duration of physiological and psychological competence. The prevention and modification of the secondary forms of aging (those not genetically determined) offer the best hope for cost effective and cost worthy strategies to face the potentially disastrous challenge of financing adequate health care for a graying America (Hazzard 1989).

This chapter explores some of the economic implications of making neuropsychiatric care more accessible to our aging population.

The pages that follow sketch the demographic and socioeconomic environment in which the problem of access to neuropsychiatric care is set. The magnitude of the problem is described, economic implications are assessed, and some policy-relevant considerations are offered.

The Socioeconomic Environment

The future of the American health care system is uncertain and its contribution to the quality of life of its citizens is being debated. Radical changes in health care delivery and financing have been implemented or proposed in the past decade both by private insurers and by the federal government. These payers are reacting to unprecedented increases in health-related expenditures (from $12.7 billion in 1950 to an estimated $590 billion in 1989, or from 4% to over 12% of gross national product) in a context of hypercompetitive global markets and an excessively large federal budget deficit. Simultaneously, there are high public expectations of the power of medicine, disillusionment with providers, wondrous technological developments, and decreasing access to health care by the poor and by minorities. Further, while a commitment to ethical and scientific concerns persists, health policy has become tantamount to budget policy in the federal realm (Walsh 1989).

The cost containment imperatives dictated by both payers and consumers attach special relevance to three trends that are reshaping the structure of the nation's population. They are a low birth rate, the increasing longevity of older adults and the maturing of an unusually large population group known as the "baby boom generation." Made up of persons born during the post-World War II period between 1946 and 1964, the baby boom generation has captured national attention and continues to command adjustments in the allocation of economic resources as the needs of its members change while they progress through life.

Public administrators remember well the exceptional pressures on educational facilities during the 1950s and 1960s. Then, the attention of these young men and women and of many politicians turned, during the 1970s and the 1980s, to jobs and housing, to being in debt, to budget deficits and interest rates, to reducing or eliminating taxes and to attaining national and personal security.

During the 1990s and the early decades of the next century, the financial position of the "baby boomers" will shift from that of net debtors to that of net creditors, and they will become concerned about the role that government services play in their lives, including Medicare and the options available for long-term care (Amara et al. 1988). While widespread public sentiment favoring the allocation of additional resources to address the unmet needs of the current generation of elderly is lacking, evidence about the size and urgency of present and forthcoming problems exists now (Windom 1988).

The Size of the Problem

The expected prevalence of neuropsychiatric morbidity and of its functional consequences can usefully be viewed in the context of sociodemographic data presented in two recent publications on the elderly (Fowles 1988; Soldo and Agree 1988). High points from the two reports are presented and discussed below.

In 1960, one in eleven Americans was at least 65 years old. Today the proportion is just over one in eight. It will be one in four by 2030. Three major groups of elderly are identified as the "young old" (65- to 74-year-old persons), the "older old" (75 to 84) and the "oldest old" (85 and older). While the dividing line of functional age is related to personal capacities and accomplishments and is only loosely correlated with chronological age, a policy-relevant definition of advanced age is set by law at age 65 (67 after the year 2000) when full Social Security retirement benefits become available to individuals. (Actually, the authors believe that too little attention is given to the 15 years preceding retirement when appropriate counseling, education, and intervention may promote higher productivity and greater well-being for aging workers.)

A combination of decreasing mortality and low fertility is increasing Americans' median age from 23 years in 1900 to 40 in the year 2020. By 2050, more than one quarter of the population over 65 will be made up of the oldest old (over 85). These demographic changes are not only of dramatic magnitudes, but are new for our society. Because of their novelty, the needs of the elderly, including their health needs, while predictable, are not necessarily perceived as urgent by the large majority of the younger generations. As already noted, public concern over the plight of the elderly will change drastically when, in 2030, approximately 75 million baby boomers will have reached their sixties.

While the absolute numbers of elderly are impressive—approximately 31 million now, 35 million in the year 2000, and 51 million in 2020, according to projections by the U.S. Census Bureau—the *relative* number of older persons in our society has greater economic significance. A rectangular shape of the "population pyramid" depicting approximately the same percentage of people in younger and older age groups, will be almost completely attained by 2030. The largest relative increase will take place between 2010 and 2030 when the baby boom generation begins crossing the 65-year mark. Since many services for the elderly are funded through intergenerational transfers (i.e., the use of contributions from younger and working individuals to pay for the needs of "dependent" age cohorts), the proportion of young versus old (the "dependency ratio") can be used as a rough index of the magnitude of society's burden in providing financial assistance to senior citizens. There were 19 retirees for every 100 workers in 1985. From conservative estimates, they will double to 38 by 2050. The situation is helped somewhat by 1983 legislation that mandates a retirement age of 67 before the baby boomers begin reaching retirement age. However, calculations by the Office of the Actuary of the Social Security Administration indicate that to maintain the dependency ratio at its 1985 level, the cut-off age for eligibility would need to be 74 by the year 2050.

Because of differences in life expectancy, membership in the older age cohorts favors women in the ratio of 1.5 to 1 among the 65 and over and by 2.5 to 1 among the 85 and over age groups. The economic importance of the survival rate differentials is considerable. The surviving female spouse usually has less earning potential or pension income than her husband. Women, in general, are more dependent on their children and on institutional health care settings such as nursing homes, in part because they are more likely to be widowed. Among other differences characterizing the 65 years and older group, the most obvious, besides age and sex, and perhaps the most ignored in research and policy, are ethnic differences. A broad definition of ethnicity distinguishes social groups on the basis of race (i.e., blacks, whites), religion (i.e., Mormon, Jewish), and national origin (i.e., Hispanics) (Gordon 1964). Ethnic minorities are increasing as a proportion of the total population and are, on the average, "younger" than their majority counterpart (in 1980 the proportion of individuals 65 years old or older was 11% for whites, 8% for blacks, 6% for Asian and Pacific Islanders, and 5% for Hispanics and native Americans). The reasons for the difference in age structure are differential fertility and mortality rates of the minority cohorts.

While minority elderly are proportionally fewer, they are more likely to need services in addition to health care (income maintenance, housing, meals, transportation) because of a condition of "double jeopardy" (Markides and Mindel 1987; Bengtson 1979; Foner 1979; Jeffries and Ransford 1980). The disadvantage of being a member of a minority group is aggravated by old age (Dowd and Bengtson 1978). The problem is multidimensional (Hazzard 1989). First, there are differences in the biophysiological manifestation of diseases among persons of ethnic minority background. Second, there are differences in the ways health care is sought and received among different sociocultural groups. Third, there are factors related to the lack of financial resources and underclass status shared by many members of ethnic minorities. Fourth, minority groups may be culturally unprepared to fully utilize available institutional services, particularly nursing home care (Valle 1989).

The economic impact of underserved elderly minorities is felt differentially in different parts of the country because of the concentration of ethnic minorities in particular regions and urban areas (e.g., the concentration of Hispanics in the states of California, Florida, Illinois, New York, and Texas). As the size of the minority population increases faster than the total, so does the regional burden of caring for individuals who, after many years of neglect, experience an intensification of their underprivileged condition due to age. The disadvantage is likely to be ignored until it leads to demand for acute and expensive health care, often of little value to the patient in terms of quality of life. The lack of adequate research data hides the magnitude and the urgency of the problem and contributes to the exclusion, in most cases, of culturally relevant services from the planning of health care delivery mechanisms. Additionally, stigma and inadequate education are particularly powerful forces among minority elderly in limiting the provision and use of appropriate neuropsychiatric services. Underservice and underutilization should never be confused with desirable cost containment efforts since the result of neglecting the health needs of the underprivileged, particularly regarding prevention and community-based assistance, produces not only a morally unacceptable condition of human suffering, but also is likely to create larger needs and expenditures in other areas of public welfare and in expensive acute medical care.

Household median income increases as the head of the household grows older, up to age 55. Then, the change in personal income is in the opposite direction, with a drop of one third to one half after age 65. The dramatic decrease pushes many individuals into the ranks of the legally poor at a most vulnerable time of their life. In 1986, one in eight elderly (3.5 million of age 65 or older) had income below the poverty level. Only one out of 10 younger persons shared a similar condition. The ratio is one out of five for individuals over age 85. In 1986, 40% of elderly income came from Social Security and 15% from wages and salaries. Only 16 years earlier, the proportions were 25% and 50%, respectively. The reduction in income during this vulnerable period of the individual's life span increases the need for assistance from the family, the community, the state, and the Federal government.

The number of days in which usual activities are restricted because of illness or injury increases with age. Older persons averaged 32 such days in 1986 (28 days for males and 35 days for females; 31 days for whites, 43 days for blacks). They spent all or most of 15 of these days in bed (12 days for males, 17 days for females; 14 days for whites, 21 days for blacks).

Most older persons have at least one chronic condition, and many have multiple conditions. In 1986, the most prevalent conditions were arthritis (48%), hypertension (39%), hearing impairments (29%), heart disease (30%), orthopedic impairments and sinusitis (17% each), cataracts (14%), diabetes and visual impairments (10% each), and tinnitus (9%).

The need for functional assistance increases sharply with age. In 1984 about 6 million (23%) older persons living in the community needed the assistance of another person to perform one or more selected personal care or home management activities. The percentage of those requiring assistance varied with age: 14% for persons 65 to 74, 26% for persons 75 to 84, and 48% for persons over 85. (Selected personal care activities included bathing, dressing, eating, toileting, getting in or out of a bed, and getting around inside. Selected home management activities included preparing meals, shopping, doing housework, using a telephone, taking medicine, getting around outside, and managing money. Persons were classified as needing assistance if they needed help from another person or a special aide to do one or more of these activities, or could not do one or more of them at all.)

The parents of the baby boom generation, entering retirement age in the 1980s and 1990s, usually can count on abundant family resources. However, when the low fertility members of the baby boom cohorts turn 65, the availability of informal care within the family will decrease and the cost of assisting the frail elderly will increasingly fall on the public sector and the home care industry (Soldo and Agree 1988). Requests for time off to care for frail parents and relatives will intensify and eventually may be legally recognized as parental leaves are now. Long-term care eventually will be a routine component of employee health care benefit programs. In conclusion, the impact of aging on industry will likely comprise more expensive health care benefit programs and higher absenteeism in addition to losses due to lower productivity and early retirement (Koff 1988).

About 20% of older persons were hospitalized during 1982. In comparison, only 9% of persons under 65 were hospitalized that year. Among those hospitalized, the elderly were more likely than younger persons to have more than one hospital stay per year (27% versus 17%) and to stay in the hospital longer (10 days versus seven days). Hospital expenditures for that year were approximately $120 billion and averaged $4,200 per year for each older person. This sum was more than three times the $1,300 spent for younger persons. About $1,000 or one fourth of the average expenditure came from "out-of-pocket" payments by or for older persons.

Hospital expenses accounted for the largest share (45%) of health expenditures for older persons in 1984. Benefits from government programs, including Medicare ($59 billion), Medicaid ($15 billion), and others ($7 billion), were estimated to cover about two thirds (67%) of the health expenditures of older persons in 1984. In contrast, only 31% of health care for persons under 65 was paid for by government resources.

Hospitalization is costly, but institutional long-term care may be even more expensive on a per case basis: in 1986, the cost of intermediate care facilities was $15,000 to $25,000 per year while that of skilled nursing facilities ranged between $22,000 and $35,000. The Office of Technology Assessment estimated that 1986 nursing home costs attributable to dementia totaled $38.9 billion.

Issues Concerning Elderly Workers

Since the 1950s, the Bureau of Labor Statistics has conducted studies of comparative job performance by age (Mark 1956, 1957, 1958; Kutscher and Walker 1960; Walker 1964; Jablonski et al. 1988). The findings, however, are limited in some cases to jobs paid on a piece-rate basis (in order to adequately measure actual contributions to output), and in others by the use of wage data as a proxy for output data (on the assumption that in a competitive economy, wages equal the value of workers' marginal products). In general, these studies found that average productivity increases at the beginning of individuals' working lives, peaks at age 45 for men and 35 for women and then begins to decline. The drop, however, is not large since productivity was found to exceed 90% of peak performance near age 60 and to exceed 80% for the group age 65 or older (Jablonski et al. 1988). Also, the studies indicate that the average age of the civilian labor force peaked around 1958, declined for most of two decades and, since 1980, began to increase once again.

The primary forces behind the earlier decline and the recent increase are the entrance into the labor market and, later, the aging of the baby boom generation.

These studies do not underscore with sufficient emphasis the challenges ahead. As the 21st century unfolds, one may expect that the double impact of fewer entry-level workers and early retirement policies will produce shortages in several critical job categories. Most companies will find themselves unprepared to optimally retain high performing senior employees either on a full-time or part-time basis. A parallel problem is that of appropriate career planning, performance assessment, and retraining for senior workers. A survey on the extent, causes, and consequences of career problems among senior employees was conducted in 1988 cooperatively by the American Society of Personnel Administration and Commerce Clearing House (ASPA/CCH 1988). The survey reveals that while the problems are already affecting some firms, health promotion programs to date have not specifically targeted aging workers nor have they given special attention to those neuropsychiatric problems that are likely to impact upon productivity qualitatively, if not quantitatively. Another important point identified by the survey is that career problems of senior employees have an impact not only on the performance and morale of the employees themselves, but may negatively affect coworkers and customers.

The labor force participation rate of men 65 years old or older decreased from 46% in 1960 to 19% in 1980 and 16% in 1986 (Fowles 1988). Participation is projected to shrink to less than 10% by the year 2000. Between 1970 and 1980, average retirement benefits (adjusted for inflation) increased faster than hourly earnings. Therefore, while it is increasingly possible to maintain aging individuals healthy and able to conduct a productive life, there have been increasing incentives for them to stop working.

Given current trends of 1) decreasing labor force participation, 2) higher retirement benefits, 3) declining self-employment, and 4) change of the population distribution from a pyramid-like to a rectangular shape, the pyramid-like job hierarchy of most organizations will become outmoded. Therefore, any major modification of the Social Security and health care systems should be accompanied by changes in attitudes and practices regarding employment for the elderly.

Decreases in productivity of older persons usually are associated with the jobs they held when they were younger. Creative restructuring of jobs to meet the special needs and strengths of the elderly may show that this increasingly large group of potential workers can be as productive as their younger counterparts. The current shift from physically demanding labor to high technology and service jobs may facilitate this strategy, but involves retraining and efforts to maintain health and motivation among the senior work force.

It is likely that timely, work site-based neuropsychiatric assessment and intervention could enhance the productivity of elderly workers. However, work site-based programs must be cost effective, and they must not infringe on the rights of individual older workers or encourage discriminatory practices. The design of these programs needs to be subtle (Rakowski et al. 1988), and they may be difficult to implement within present industry-sponsored wellness programs. However, the potential economic benefits justify their exploration.

Real Versus Illusory Issues

In 1986, 122 million workers contributed 5.7% of total earnings or about $215.5 billion to various Social Security Trust Funds. Most of the money was used in monthly payments to 2.8 million disabled persons and 23 million retirees. Transferring money from younger to older generations is what the Social Security System was designed to do in spite of a popular misconception that it is some type of public annuity program fully funded by workers' paid contributions. Benefits were tied in 1972 to the consumer price index to protect retirees from inflation. At that time, wages had been increasing faster than the general price level for almost three decades. Unexpectedly, beginning in 1973, inflation-adjusted wages declined for more than a decade (Levy 1987). As a consequence of this and other considerations, a sometimes bitter debate around the issue of intergenerational equity has taken place (Chakravarty and Weisman 1988; Soldo and Agree 1988).

Projections of a combined employer-employee tax rate increase between 25% and 45% by 2030 were followed by the 1983 Social Security amendments, such as the increase in employees' tax to the rate of 7.65% and the increase in the full benefit retirement age to 67 years by 2026.

The crucial issue here is neither the solvency of the Social Security system, which can be maintained with modest growth in real wages and productivity (U.S. Senate 1987), nor is it the transfer of wealth from younger to older generations. Social Security benefits pay bills that otherwise would have to be paid by the younger family members or by the community and society at large in the form of decreased living standards or inadequate public assistance not based on Social Security. Also, the young cohorts of today will be the old cohorts of tomorrow. Cuts in benefits for today's elderly probably would imply that tomorrow's elderly would receive less assistance.

The real issue is that the quality and the composition of the labor force in the 21st century will be dramatically different from the one upon which present public and private policies of human resource development are based. Instead of viewing aging workers as threats to productivity and competitiveness, we must learn to harness their experience, dependability, and commitment. Economic incentives to earlier retirement may be reversed and an environment of security and personal growth may be created to induce older individuals to be economically productive until very advanced age or chronic disability set in.

Another observation may be made at this point. Erroneously, the disability of elderly people has been attributed primarily to the aging process. This ageist phenomenon has created self-fulfilling prophecies of impairment for some elderly persons. More commonly now, disability in old age is ascribed to physical health status. However, it has been argued that loss of income, employment, spouse, friends, and socioeconomic status may be at times more relevant than either age or physical health status in determining disability (Ginzberg 1985). We would add that the cognitive and emotional status of the individual experiencing the inevitable losses of later life may be a crucial determinant in many cases. While no one escapes old age without some losses, and the rare person escapes without some chronic illness, the neuropsychiatric complications of loss, bereavement, and physical illness are treatable and often reversible. A sense of fatalism, and a view that depression, dementia and social withdrawal are inevitable consequences of old age and physical illness, contribute to disability as much as overt ageism.

Accumulated *clinical* experience suggests that the patients who benefit most from accurate neuropsychiatric diagnosis and treatment are those with less severe and overwhelming functional impairment, and those who still have meaningful social support from family or community (Brody and Ruff 1986). It is far more difficult and expensive to reverse a severe disability in a chronically institutionalized or socially isolated individual than it is to prevent a loss of function, or to improve quality of life for an individual with many preserved assets. When programs focus primarily on the most impaired, they may provide a disappointing return on investment. For example, most Medicare hospital dollars are spent on patients in the last year of life (Waldo and Lazenby 1984). Timely and competent neuropsychiatric care, when offered without stigma, to treat, delay or avert disorders of mood, cognition, and behavior accompanying or preceding physical illness in aging workers, early retirees, or senior retired persons, promises to offer a more satisfactory return.

Implications of Economic Growth Rates

True cost containment is defined as "a reduced inflow of real resources (into the health care system) without a diminution in useful output that would adversely affect the satisfaction of patients or their health status" (Ginzberg 1985). In other words, decreases in the utilization of health services should not be accomplished at the cost of poor health and quality of life for consumers. Limits to coverage in the attempt to eliminate overtreatment or the application of life-extending high technology to hopeless cases (Callahan 1989; Ginzberg 1985) need to be judged with a commitment to rationality and a global (as opposed to a piecemeal) view of the problem (Schneider 1989). Also, as part of rethinking the future of health care, one must consider that the "Medicare program creates a cruel imbalance between support for life-extending, high technology medicine and that medical care necessary for a decent quality of life, most notably, affordable long term institutional care and decent home care" (Callahan 1989).

The other authors in this volume present a range of proposals for enhancing specific forms of care for the elderly. However, any solution to the needs of the elderly must be amenable to being integrated into one of two probable scenarios of the next ten years (Amara et al. 1988).

First, the economy might grow through the year 2000 at the modest average rate of 2.5% yearly in real terms. If one expects this scenario to unfold, preoccupation over the budget deficit will limit public policy choices. Competition for shares of government spending will be intense and dominated by the mid-life baby boomers' concerns of educating their children, providing safety and physical security, and hopefully offering some assistance to underprivileged minorities. Cost containment would become a single major imperative strongly supported by the business community which must retain competitiveness in increasingly global markets. Pressures to apply drastic cost containment measures to specific sectors without preceding comprehensive and strategic planning would abound. In that environment, the emergence of a major role for health care managers is likely and large numbers of people, about 30% of the population (Amara et al. 1988), might be enrolled in some form of capitated payment system. Under this scenario, the financing of elderly care as the baby boom generation becomes old would be a formidable challenge.

The second scenario allows a healthier average economic growth of 3% annually and with it "a wider range of health care services to an aging and technologically sophisticated population" (Amara et al. 1988). Total spending on health care would be likely to rise by 4.2% yearly (faster than the economy as a whole) as medical high technology diffuses and its measurable benefits are sought more widely. These prevailing attitudes would also favor the expansion of institutional chronic care, acute care, and rehabilitative services. When the "bigger and most sophisticated" also is better and is affordable, cost containment ceases to be an immediate priority.

Both scenarios will offer unique, if different, opportunities for integrating neuropsychiatric interventions into a more comprehensive approach to affordable health care. In the slow growth scenario, the role of neuropsychiatric assessment and treatment in *rationalizing care* would be emphasized. In the more optimistic scenario, because of greater prosperity, the potential of neuropsychiatric care for *enhancing the quality of life* would find a better reception.

References

ASPA/CCH: 1988 ASPA/CCH Survey. Chicago, Commerce Clearing House, Inc, June 28, 1988

Amara R, Harrison JI, Schmid G: Looking Ahead at American Health Care. Washington, DC, McGraw Hill, 1988, p 33

Bengtson VL: Ethnicity and aging: problems and issues in current social science inquiry, in Ethnicity and Aging: Theory, Research and Policy. Edited by Gelfand DE, Kutzik AJ. New York, Springer, 1979

Brody SJ, Ruff GE: Aging and Rehabilitation: Advances in the State of the Art. New York, Springer, 1986

Callahan D: Old Age and new policy. JAMA 261:905-906, 1989

Chakravarty SN, Weisman K: Consuming our children? Forbes, November 14, 1988

Cutler J, Fine T: Federal health care financing of mental illness: a failure of public policy, in The New Economics of Psychiatric Care. Edited by Sharfstein S, Beigel A. Washington, DC, American Psychiatric Press, 1985

Dowd JJ, Bengtson VL: Aging in minority populations: an examination of the double jeopardy hypothesis. Journal of Gerontology 30:427 436, 1978

Foner A: Ascribed and achieved bases of stratification, in Annual Review of Sociology. Edited by Inkeles A. Palo Alto, CA, 1979, pp 219-242

Fowles DG: A Profile of Older Americans: 1987. Washington, DC, American Association of Retired Persons, 1988

Gallagher RM: Rehabilitative Adult Day Care: Cost Effective Care for the Elderly. NLN Publication (20 2191). New York, National League for Nursing, December 1987, pp 389-402

Ginzberg E: American Medicine: The Power Shift. Totowa, NJ, Rowman and Allanheld, 1985, p 159

Gordon MM: Assimilation in American Life. New York, Oxford University Press, 1964

Gottlieb GL: Cost implication of depression in older adults. Int J Ger Psychiat 3:191-200, 1988

Harwood HJ, Napolitano DM, Dristiansen PL, et al: Economic Costs to Society of Alcohol, Drug Abuse and Mental Illness. Unpublished document submitted to ADAMHA by Research Triangle Institute, June 1984

Hazzard WR: Geriatric medicine: life in the crucible of the struggle to contain health care costs, in The Medical Cost Containment Crisis. Edited by McCue JD. Ann Arbor, MI, Health Administration Press, 1989, pp 263-264

Jablonski M, Kunze K, Rosenblum L: Productivity, Age, and Labor Composition Changes in the U.S. Work Force. Paper presented at the Conference on the Aging Workforce: Agenda for Action, Washington, DC, March 10-11, 1988

Jeffries V, Ransford HE: Social Stratification: A Multiple Hierarchy Approach. Boston, MA, Allyn and Bacon, 1980

Koff TH: New Approaches to Health Care for An Aging Population. San Francisco, CA, Jossey Bass Publishers, 1988

Kutscher RE, Walker JF: Comparative job performance of office workers by age. Monthly Labor Review, January 1960

Lavizzo-Mourey R, Day SC, Diserens D, et al (eds): Practicing Prevention for the Elderly. Philadelphia, C. V. Mosby, 1988

Levy F: The middle class: is it really vanishing? in The Brookings Review. Washington, DC, The Brookings Institution, 1987

Luce BR, Schweitzer SO: Smoking and alcohol abuse: a comparison of their economic consequences. N Engl J Med 298:569-571, 1978

Mark JA: Measurement of job performance and age. Monthly Labor Review, December 1956

Mark JA: Comparative job performance by age. Monthly Labor Review, December 1957

Mark JA: Older Worker Productivity in Manufacturing. Paper presented at the Pennsylvania Department of Labor and Industry Conference on Older Workers, Philadelphia, PA, May 15, 1958

Markides KS, Mindel CH: Aging and Ethnicity. Newbury Park, CA, SAGE Publications, 1987

Millard PH: Depression in old age. Br Med J 287:375-376, 1983

Rakowski W, Carl F, Flora J: Health education for older workers: interests and preferences of university employees aged 55 and over. Family and Community Health 11:65-73, 1988

Schneider EL: Options to control the rising health care costs of older Americans. JAMA 261:907-908, 1989

Soldo BJ, Agree EM: America's elderly. Population Bulletin 43:3, 1988

U.S. Senate, Special Committee on Aging: Developments in Aging, Vol 1. Washington, DC, U.S. Government Printing Office, 1987

Valle R: U.S. ethnic minority group access to long term care, in Caring for An Aging World: International Models for Long Term Care, Financing, and Delivery. Edited by Schwab T. New York, McGraw Hill, 1989

Waldo DR, Lazenby HC: Demographic Characteristics and Health Care Use and Expenditures by the Aged in the United States: 1977-1984. Health Care Financing Review 6:1-29, 1984

Walker JF: The job performance of federal mail sorters by age. Monthly Labor Review, March 1964

Walman HM, Carver EA, Klein M: Underutilization of mental health professionals by community elderly. Gerontologist 24:23-30, 1984

Walsh WB: Publisher's letter. Health Affairs, Spring 1989, p 3

Waxman HM, Carner EA: Physicians' recognition diagnosis and treatment of the mental disorders in elderly medical patients. Gerontologist 24:593-597, 1984

Windom RE: An aging nation presents new challenges to the health care system. Public Health Reports 103(1):1-2, 1988

3

The Nature and Efficacy of Interventions for Depression and Dementia

Barbara Kamholz, M.D.
Gary L. Gottlieb, M.D., M.B.A.

Mental function explicitly influences all other areas of individual function. The abilities to interact socially, to communicate and to autonomously manage personal affairs depend upon higher cortical functions and the cerebral cortex. Virtually all activities of daily living (ADL) may be impaired if cognitive or emotional status is disturbed. Similarly, medical well-being and health promotion are severely undermined by psychiatric disorders; individuals with minor impairments in memory and learning are less likely to be able to follow prescribed medical protocols (Foster and Kay 1986).

Treatment of the neuropsychiatric disorders of late life and palliation of their behavioral manifestations may improve function and autonomy substantially. This chapter reviews the currently existing treatments for depression and dementia, the most prevalent and well-defined psychiatric and neuropsychiatric disorders in the elderly (Gottlieb 1988).

Finally, some implications of these clinical findings for the organization and financing of health services for the elderly are presented.

Prevalence and Consequences of Depression and Dementia

Depressive symptoms are highly prevalent among the elderly. Two groups of investigators found a 13%–18% point prevalence of depression in large samples of community-residing elderly (Gurland et al. 1980; Murrell et al. 1983). Studies of elderly medical patients

37

reveal rates of up to 20% (Waxman et al. 1984; Kathol and Petty 1981). Elderly people who perceive their health as poor are at particular risk for depression (Levkoff et al. 1988); Kennedy et al. (1989) found depressive symptomatology in 54% of such community-residing older adults. Older patients with even mild depressive symptoms express a negative perception of their own health status, they have more physical complaints, and they make significantly more physician visits than do normal elderly patients (Kennedy et al. 1989; Waxman et al. 1983). There also appear to be close connections between depression and functional disability in the setting of chronic illness (Borson et al. 1986; Gurland et al. 1988). The presence of depression may predict a higher rate of failure to recover from disability, and thus the development of long-term disability (Gurland et al. 1988). In addition, Gurland (1988) and Murphy (1983) found higher death rates and shorter life expectancies associated with depression. Depression is also the single greatest risk factor for completed suicide (Stevenson 1988). Suicide rates among the elderly are disproportionately high. This population comprises only 11.9% of the population but accounts for nearly a quarter of all suicides. For example, whereas the suicide rate for the general population is approximately 13 per 100,000, the rate for men in their eighties is close to three times that level. The exact prevalence of dementia is unknown. Community surveys estimate that severe forms of dementia affect more than 5% of people over 65 years of age. Another 10%–15% of older adults are thought to suffer mild moderate dementia (Schneck et al. 1982; Reifler et al. 1982). In a survey of outpatient Medicare recipients selected randomly, Kennedy et al. (1989) found that 23% of the sample were cognitively impaired to a moderately severe degree. Nearly 70% of primary care medical patients who present with evidence of significant cognitive impairment may have senile dementia of the Alzheimer's type (DAT) (Larson et al. 1985).

A substantial number of patients present with severe disability due to a mixed syndrome of depression and dementia (McAllister et al. 1982; Malhendra 1985). Miller (1980) found that ambulatory elderly patients with "senile dementias" of various etiologies had Hamilton Rating Scale for Depression (HAM-D) (Hamilton 1967) scores in the mild to moderately depressed range. Reifler et al. (1982; 1986) found 19% and 31% prevalence rates of Major Depressive Disorder in samples of cognitively impaired geriatric outpatients. Lazarus et al. (1987) and Merriam et al. (1988) studied well-diagnosed populations of ambulatory patients with probable DAT. Cross-sectional assessments in those studies yielded inferred prevalence rates for depression of 40% and 86%, respectively. Other studies have reported clinical depression in 15% to 57% of DAT patients (Kral 1983).

Depressive symptoms may be difficult to distinguish from a clinically recognizable depressive syndrome in patients with dementia. Patients with major depressive disorder and/or DAT often manifest psychomotor retardation, sleep disturbances, anorexia, apathy and constricted affect (Miller 1980). While epidemiologic studies confirm the importance of depression in DAT, the difficulties in diagnosis may be responsible for the range of prevalence estimates. For some patients, depressive symptoms may be part of the global process of deterioration in DAT. For others, clear episodes of major depression may be superimposed on the degenerative process. Thus, dysphoria, or unpleasant mood, is an integral part of some syndromes of dementia, and may be a direct consequence of brain damage (Reifler et al. 1982; Reifler et al. 1986; Meyers and Alexopoulos 1988) This effect has been demonstrated clearly in the case of post-stroke (cerebrovascular accident [CVA]) depressive syndromes (Robinson et al. 1983; Robinson et al. 1985).

Depression is known to cause difficulties with motivation in physical rehabilitation programs (Kemp 1986). This is further complicated by difficulty obtaining certification for third-party reimbursement of rehabilitation services for "poorly motivated" patients. These patients may then become stranded at a dependent level of function. Adequate treatment for the most common mental disorders in the elderly requires their recognition and their differentiation from one another and from other conditions. Painstaking analysis and observation are required to identify the pathological or syndromal etiology of disturbed behavior in elderly, debilitated patients (Morstyn et al. 1982; Jorm 1986).

Without systematic assessment, cognitive impairment and depression may go unrecognized and appropriate interventions may be overlooked. Effective treatments for depression and the behavioral manifestations of dementia are available. Additionally, comprehensive evaluation allows the identification and management of nonpsychiatric reversible etiologies of cognitive impairment, depression and excess disability. Delayed intervention increases the risk of chronic deterioration (Murphy 1983; Stoudemire and Thompson 1981; Butler 1975).

Older patients and their families depend on primary care providers almost universally to recognize and address complaints related to intellectual and emotional function (Brody and Kleban 1981).

Furthermore, even when psychiatric disorders are identified, older adults have an extreme preference for treatment by medical providers (Waxman et al. 1984). Unfortunately, the subtlety of mental impairment in this population severely limits the ability of primary physicians to recognize and to treat these disorders appropriately (Kathol and Petty 1981). The cost ramifications of prompt intervention in psychiatric complications of dementia syndromes are apparent: improvement in disorientation, psychosis, and in self care can prolong productive and autonomous function and postpone or prevent the need for acute or long-term institutionalization (Brody et al. 1984). The human cost may be measured in despair, excess disability, and the potential for neglect, poor health, or abuse. Moreover, families report that difficulty in managing the behavior of an impaired older adult is of substantial importance in the decision to seek nursing home placement for the affected individual (Secretary's Task Force 1984; Ross and Kedward 1977; Teri et al. 1989).

Behavioral disturbance is also strongly associated with caregiver stress even when controlling for the level of cognitive impairment (Teri et al. 1989). Sleep disturbances and poor physical self maintenance have been shown to be more stressful for caregivers than physical impairment (Sommers et al. 1988; Greene et al. 1982). A combination of severe sleep disorder and the need for around-the-clock supervision due to wandering or impaired judgment can exhaust even the most stable and caring of caregivers (Chenoweth amd Spencer 1986). This may reduce caregiver productivity, function and general health status. "Nonaggressive" agitated behaviors, including wandering and repeated requests for attention have been found to be more prevalent than violent behavior (Cohen-Mansfield 1986; Reisberg et al. 1987; Rovner et al. 1986). Additionally, most studies reveal lower incidence rates of physical violence and aggression in home care settings than in institutions. However, when aggressive behaviors occur in the home, they may have serious consequences (Chenoweth and Spencer 1986; Rabins et al. 1982). Likewise, violent behaviors in institutional settings may impose substantial limitations in function. For example, Chandler and Chandler (1988) found that 48% of patients in a community nursing home exhibited violent behaviors and that 50% of all patients required physical restraints at some point during their residence. The physical immobility imposed by restraints predisposes to decreased function, which in turn predisposes to chronicity of illness and the potential need for prolonged institutionalization. Similarly, Cohen-Mansfield (1986) demonstrated that falls, commonly associated with substantial morbidity and mortality, are common in agitated elderly patients. Disordered behavior predisposes to institutionalization, which in turn predicts mortality and chronic disability.

Ross and Kedward (1977) followed patients for one year after discharge from an acute care psychogeriatric unit. They found that institutionally placed patients were significantly more likely than community-placed patients to be dead, still hospitalized, or in other institutions. Psychiatric problems affect the placement process adversely. Patients who have histories of confusion, behavior problems, psychiatric institutionalization and/or alcoholism are often very difficult to place after hospitalization (Brody et al. 1984). This difficulty may promote costly overutilization of the acute care hospital system, and may stress family caregivers emotionally and financially (Markson et al. 1983). The implementation of the preadmission screening provision of the 1987 Omnibus Budget Reconciliation Act may further aggravate this problem.

Despite barriers to institutional admission, neuropsychiatric disorders are the most frequently diagnosed clinical problems in long-term care settings (Teri et al. 1989; Rovner et al. 1986; Chandler and Chandler 1988; Markson et al. 1983; Hegeman and Tobin 1988; Teeter et al. 1976). Available epidemiologic data indicate that the largest proportion of mentally disabled elderly in nursing homes suffer dementia (see Chapter 4). However, other more acute disorders are also highly prevalent: Chandler and Chandler (1988) found that 12.3% of a community nursing home sample met DSM-III-R (American Psychiatric Association 1987) criteria for organic delusional disorder or organic hallucinosis. Twenty-two percent (Chandler and Chandler 1988) of the sample had evidence of other psychoses. Rovner et al. (1986) found that 38% of a randomly selected sample of community nursing home residents had delusions or hallucinations. They also found that problematic behaviors correlated significantly with total nursing care time. Therefore, improving the target symptoms of psychosis (delusions and hallucinations) may impact directly on costs of care as well as staff relations and the life quality of patients. In this regard, Teeter et al. (1976) found that hostility and infantilization were common staff reactions toward psychiatrically disturbed nursing home residents.

Treatments for Depression and the
Psychiatric Complications of Dementia

Over the past twenty years, there has been substantial progress in the development of relatively safe and effective treatments for depression and the behavioral disorders associated with dementia. These treatments offer extraordinary opportunities for reduction of morbidity and improvement of functional outcomes.

Depression

Geriatric depression is a subtle and peculiar entity. In many cases, the disorder is diagnosed in the absence of subjectively depressed mood (Busse and Simpson 1983; Fogel and Fretwell 1985). The disorder is easily confused with numerous medical conditions. Nearly 20% of elderly depressives present with complaints that they attribute to medical illness (Busse and Simpson 1983). Somatic complaints, disturbances of sleep and appetite, anxiety and apathy often predominate. Subjectively depressed mood, guilt, and suicidal ideation are rarely expressed. Patients insist that the disorder is physical in nature. Exhaustive medical workups, even when completely negative, rarely convince patients that their symptoms are psychological in origin. Appropriate diagnosis requires appreciation of constricted affect, vegetative symptoms, apathy, and pervasive dissatisfaction. Cognitive impairment can also be produced or exacerbated by depression in the elderly (Reifler et al. 1982; McAllister and Price 1982; Malhendra 1985; Jorm 1986; Kramer 1982). Some of the memory impairment associated with major depression may be reversible (McAllister and Price 1982). While dementing symptoms in elderly depressives with cognitive impairment may not reverse completely, cognitive function may improve measurably with improvement in depression, even in patients with mild-to-moderate dementia of organic etiology (McAllister and Price 1982; Kramer 1982). These improvements often are highly relevant to every day function, particularly in the instrumental activities of daily living (IADL).

General Approach to Treatment of
Depression in the Medically Ill Elderly

Treatment of late-life depression begins with a careful comprehensive assessment of the patient's medical problems, and the complete list of medications the patient is taking. Numerous common medical problems of late life may cause or aggravate depression, and a variety of commonly prescribed medications can do the same (Lavizzo-Mourey 1988). Furthermore, medical status must be taken into account in selecting a biologic treatment for depression. For example, certain types of heart block are contraindications to the use of tricyclic antidepressants. Also, the dosage of drugs used in the treatment of depression may need to be modified depending on the patient's medical status, and special techniques may be needed for anesthesia if electroconvulsive therapy (ECT) is to be administered. After identification of the patient's medical problems and review of the drug list, medical problems are corrected to the greatest possible extent, and offending drugs eliminated or less psychotoxic substituted whenever possible. Once this is done, the depression may improve with no further specific psychiatric treatment. However, in many cases, perhaps the majority, specific antidepressant therapy is necessary.

Another early step is the detailed evaluation of cognitive status. Not only is cognitive status relevant to the differential diagnosis between depression and other disorders, but it may be a limiting factor in the use of psychotherapeutic treatments. A patient with severe impairments in memory or abstract reasoning could be expected to benefit from general emotional support, but probably would not respond to a cognitive therapy intervention.

A full service component of the treatment of late-life depression is assessment and intervention with the family and social environment. Particularly in cases of isolation, deprivation, abuse, or severe and specific family conflicts, correction of an aggravating factor in the social environment is a precondition for sustained remission from depression.

The following sections discuss specific biologic and psychotherapeutic treatments of demonstrated effectiveness in the therapy of late-life depression.

Specific Antidepressant Treatments

Pharmacotherapy

Gerson et al. (1988) comprehensively reviewed a generation of literature regarding the pharmacotherapy of depression in the elderly. Despite numerous methodological criticisms, they concluded that, given appropriate treatment, "the elderly patient is just as likely as the younger patient to go into remission" (p. 319). However, successful drug treatment of depressed patients requires careful scrutiny of their medical problems. Antidepressant interventions must be tailored carefully with full knowledge of medication side effects as they may positively or negatively affect the patient's physical condition (Stoudemire and Fogel 1987).

Tricyclic agents. The tricyclic antidepressants (TCAs) are the most prescribed antidepressants (Talbott et al. 1988) Three decades of experience with these agents have yielded numerous clinical trials supporting their efficacy. However, there have been only a small number of well-controlled studies in the elderly (Gerson et al. 1988). These studies support the notion that, when tolerated and employed appropriately, the tricyclic agents are effective in the treatment of major depression. However, the range of improvement reported varies greatly. The tertiary amine tricyclics (amitriptyline, imipramine, doxepin, and trimipramine) have been studied most extensively in the geriatric population. These agents are employed extensively by primary care providers. Unfortunately, they are quite anticholinergic, and the elderly are particularly vulnerable to urinary retention, constipation, and confusion as a consequence of this property. Additionally, through effects on the alpha-adrenergic and histaminic systems, tertiary amine agents are likely to cause postural hypotension and sedation, important risk factors for falls in the elderly (Jenike 1988b). Their principal metabolites, the secondary amine tricyclics (nortriptyline, desipramine, and protriptyline) are considerably less anticholinergic and they are better tolerated by older patients. They appear to be equally effective, so they are emerging as the tricyclics of choice for depressed elderly patients.

The TCAs have been used successfully for depression associated with a number of medical and neurological conditions. For example, one placebo-controlled study demonstrated that trimipramine was superior to placebo in treating depression in patients with concomitant medical illness (Rifkin et al. 1985). Similarly, nortriptyline has been shown to be effective in the treatment of depression following stroke (Lipsey et al. 1984).

TCAs have also been used successfully in rehabilitation settings. Lakshmanan et al. (1986) performed a placebo-controlled study of low doses of doxepin (10 to 20 mg/day) in elderly depressives during physical rehabilitation for a number of disorders. Doxepin-treated patients showed a significant improvement in mood ratings. Improvement was evident after only one week of treatment. The physical function of patients treated with doxepin and with placebo improved significantly over the three-week study period. This study is important because it demonstrated that very low dose TCA therapy in the elderly could be effective without causing clinically significant side effects. Further research is needed to identify low-dose responders for whom tertiary amine tricyclics would be effective and to distinguish them from patients who would do better on higher doses of secondary amine tricyclics.

Monoamine oxidase inhibitors. Until about ten years ago, clinicians were generally reluctant to employ monoamine oxidase inhibitors (MAOIs) because of reported hypertensive crises associated with dietary and pharmacologic interactions. However, those reactions appear to be relatively rare in practice. For example, Neil et al. (1979) found that many patients treated with MAOIs may commit significant dietary violations without problems. MAOIs may be considerably better tolerated than tricyclics for some older patients: They are far less anticholinergic and less sedating than TCAs and they have little demonstrable effect on cardiac conduction (Jenike 1984). However, they may cause considerable supine and postural hypotension (Jenike 1988b). This effect may be complicated by idiosyncratic hyponatremia (Sandifer 1983; Matuk and Kalyanaraman 1977).

Recent reviews and studies of the efficacy and tolerance of MAOIs in the elderly suggest extraordinary clinical utility, particularly in treatment-resistant depressions (Georgotas et al. 1983; Georgotas et al. 1986; Pare 1985;). Georgotas et al. (1983) treated 30 chronically depressed and medically ill elderly patients with MAOIs. These patients had not responded to previous treatment regimens, including TCAs, and ECT. After uncontrolled MAOI treatment for two to seven weeks, 65% of the patients improved. The side effects reported most frequently were dizziness, weight gain, and orthostasis. Georgotas et al. (1986) also completed a randomized double blind placebo controlled comparison of phenelzine (a MAOI) and nortriptyline in elderly depressives. Both active treatments were significantly superior to placebo. Approximately 60% of patients in the medication groups responded to treatment. The authors concluded that "...with a careful selection of patients and of drugs, proper dosing based on optimal serum levels, few readjustments of the dose, an adequate treatment time, and the elimination of unnecessary concurrent medications, both TCAs and MAOIs are easily tolerated by the elderly (p. 1,165)." An earlier study by Ashford and Ford (1979) showed similarly favorable results. In this uncontrolled trial, MAOIs were useful for treatment of simple geriatric depression and for treatment of depression in a small group of depressed DAT patients.

Psychostimulants. In his review of treatments for affective illness in the elderly, Jenike (1988b) argues that stimulants (i.e., dextroamphetamine, methylphenidate) are useful in the treatment of medically ill and postoperative geriatric patients with apathy, withdrawal, or anergy. He maintains that these agents are also useful for the treatment of depressed demented patients who have substantial psychomotor retardation. Katon and Raskind (1980) treated a series of elderly depressives who had been unable to tolerate TCAs. Two- to four-month methylphenidate treatment effected improvement. Remission of symptoms persisted at one year follow-up in three patients. None of the patients experienced significant adverse effects. A series of randomized clinical trials is necessary to clarify the role of these agents in geriatric psychopharmacology.

Fluoxetine. Fluoxetine, a bicyclic antidepressant, is a highly selective serotonin reuptake inhibitor which has virtually no anticholinergic or adrenergic effects. It has enjoyed rapid clinical acceptance with few reported toxic effects since its introduction in the United States in January 1988. While the efficacy and safety of fluoxetine has been established by several double blind placebo-controlled studies (Feighner et al. 1985; Stark et al. 1985; Feighner 1985), the agent has not been evaluated systematically in the elderly.

Trazodone. Trazodone is a heterocyclic antidepressant which is only mildly anticholinergic. However, this agent causes substantial sedation and orthostatic hypotension, particularly in the elderly. Gerner et al. (1980) described several clinical trials demonstrating that trazodone is similar in efficacy to imipramine, amitriptyline and desipramine. Its lack of anticholinergic effect implies a lesser risk of urinary retention, constipation, and confusion. While it may not always be effective for patients who would respond to TCAs, its safety and tolerability have supported its use in elderly depressives and in patients with concomitant depression and dementia (Winograd et al. 1986).

Benzodiazepines. Alprazolam, a benzodiazepine agent introduced for the treatment of anxiety, has been shown to have antidepressant efficacy (Feighner et al. 1983; Rickels et al. 1987). However, there are few reports of its use in elderly populations (Levy et al. 1984). In our experience, it may be useful in a small group of agitated depressed patients who are medically unable to tolerate any other somatic intervention. Unfortunately, we have not yet treated enough cases to develop a clinical typology to identify responders. Important adverse effects include dependence, central nervous system depression, postural instability and paradoxical agitation.

Lithium. A number of antidepressant adjuvants have been suggested and some have been tested. Synthesizing their literature review, Goff and Jenike (1986) suggest that addition of lithium carbonate may improve clinical response to MAOIs and to TCAs. In one controlled trial, one third of patients treated with amitriptyline, desipramine, or mianserin improved within 48 hours of the addition of lithium. The remaining patients studied showed some positive response within eight days of lithium enhancement. However, the age-associated decrease in renal function and increase in neurologic sensitivity to lithium requires conservative dosage and close monitoring (Himmelhoch et al. 1980).

Electroconvulsive Therapy

Electroconvulsive Therapy (ECT) has been used extensively in the elderly since its introduction in the United States more than fifty years ago. It remains among the safest and most effective treatments for depression in the elderly (Jenike 1988b; Fogel 1988). Even among previously treatment-resistant patients, remission rates as high as 80%–85% have been demonstrated. Additionally, ECT has been shown consistently to be superior to antidepressants of all classes (Jenike 1988b). ECT is well tolerated in a large number of medical and neurological conditions and in the elderly (Dubovsky 1986; Price and McAllister 1989). ECT is particularly useful in the treatment of severe depressions characterized by delusional ideation or agitation. ECT can produce remarkable transformations of elderly patients functionally disabled by depression who have had tortuous clinical courses marked by treatment failures. In these patients, aggressive treatment improves functional outcomes and it may allow greater autonomy and deinstitutionalization. Although ECT has the predictable side-effect of time-limited anterograde and retrograde amnesia, this effect *rarely* impairs function or causes lasting distress. The temporary reduction in function caused by cognitive impairment is often outweighed by affective improvement. A review by Fogel (1988) describes a number of innovative protocols for safe use of ECT in the elderly.

Psychotherapy

Psychotherapy may be employed as a primary or concomitant treatment for depression in the elderly. While there have been few systematic evaluations of specific psychotherapies for geriatric depression, a number of treatments appear to be useful in the treatment of mild to moderate depressive disorders. Cognitive therapy and brief dynamic psychotherapy may be useful in reducing depressive symptoms and in improving function (Gallagher and Thompson 1982). A number of ongoing clinical trials will be useful in assessing the efficacy of psychotherapy in geriatric depressives.

Inferences Concerning Service Delivery

The preceding review has demonstrated that specific treatment for late-life depression is usually effective, but frequently may involve the simultaneous or sequential application of several medical interventions, including stabilization of concurrent medical problems and the administration of drug trials. A large portion of the treatment rendered must necessarily be under a physician's direction. More severe or refractory cases may require treatments such as drug combinations or electroconvulsive therapy that generally are administered jointly by specialists in psychiatry. Components of the initial evaluation, particularly concerning evaluation of cognitive status and the social environment can be carried out by nonmedical personnel. Cognitive therapy certainly can be rendered by nonphysician therapists, and monitoring of drug therapy in the maintenance phase can be carried out by nurses or physicians' assistants under a physician's supervision. The medical component of treatment can in most cases be provided by the primary care physician, but depending on the physician's knowledge and skills in the treatment of depression, a threshold will be reached where psychiatric consultation will be necessary. If the depression is recognized as a serious and ultimately treatable condition by both the primary care physician and the patient or family, psychiatric consultation usually takes place and the ultimate results are generally gratifying. When the diagnosis of depression is less firm and its implications and treatability less well appreciated, the physician or patient may abandon treatment after an initially unsuccessful drug trial, without obtaining specialist consultation. This occurrence, which in our experience is fairly common, ranks second to nonrecognition of depression as a cause of unsatisfactory outcomes in depressed elderly patients. The interventions described above usually can be carried out on an outpatient basis. Reasons for hospitalization would include suicidal risk, severe agitation or uncooperativeness precluding compliance with outpatient treatment, extreme physical frailty of the patient, or concurrent medical problems requiring a hospital level of monitoring or intervention to allow safe treatment of the depression.

Dementia

A wide range of behavioral and functional problems complicate the management of people with dementia. The vulnerability of older adults, especially those who are impaired cognitively, to even the rarest toxic effects of medications must be recognized (Lavizzo-Mourey 1988). Therefore, the sparsest pharmaceutical regimen possible—one lacking direct central nervous system (CNS) toxins—is always recommended.

General Approach to Treatment

Any change in cognitive function or in behavior warrants a comprehensive medical and neurological examination. The purpose of the evaluation is to determine the etiology and potential reversibility of cognitive dysfunction. If an irreversible dementing process is found, a tertiary rehabilitative approach to slowing deterioration and optimizing function is necessary (Larson et al. 1984). The rigorous work-up recommended by a National Institute on Aging task force is justified by numerous reports that between 10 and 30% of cognitively impaired patients suffer from potentially treatable entities (National Institute on Aging Task Force 1980). Additionally, Larson and his colleagues (1985) found that over 30% of a large series of patients presenting with cognitive impairment had more than one illness contributing to the dementia state. Treatment of concomitant medical, neurological, and psychiatric disorders provided at least temporary improvement in 27.5% of the patients. Improvement was sustained for at least one year in 14% of the study group. While improvement was not defined as reversibility, amelioration in quality of life was appreciated by patients and their families (Larson et al. 1985). Although cost outcomes were not evaluated in this study, treatment of concomitant disorders may have direct effects on function and on health care utilization. (For a more conservative viewpoint on dementia evaluation, see Chapter 10.) The relatively high rate of reversible problems found by Larson et al. (1985) may reflect the bias of selection for referral to a specialty program.

Specific Treatments

Treatments for the Primary Illness

Considerable research is underway to understand the etiology, neuropathology and physiology of DAT and other common dementias (i.e., multi-infarct dementia [MID] and the dementia associated with Parkinson's disease [PD]). For example, since DAT was associated with reductions in brain levels of the enzymes choline acetyltransferase and acetylcholinesterase, investigators have made minor progress in evaluating treatments for the degenerative process (Summers et al. 1986; Jenike 1988a). Other investigators have identified potentially important biological markers (Martin 1987) while others have advanced the understanding of genetic contributions to DAT (Finch 1987). However, treatment of the cognitive decline associated with progressive dementia remains experimental. There has been greater progress in the management of the behavioral and personality alterations associated with dementia. Symptoms including depression, night-time restlessness, emotional lability, combativeness, psychosis, social disinhibition, and wandering comprise a potentially remediable "excess disability."

Many patients who appear to have "treatment-resistant" depression may be suffering depression superimposed on underlying dementia. Reding et al. (1985) found that elderly patients treated for depression who did not tolerate or respond to somatic treatments were likelier to "develop" dementia within three years of presentation than were treatment-responsive patients. The literature regarding treatment of depression in dementia is growing rapidly. While it is premature to draw conclusions from the small number of available clinical trials, there is some evidence that affective symptoms improve with treatment of depression in DAT (Reifler et al. 1986). In more advanced cases of dementia, cognitive function has not been shown to improve significantly with remission of depressive symptoms. However, family satisfaction and patient well-being and motivation improve with diminution of depressive symptoms.

Reifler et al. (1989) recently completed a double blind placebo controlled trial of imipramine in depressed and nondepressed DAT patients that failed to show superiority of imipramine over placebos, though both groups improved. Thus, while there is consensus that *treatment of depression in general is desirable and effective*, further research will be needed to address issues of specialty.

Behavioral symptoms in dementia appear to have two origins: 1) primary neurological deficits inherent in the disease which may cause disturbance of behavior; 2) overtly psychotic phenomena such as delusions and hallucinations which may be associated with impaired interpretations of reality caused by cognitive deficits (Swearer et al. 1988).

Teri et al. (1989) recently found that severity of cognitive impairment in outpatients with DAT was not correlated with specific behavioral problems. Further, Merriam et al. (1988) found that caregivers of community-residing DAT patients reported significant agitation in 61% of the patients whom they cared for. Agitation was not correlated with severity of the patient's depression or dementia. However, the study indicated that perceptual disorders (auditory and visual hallucinations, and misrecognition of stimuli) were highly correlated with severity of cognitive dysfunction. In a study of a heterogeneous group of outpatients with dementia, Swearer et al. (1988) found "a significant relationship between the severity of dementia and the presence and severity of behavioral disturbances" (p. 786). This finding was supported by Rovner et al. (1986). In their landmark study of patients in a community nursing home, they found that hallucinations and delusions were significantly correlated with severity of dementia and with behavioral disturbance. Controlling for severity of dementia, they also found that patients with delusions and hallucinations were significantly more disordered behaviorally than were patients without these disturbances. Additionally, at least one study has demonstrated an association between severity of psychosis in patients with DAT and functional and intellectual deterioration (Mayeux et al. 1985).

Rovner et al. (1986) concluded that psychotic symptoms may be more important determinants of behavioral problems than severity of cognitive impairment. This supports the notion that specific psychiatric interventions aimed at ameliorating psychotic symptoms may be useful in reducing morbidity in this population. Further research is necessary to clarify this issue.

Specific Treatments for Behavioral Disorder in Dementia

Neuroleptics

Neuroleptic medications are used extensively by primary care physicians and by psychiatrists for treatment of behavioral disorders in the elderly. Comprehensive reviews of the literature (Devanand et al. 1988; Helms 1985; Risse and Barnes 1986) indicate that there is little scientific support for the widespread use of these agents: few controlled clinical trials have been performed; diagnostically homogeneous patient samples have not been used; the effects of neuroleptics on cognition and function have not been assessed; and most studies have been performed in institutional settings. However, all of the well-controlled studies in the literature demonstrate that while effects are modest, neuroleptics are superior to placebo in controlling anxiety, suspiciousness, uncooperativeness and hallucinatory behaviors (Devanand et al. 1988; Barnes et al. 1982; Petrie et al. 1982). Neuroleptics have little effect on poor self care, social withdrawal, wandering, and cognition (Barnes et al. 1982).

Neuroleptics have some utility in managing behavioral disorders associated with dementia particularly when specific psychiatric symptoms are present. Appropriately prescribed neuroleptics may reduce caregiver stress, delay the need for institutional management and improve adaptation to new environments. However, extrapyramidal side effects, tardive dyskinesia, sedation, and anticholinergic effects may obscure potential functional improvements. Therefore, tiny doses should be employed for short periods of time in the most necessary circumstances. The indications for neuroleptic use in dementia are best summarized by Raskind et al.:

> In summary, the available studies of antipsychotic drugs in demented patients support the concept of using these drugs only if signs and symptoms of psychosis or significant excitement and agitation complicate the dementia syndrome. Repetitive, bothersome behaviors, such as aimless wandering, pacing, and calling out, are usually less responsive to antipsychotic treatment and the adverse drug effect akathisia can exacerbate pacing behavior. (Raskind et al. 1986, p. 20)

Nonneuroleptics

Benzodiazepines have been used extensively in attempts to diminish agitated behavior in cognitively impaired older patients. For example, diazepam may have a calming effect on agitated patients. However, it appears to be less effective in controlling agitation than phenothiazines (Kirven and Mantero 1973). Similarly, oxazepam, a shorter acting agent, has been shown to diminish psychomotor agitation and aggressive behavior (Salzman 1984). The effects of benzodiazepines on agitation in patients with dementia are modest. Additionally, their CNS depressant properties can exacerbate cognitive impairment and diminish function.

A case report and a case series (Yudofsky et al. 1981; Jenike 1983) suggest that beta blockers may be useful in controlling agitation associated with the dementing process. In these reports, severely combative agitated behavior responded to relatively low doses of propranolol. However, well-controlled clinical trials are necessary to assess the overall benefit of these agents.

A few small studies suggest that trazodone is useful for treatment of agitated behavior in elderly demented patients (Simpson and Foster 1986; Nair et al. 1973; Greenwald et al. 1986). This may be due to trazodone's ability to block serotonin reuptake. This property appears to be common to certain medications which can ameliorate violent behavior (Eichelman 1987). Because of its antidepressant effects, this agent may be useful for agitated patients with dementia who are particularly dysphoric.

Other Therapies

Certain behaviors common to demented patients may be remediable by environmental manipulation. Wandering is a problem which is difficult to manage at home and in institutional settings. Wandering does not diminish in response to pharmacotherapies. Neuroleptics may actually aggravate this symptom by causing akathisia, a particularly severe form of drug-induced restlessness. Therefore, nonpharmacologic strategies may be more valuable.

Dawson and Reid (1987) evaluated a series of institutionalized patients and concluded that wanderers were more active physically premorbidly than nonwanderers. They suggested that wandering may represent an attempt to reduce a specific distressing symptom adaptively. Addressing the "source" of the wandering may diminish the behavior. Additionally, Dawson and Reid found that wanderers had greater difficulties with speech, reading, and orientation. They recommend providing special activities that can be mastered, providing "room to roam," and attempting to optimize cognitive function. Similarly, Rader et al. (1985) and Rader (1987) stress a humanistic approach to management of agitation and wandering. They characterize wandering as an "agenda behavior" and they argue eloquently for an empathic, individually focused approach. Rader et al. (1985) and Rader (1987) maintain that these behaviors are not merely neurological aberrations. Instead, they represent attempts by patients to recapitulate some aspects of their former lives. In order to test this hypothesis, the authors constructed a long-term care unit with a high staff-to-patient ratio. Staff were systematically sensitized to the patience and attention required to identify and address patient needs. The investigators placed subtle identification badges on the residents, they allowed much more freedom of movement and they developed an emergency procedure to find patients if they got lost. Rader (1987) presents evidence that this approach resulted in fewer combative episodes and injuries to staff over a three-year period. Wandering patients were located quickly, and no patient injuries were attributable to wandering. Their intuitively appealing approach should be evaluated with a controlled clinical trial. Outcomes should include patient function and morbidity as well as the costs and benefits of increased staff time and changes in levels of staff stress.

In another innovative approach, Cleary et al. (1988) developed a "reduced stimulation" unit for patients with DAT. This 16-bed closed unit with a neutral color scheme has no televisions, radios, or telephones. This milieu provides freedom for walking, eating, and resting in any location desired. Consistent daily rest periods and defined small-group activities are employed to structure time. Staff and families are trained to speak slowly and quietly and to provide choices rather than confrontation. Patients, their families, and staff were assessed before the unit opened and three months later. Patients sustained a significant improvement in the ability to perform ADL. While overall behavioral ratings were unchanged, there was evidence of improved nutritional status and a reduction in the use of restraints and tranquilizing medications. Additionally, family satisfaction improved significantly. Staff attitudes and knowledge did not change over the study period. This innovative model addresses patient, family, and staff issues regarding management of dementia patients. It is too small to generalize. However, pilot data are adequately encouraging to suggest the need for a clinical trial.

In an effort to better understand innovative behavioral management programs, Hegeman and Tobin (1988) solicited 111 nonprofit long-term care programs via questionnaire to describe their efforts. They found that 1) specialized locked-door units for "mentally impaired" residents increased autonomy, decreased the need for chemical or physical restraint, and increased ADLs of many residents; 2) allowing space to "wander" improved function, self-esteem, and increased staff respect for patients' dignity; 3) a "creative dining" program in one location improved autonomy, function, behavior, and nutrition by enabling the patients to be more directly involved in meal planning; 4) training and information sessions for families resulted in greater staff-family understanding and a greater ability for families to help enhance the function of residents. These descriptive data are useful and they provide a framework for future formal demonstrations and research.

These innovative programs and concepts are exciting contributions to rehabilitation of patients with dementia. Larger demonstration projects to assess the generalizability of these models and their outcomes must be pursued.

Inferences Regarding Service Delivery

Of the interventions described above, the ones that necessarily require physician involvement are the differential diagnosis of reversible causes and aggravating factors for the dementia, and the drug therapy of psychiatric complications including agitation, paranoid behavior, and depression. Regarding the latter, subspecialist geriatric physicians and geriatric psychiatrists both claim expertise in the selection of appropriate drug therapy for psychosis and agitation in demented patients. While neither of these specialties has an empirically based claim to superiority, it is clear that the practice of general physicians in treating these problems may be unsatisfactory, particularly with institutionalized patients. Several recent studies of the use of psychotropic drugs with demented patients in nursing homes revealed a widespread use of neuroleptic drugs, often without appropriate indications (Avorn et al. 1989;

Beers et al. 1988). Also, benzodiazepines are used to treat sleep disorders in demented patients, even though they are unlikely to yield a lasting benefit and they increase the risk of falls and fractures.

The foregoing review indicates that less than half of demented individuals with agitation or psychosis will respond to neuroleptics, and response to alternative nonneuroleptic agents is at present unpredictable. Since each of these agents has potential toxicities, close medical monitoring for effects and side effects is essential. While this is theoretically possible for the primary physician, it would be reasonable at this point to suggest that referral be made to a geriatric specialist or psychiatrist if a demented patient showed psychosis or agitated behavior that was not responsive to elimination of psychotoxic medications, and the use of modest doses of neuroleptic drugs.

The behavioral and environmental interventions described above for wandering and agitation clearly can be implemented by nonmedical personnel, although program design would seem to require a mental health professional with knowledge of applied behavioral analysis. No one behavioral management program has as yet evolved to the point where it could be carried out from a manual without professional involvement.

The drug therapies described can safely be given to outpatients, unless there are overwhelming safety considerations, as might exist with a frail person living alone, or in the rare case of an extremely violent patient. Behavioral interventions do require a structured setting, although not necessarily a hospital or nursing home. Some interventions might be applicable to day treatment. Further, it is conceivable that environmental modifications can be made in patients' homes, and that family or nonprofessional personal care attendants could be trained in the administration of behavioral therapies.

Conclusion

Dementia and depression are highly prevalent geriatric neuropsychiatric disorders. These disorders impart substantial disability and they may create a severe burden for affected individuals and their families and for society. Over the last twenty years, substantial progress has been made in diagnosis and management of these conditions. The evidence presented in this chapter shows that a substantial proportion of the morbidity and disability related to these clinical entities can be reduced. However, rehabilitation and treatment require special skills and persistent incentives to provide care. The continued implementation of innovative strategies will require creative solutions in funding, training, and research and in the organization of service delivery.

In both depression and dementia, specific elements of care require the involvement of physicians, and at times, specialists in psychiatry or geriatrics. On the other hand, the bulk of longer-term care for both conditions can be provided by nonmedical personnel, usually in outpatient or nonhospital settings. For both conditions, specialist medical intervention appears most relevant "up front," during the initial evaluation of the patient for treatable medical factors and drug toxicity, and in the selection of appropriate pharmacologic treatment. The second key role for specialist medical intervention is when patients fail to respond to treatment as expected, or develop significant adverse reactions to treatment. After the diagnostic phase, and once a basically satisfactory treatment regimen has been developed, supervision and maintenance can usually be carried out by nonphysician care providers.

References

American Psychiatric Association: Diagnostic and Statistical Manual of Mental Disorders, 3rd ed, revised. Washington, DC, American Psychiatric Association, 1987

Ashford JW, Ford CV: Use of MAO inhibitors in elderly patients. Am J Psychiatry 136:1466-1467, 1979

Avorn J, Dreyer P, Conelly K, et al: Use of psychoactive medication and the quality of care in rest homes: findings and policy implications of a nationwide study. N Engl J Med 320:227-232, 1989

Barnes R, Veith R, Okimoto J, et al: Efficacy of antipsychotic medications in behaviorally disturbed dementia patients. Am J Psychiatry 139:1170-1174, 1982

Beers M, Avorn J, Soumerai S, et al: Psychoactive medication use in intermediate care facility residents. JAMA 260:3016-3020, 1988

Borson S, Barnes RA, Kukull WA, et al: Symptomatic depression in elderly medical outpatients. J Am Geriatr Soc 34:341-347, 1986

Brody EM, Kleban MH: Physical and mental health symptoms in older people: who do they tell? J Am Geriatr Soc 29:442-449, 1981

Brody EM, Lawton MP, Liebowitz B: Senile dementia: public policy and adequate institutional care. Am J Public Health 74:1381-1383, 1984

Busse EW, Simpson D: Depression and antidepressants and the elderly. J Clin Psychiatry 44:35-39, 1983

Butler RN: Psychiatry and the elderly: an overview. Am J Psychiatry 32:899-900, 1975

Chandler JD, Chandler JE: The prevalence of neuropsychiatric disorders in a nursing home population. J Geriatr Psychiatry Neur 1:71-76, 1988

Chenoweth B, Spencer B: Dementia: the experience of family caregivers. Gerontologist 26:267-272, 1986

Cleary TA, Clamon C, Price M, et al: A reduced stimulation unit: effects on patients with Alzheimer's disease and related disorders. Gerontologist 28:511-514, 1988

Cohen-Mansfield J: Agitated behaviors in the elderly, II: preliminary results in the cognitively deteriorated. J Am Geriatr Soc 34:722-727, 1986

Dawson P, Reid DW: Behavioral dimensions of patients at risk of wandering. Gerontologist 27:104-107, 1987

Devanand DP, Sackeim HA, Mayeux R: Psychosis, behavioral disturbance, and the use of neuroleptics in dementia. Comp Psychiatry 29:387-401, 1988

Dubovsky SL: Using electroconvulsive therapy for patients with neurological disease. Hosp Comm Psychiatry 37:819-825, 1986

Eichelman BV: Neurochemical and psychopharmacologic aspects of aggressive behavior, in Psychopharmacology: The Third Generation of Progress. Edited by Meltzer H. New York, Raven Press, 1987

Feighner JP: A comparative trial of fluoxetine and amitriptyline in patients with major depressive disorder. J Clin Psychiatry 46:369-372, 1985

Feighner JP, Cohn JB: Double-blind comparative trials of fluoxetine and doxepin in geriatric patients with major depressive disorder. Am J Psychiatry 46:20-25, 1985

Feighner JP, Aden GC, Fabre LF, et al: Comparison of alprazolam, imipramine, and placebo in the treatment of depression. JAMA 249:3057-3064, 1983

Finch CE: Biochemical markers in the diagnosis of the dementias. Paper presented at the NIH Consensus Development Conference on Differential Diagnosis of Dementing Diseases, Bethesda, MD, July 6-8, 1987

Fogel BS: Electroconvulsive therapy in the elderly: a clinical research agenda. Int J Geriatr Psychiatry 3:181-190, 1988

Fogel BS, Fretwell M: Reclassification of depression in the medically ill elderly. J Am Geriatr Soc 33:446-448, 1985

Foster EM, Kay DW: The characteristics of old people receiving and needing domiciliary services: the relevance of psychiatric diagnosis. Age/Ageing 5:245-255, 1976

Gallagher D, Thompson LW: Differential effects of psychotherapies for the treatment of major depressive disorders in older adult patients. Psychotherapy: Theory, Research and Practice 19:482-490, 1982

Georgotas A, Friedman E, McCarthy M, et al: Resistant geriatric depressions and therapeutic response to monoamine oxidase inhibitors. Biol Psychiatry 18:195-205, 1983

Georgotas A, McCrue RE, Hapworth W, et al: Comparative efficacy and safety of MAOIs versus TCAs in treating depression in the elderly. Biol Psychiatry 21:1155-1166, 1986

Gerner R, Estabrook W, Steuer J, et al: A placebo-controlled double-blind study of imipramine and trazodone in geriatric depression, in Psychopathology in the Aged. Edited by Cole JO, Barrett JE. New York, Raven Press, 1980

Gerson SC, Plotkin KA, Jarvik LF: Antidepressant drug studies, 1964 to 1986: empirical evidence for aging patients. J Clin Psychopharm 8:5:311-322, 1988

Goff DC, Jenike MA: Treatment-resistant depression in the elderly. J Am Geriatr Soc 34:63-70, 1986

Gottlieb, GL: Optimizing mental function in the elderly, in Practicing Prevention for the Elderly. Edited by Lavizzo-Mourey R, Day SC, Diserens D, et al. Philadelphia, C. V. Mosby, 1988

Greene JG, Smith K, Gardiner M, et al: Measuring behavioral disturbance of elderly demented patients in the community and its effects on relatives: a factor analytic study. Age Ageing 11:121-126, 1982

Greenwald BS, Marin DB, Silverman SM: Serotonergic treatment of screaming and banging in dementia. Lancet 8521(22):1464-1465, 1986

Gurland B, Dean L, Cross B: The epidemiology of depression and dementia in the elderly: the use of multiple indicators of these conditions, in Psychopathology in the Aged. Edited by Cole JD, Barrett JE. New York, Raven Press, 1980

Gurland BJ, Wilder DE, Berkman C: Depression and disability in the elderly: reciprocal relations and changes with age. Int J Geriatr Psychiatry 3:163-179, 1988

Hamilton M: Development of a rating scale for primary depressive illness. Br J Soc Clin Psychol 6:278-296, 1967

Hegeman C, Tobin S: Enhancing the autonomy of mentally impaired nursing home residents. Gerontologist 28(Suppl):71-75, 1988

Helms PM: Efficacy of antipsychotics in the treatment of the behavioral complications of dementia: a review of the literature. J Amer Geriatr Soc 33:206-209, 1985

Himmelhoch JM, Neil JF, May SJ, et al: Age dementia, dyskinesias, and lithium response. Am J Psychiatry 137:941-945, 1980

Jenike MA: Treating the violent elderly patient with propranolol. Geriatrics 38:29-31, 1983

Jenike MA: The use of monoamine oxidase inhibitors in the treatment of elderly, depressed patients. J Am Geriatr Soc 32:571-575, 1984

Jenike MA: Alzheimer's disease—what the practicing clinician needs to know. J Geriatr Psychiatry Neur 1:37-46, 1988a

Jenike MA: Assessment and treatment of affective illness in the elderly. J Geriatr Psychiatry Neur 1:89-106, 1988b

Jorm AF: Cognitive deficit in the depressed elderly: a review of some basic unresolved issues. Australia and New Zealand Journal of Psychiatry 20:11-22, 1986

Kathol RG, Petty F: Relationship of depression to medical. J Affective Dis 3:11-121, 1981

Katon W, Raskind M: Treatment of depression in the medically ill elderly with methylphenidate. Am J Psychiatry 137:963-965, 1980

Kemp B: Psychosocial and mental health issues in rehabilitation of older persons, in Aging and Rehabilitation: Advances in the State of the Art. Edited by Brody SJ, Ruff GE. New York, Springer, 1986

Kennedy GJ, Kelman HR, Thomas C, et al: Hierachy of characteristics associated with depressive symptoms in an urban elderly sample. Am J Psychiatry 146:2:220-225, 1989

Kirven LE, Mantero EF: Comparison of thioridazine and diazepam in the control of nonpsychotic symptoms associated with senility: double-blind study. J Am Geriatr Soc 21:546-551, 1973

Kral VA: The relationship between senile dementia (Alzheimer type) and depression. Can J Psychiatry 28:304-306, 1983

Kramer BA: Depressive pseudodementia. Psychiatry 23:538, 1982

Lakshmanan M, Mion LC, Frengley JD: Effective low-dose tricyclic antidepressant treatment for depressed geriatric rehabilitation patients: a double blind study. J Am Geriatr Soc 34:421-426, 1986

Larson EB, Reifler BV, Featherstone HJ, et al: Dementia in elderly outpatients: a prospective study. Ann Intern Med 100:417-423, 1984

Larson EB, Reifler BV, Sumi SM, et al: Diagnostic evaluation of 200 elderly outpatients with suspected dementia. J Gerontol 40:536-543, 1985

Lavizza-Mourey R: Preventing adverse drug reaction in the elderly, in Practicing Prevention for the Elderly. Edited by Lavizzo-Mourey R, Day SC, Diserens D, et al. Philadelphia, Hanley and Belfus, 1988

Lazarus LW, Newton N, Cohler B, et al: Frequency and presentation of depressive symptoms in patients with primary degenerative dementia. Am J Psychiatry 144:41-45, 1987

Levkoff SE, Cleary PD, Wetle T, et al: Illness behavior in the aged. J Am Geriatr Soc 36:622-629, 1988

Levy AB, Davis J, Bidder TG: Treatment of endogenous depression with alprazolam in a patient with recent cardiac disease: case report. J Clin Psychiatry 45:480-481, 1984

Lipsey JR, Robinson RG, Pearlson GD, et al: Nortriptyline treatment of post-stroke depression: a double-blind study. Lancet 1:297-300, 1984

Malhendra B: Depression and dementia: the multi-faceted relationship. Psychological Med 15:227-236, 1985

Markson EW, Steel K, Kane E: Administratively necessary days: more than an administrative problem. Gerontologist 23:486-492, 1983

Martin JB: Genetic markers in the diagnosis of the dementias. Paper presented at the NIH Consensus Development Conference on Differential Diagnosis of Dementing Diseases, Bethesda, MD, July 6-8, 1987

Matuk F, Kalyanaraman K: Syndrome of inappropriate secretion of antidiuretic hormone in patients treated with psychotropic drugs. Arch Neurol 34:374-375, 1977

Mayeux R, Stern Y, Sano M: Heterogeneity and prognosis in dementia of the Alzheimer type. Bull Clin Neurosci 50:7-10, 1985

McAllister TW, Price TR: Severe depressive pseudodementia with and without dementia. Am J Psychiatry 139:626-628, 1982

Merriam AE, Aronson MK, Gaston P, et al: The psychiatric symptoms of Alzheimer's disease. J Am Geriatr Soc 36:7-12, 1988

Meyers BS, Alexopoulos G: Age of onset and studies of late-life depression. Int J Geriatr Psychiatry 3:219-228, 1988

Miller NE: The measurement of mood in senile brain disease: examiner ratings and self reports, in Psychopathology in the Aged. Edited by Cole JO, Barrett JE. New York, Raven Press, 1980

Morstyn R, Hochanadel G, Kaplan E: Depression vs pseudodepression in dementia. J Clin Psychiatry 43:5:197-199, 1982

Murphy E: The prognosis of depression in old age. Br J Psychiatry 142:11-119, 1983

Murrell SA, Himmelfarb S, Wright K: Prevalence of depression and its correlates in older adults. Am J Epidemiol 117:173, 1983

Nair NPV, Ban TA, Hontela S, et al: Trazodone in the treatment of organic brain syndromes with special reference to psychogeriatrics. Curr Ther Res 15:769-775, 1973

National Institute on Aging Task Force: Senility reconsidered: treatment possibilities for mental impairment in the elderly. JAMA 244:259-263, 1980

Neil JF, Licata SM, May SJ, et al: Dietary noncompliance during treatment with tranylcypromine. J Clin Psychiatry 40:33-37, 1979

Pare CMB: The present status of monoamine oxidase inhibitors. Br J Psychiatry 146:576-584, 1985

Petrie WM, Ban TA, Berney S, et al: Loxapine in psychogeriatrics: a placebo- and standard-controlled clinical investigation. J Clin Psychopharmacol 2:122-126, 1982

Price TRP, McAllister TW: Safety and efficacy of ECT in depressed patients with dementia: a review of clinical experience. Convulsive Therapy 5:61-74, 1989

Rabins PV, Mace NL, Lucas MJ: The impact of dementia on the family. JAMA 248:333-335, 1982

Rader J: A comprehensive staff approach to problem wandering. Gerontologist 27:756-760, 1987

Rader J, Doan J, Schwab M: How to decrease wandering: a form of agenda behavior. Geriatr Nurs 6:196-199, 1985

Raskind MA, Risse SC: Antipsychotic drugs and the elderly. J Clin Psychiatry 47(Suppl):17-22, 1986

Reding M, Haycox J, Blass J: Depression in patients referred to a dementia clinic: a three year prospective study. Arch Neurol 42:894-896, 1985

Reifler BV, Larson E, Hanley R: Coexistence of cognitive impairment and depression in geriatric outpatients. Am J Psychiatry 139:623-626, 1982

Reifler BV, Larson E, Teri L, et al: Dementia of the Alzheimer's type and depression. J Am Geriatr Soc 34:855-859, 1986

Reifler BV, Teri L, Raskind M, et al: Double-blind trial of imipramine in Alzheimer's disease patients with and without depression. Am J Psychiatry 146:45-49, 1989

Reisberg B, Borenstein J, Salob S, et al: Behavioral symptoms in Alzheimer's disease: phenomenology and treatment. J Clin Psychiatry 48(Suppl):9-15, 1987

Rickels K, Chung HR, Csanalosi IB, et al: Alprazolam, diazepam, imipramine and placebo in outpatients with major depression. Arch Gen Psychiatry 44:862-866, 1987

Rifkin A, Reardon G, Siris S, et al: Trimipramine in physical illness with depression. J Clin Psychiatry 46:4-6, 1985

Risse SC, Barnes R: Pharmacologic treatment of agitation associated with dementia. J Amer Geriatr Soc 34:368-376, 1986

Robinson RG, Starr, LB, Kubos KL: A two-year longitudinal study of post-stroke mood disorders: Findings during the initial evaluation. Stroke 14:736-741, 1983

Robinson RG, Lipsey JR, Price TR: Diagnosis and clinical management of post-stroke depression. Psychosomatics 26:10:769-778, 1985

Ross HE, Kedward HB: Psychogeriatric hospital admissions from the community and institutions. J Gerontology 32:420-427, 1977

Rovner BW, Kafonek S, Filipp L, et al: Prevalence of mental illness in a community nursing home. Am J Psychiatry 143:1446-1449, 1986

Salzman C: Treatment of anxiety, in Clinical Geriatric Psychopharmacology. Edited by Salzman C. New York, McGraw-Hill, 1984

Sandifer MG: Hyponatremia due to psychotropic drugs. J Clin Psychiatry 44:301-303, 1983

Schneck MK, Reisberg B, Ferris SH: An overview of current concepts of Alzheimer's disease. Am J Psychiatry 139:165-173, 1982

Secretary's Task Force: Secretary's Task Force on Alzheimer's Disease, U.S. Department of Health and Human Services. DHHS Publication No. (ADM) 84-1323. Washington, DC, Department of Health and Human Services, 1984

Simpson DM, Foster D: Improvement in organically disturbed behavior with trazodone treatment. J Clin Psychiatry 47:191-193, 1986

Sommers I, Baskin D, Specht D, et al: Deinstitutionalization of the elderly mentally ill: factors affecting discharge to alternative living arrangements. Gerontologist 28:653-658, 1988

Stark P, Hardison CD: A review of multicenter controlled studies of fluoxetine vs imipramine and placebo in outpatients with major depressive disorder. J Clin Psychiatry 46:53-58, 1985

Stevenson J: Suicide, in The American Psychiatric Press Textbook of Psychiatry. Edited by Talbott JA, Hales RE, Yudofsky SC. Washington, DC, American Psychiatric Press, 1988

Stoudemire A, Fogel B: Psychopharmacology in the medically ill, in Principles of Medical Psychiatry. Edited by Stoudemire A, Fogel B. Orlando, Grune and Stratton, 1987

Stoudemire A, Thompson TL: Recognizing and treating dementia. Geriatrics 36:112-120, 1981

Summers WK, Majovski LV, Marsh GM: Oral tetrahydroaminoacridine in long-term treatment of senile dementia, Alzheimer type. N Engl J Med 315:1241-1245, 1986

Swearer Jm, Drachman DA, O'Donnell BF, et al: Troublesome and disruptive behaviors in dementia: relationships to diagnosis and disease severity. J Amer Geriatr Soc 36:784-790, 1988

Talbott JA, Hales RE, Yudofsky SC (eds): American Psychiatric Press Textbook of Psychiatry. Washington, DC, American Psychiatric Press, 1988

Teeter RB, Garetz F, Miller WR, et al: Psychiatric disturbances of aged patients in skilled nursing homes. Am J Psychiatry 133:1430-1434, 1976

Teri L, Borson S, Kiyak HS, et al: Behavioral disturbance, cognitive dysfunction, and functional skill. J Am Geriatr Soc 37:109-116, 1989

Waxman HM, Carner EA: Physicians' recognition, diagnosis and treatment of mental disorders in elderly medical patients. Gerontologist 24:593-597, 1984

Waxman HM, Carner EA, Blum A: Depressive symptoms and health service utilization among community elderly. J Am Geriatr Soc 31:145-149, 1983

Waxman HM, Carner EA, Klein M: Underutilization of mental health professionals by community elderly. The Gerontologist 24:23-30, 1984

Winograd CH, Jarvik LF: Physician management of the demented patient. J Am Geriatr Soc 34:295-308, 1986

Yudofsky S, Williams D, Gorman J: Propranolol in the treatment of rage and violent behavior in patients with chronic brain syndrome. Am J Psychiatry 138:218-220, 1981

4

Mental Health Services in General Medical Care and in Nursing Homes

Barbara J. Burns, Ph.D.
Carl A. Taube, Ph.D.

The general health sector functions as the de facto mental health service system for all age groups (Regier et al. 1978), and even more so for the elderly (Schurman et al. 1985). From the perspective of considering future alternatives for the mentally ill elderly, it is important to understand the configuration of the current system of care and the forces which influence it. In this chapter, the role of the general health sector will be examined in relation to the following topics:

1. Estimates of need for mental health services.
2. The prevailing philosophy of health care and its policy manifestations.
3. The continuum of care.
4. Use of the total service system—mental health, health and social services.
5. Service system problems and options for change in the general health sector.

The intent is to identify a mental health role for the general health sector that is consonant with and coordinated with the roles of specialty mental health and other human services. The chapter concludes by offering options for strengthening the mental health service capability of the general health sector.

Need for Mental Health Services

Estimates of need for treatment are traditionally derived from rates of distress or mental illness in the population. Rates of illness are

63

then used to project the amount and type of services needed. The resulting estimates can then be used to allocate resources and to design service systems to meet needs. Although planners need estimates, developing credible estimates is difficult.

First, prior to the present decade, epidemiological estimates for mental disorder in the elderly have tended to be high (15 to 25%) (Cohen 1976; U.S. Department of HEW 1979), and thus not considered to be very reliable or useful by planners and policy makers. (Health budgets would be quickly exhausted if a quarter of the elderly used specialty mental health services.) Estimates often included psychological distress as well as diagnosable illness. Although treatment could be beneficial for the former problem, attention to severity of illness is necessary for planning purposes when resources are limited.

Second, the large gap between estimated need and use of specialty services (even with lower estimates) is not fully explained by service system problems such as accessibility and availability of services. Even under ideal circumstances with few system barriers to service use, rates of service use for the elderly remain low relative to the prevalence of illness (Goldstrom et al. 1987). This may be explained largely by a cohort effect, whereby concerns about stigma inhibit service use by the current elderly population. With a more sophisticated and better educated aging population coming along, predictions of future service use should not be based on current utilization patterns.

A third factor related to the failure of policymakers to take epidemiological estimates seriously is policymakers' doubt about the effectiveness of mental health treatment for older persons. Older persons' mental health problems are often seen as a function of normal aging, or as essentially untreatable. Accumulating evidence on the efficacy of psychiatric treatment in the elderly—for example, psychoactive drugs for depression (Zung 1980) and for some symptoms of dementia (Crook 1988; Salzman 1988), and the use of psychotherapy for selected conditions (Butler and Lewis 1982)—may encourage policymakers to take sound epidemiological estimates more seriously (see Chapter 3 for further details).

Fourth, since physical illnesses and the medications used to treat them can produce psychological symptoms, the differential diagnosis of psychological symptoms is a particular challenge for the elderly, who are subject to chronic physical illness. Clinically, it is important to identify all treatable psychiatric complications of physical illness. Epidemiologically, conservative practice in counting cases of mental illness excludes those in which symptoms are produced by physical illness.

The Epidemiology Catchment Areas (ECA) program supported by the National Institute of Mental Health (NIMH) during the early 1980s offers a state-of-the-art approach to the estimation of mental disorder in the U.S. elderly population. Population-based studies conducted in five communities (New Haven, Baltimore, St. Louis, Durham, and Los Angeles), which added an oversample of elderly persons in three of these communities, enable estimates of mental illness in older persons. The one-month prevalence rates have been weighted to provide estimates of the U.S. population (Regier et al., in press).[1]

The methods and measures used in the ECA address the major criticisms of prior epidemiological studies. With the Diagnostic Interview Schedule (DIS) (Robins et al. 1981), disorders are identified based on a structured interview which applies DSM-III criteria (American Psychiatric Association 1980). Thus, distress or problems in living, apart from a specific mental disorder, are not included in the estimates, and severity is to some extent assessed. The DIS also attempts to rule out physical causes for individual symptoms, to avoid confounding mental and physical illness. (In other words, symptoms possibly due to the patient's physical illness are not counted toward the diagnosis of mental disorder. This exclusive approach has the virtue of simplicity and reliability, but may underestimate psychiatric comorbidity in severely physically ill people [Cohen-Cole and Harpe 1987].)

Community Estimate of Mental Illness

The overall ECA estimate of mental illness in the elderly population is 12.3%. This estimate may be more reasonable than prior estimates as a basis for discussing the need for mental health services. Selected one-month prevalence rates for the elderly in the community developed by Regier et al. (1988) are presented in Table 4-1. The most frequently occurring conditions are anxiety disorders, severe cognitive impairment, phobias, and affective disorders (12.5%). A more conservative (8.7%) estimate of mental illness in the elderly could be obtained by eliminating phobias, as questions have been raised about how effectively this category was assessed by the DIS (Thompson et al. 1988). However, since it is not feasible to determine what proportion of persons with phobias had conditions sufficiently disabling to require treatment, it is not clear that the lower estimate would be more accurate.

While the ECA did not attempt to predict or to assess attitudes about service use, service use was documented at three points in time to link episodes of illness with service use in different sectors

Table 4–1. One month prevalence of DIS/DSM-III disorders in the community by age 65+

Type of disorder	Percentage
Any DIS disorder	12.3
Any DIS disorder except phobia	8.7
Alcohol abuse/dependence	0.9
Schizophrenia	0.1
Affective disorders	2.5
Anxiety disorders	5.5
Phobia	4.8
Panic disorder	0.1
Obsessive-compulsive disorder	0.8
Somatization disorder	0.1
Severe cognitive impairment	4.9
65–74	2.9
75–84	6.8
≥85	15.8

Note. Disorders with a rate of 0.0 were not listed.

and settings. These data permit the estimation of the need for mental health services, as illustrated by Shapiro et al. (1985) with Baltimore ECA data. To be classified as being in need of mental health services, individuals either had to report that they visited a general health or mental health professional for a mental health complaint in the 6-month period prior to the interview, or had to have at least two of the three following manifestations of emotional problems: 1) a DIS/DSM disorder in the past 6 months; 2) a General Health Questionnaire score of 4 or more; or 3) disability attributed by the individual to emotional problems which impaired usual functioning for at least one day during the prior 3 months. Using these criteria, 7.8% of persons 65 and over were estimated to need mental health care. This approach contrasts in two ways with the prior one which relies exclusively on the presence of a diagnosable condition:

1. All persons who received mental health treatment are included irrespective of a DIS/DSM diagnosis.
2. The criteria for need are more restrictive, requiring two out of three criteria, one of which may be a diagnosable condition.

This method of assessing need was further validated using ECA Wave II data, which yielded similar population rates for service need (Shapiro et al. 1986). However, since age-specific estimates of need were not reported in the Wave II study, the Wave I rate of 7.8% of the elderly population is used here. The 7.8% estimate, projected to the entire U.S. elderly population (Rosenstein et al. 1987) identifies 1,888,316 noninstitutionalized older persons in need of services.[2] Shapiro and colleagues also provide an estimate of *unmet* need (percent meeting criteria for needing mental health treatment who did not receive any in the prior 6 months) of 62.6% of cases, or 5.7% of the total population aged 65 or over.

Institutional Estimate of Mental Illness

Obtaining an estimate of mental illness in institutional settings is more complicated and potentially less reliable. Although the ECA sampled long-term care institutions, such as state hospitals and nursing homes, these data have not been analyzed to date. Thus, it is necessary at present to rely on medical record diagnoses of persons in these facilities in order to obtain information. Medical record diagnoses probably underestimate prevalence, as there are disincentives for nursing homes to record mental illness diagnoses. Table 4-2 presents an estimate based on data from 1980 and later.

The overall rate of mental illness among the institutionalized elderly is estimated to be 65%; there were 840,198 institutionalized mentally ill elderly persons in 1980. Their dominant locus is the nursing home, which provides care for 94% of them. Mental hospitals, treating 6%, are not even a close second.

When diagnostic distributions are considered by setting, dementia accounts for 73% of all mental diagnoses in nursing homes, so that 47% of all residents suffer from dementia while another 17% have one of a wide range of other mental disorders (U.S. Department of HHS 1980). Older patients in mental hospitals are also most likely to receive a dementia diagnosis, but substantial minorities suffer from affective disorders or schizophrenia (as determined by an analysis of the 1985 National Nursing Home Survey by one of the authors [B.J.B.]). Thus, the need for active treatment of conditions other than dementia and its complications will be greater in mental hospitals. Nonetheless, since demented as well as nondemented patients can benefit from some form of mental health treatment (an evaluation and/or medication, at a minimum), the total diagnosed population can be considered to need services.

Combined Community and Institutional Estimate

When the estimated 7.8% of the community elderly needing treatment, or 1,888,316 persons, is added to 65% of the institutionalized elderly, or 840,198 persons, a total of 2,728,514 persons are estimated to need treatment. Dividing this number by the total commu-

Table 4–2. Persons 65 + with mental illness (including dementia) in long-term care institutions, 1980

Facility type	Population aged ≥65	Percentage mentally ill	Number mentally ill	Percentage of all institutionalized mentally ill
Mental Hospitals	51,105	100.0	51,105	6.0
Nursing Homes	1,232,958	64.0	789,093	94.0
All Institutions	1,284,063	65.0	840,198	100.0

Note. The institutionalized elderly population is defined by the 1980 census categories of mental hospitals and nursing homes (Bureau of Census 1983). Mental hospitals include public and private psychiatric hospitals and psychiatric wards of general hospitals. Rates of mental illness are applied to each category based on the other surveys, the 1980 NIMH surveys of state and county hospitals and V.A. Medical Centers (Rosenstein et al. 1987), and the 1985 National Nursing Home Survey (Burns 1988). All ICD (U.S. Department of Health and Human Services 1980) and DSM-III categories 290–315 (American Psychiatric Association 1980) are included. The number of persons in each setting is multiplied by the estimated rate of mental illness to obtain the number of mentally ill in each setting. The percentage of all mentally ill is obtained by dividing the number in each setting by the total mentally ill in all institutions. Other institutions (prisons, chronic disease and tuberculosis hospitals, and homes for the physically and mentally handicapped) were not included in the totals or calculations because their combined total is less than one-half of a percent of the over-65 population, and data estimating their mental conditions and treatment are not available.

Source. Bureau of Census: 1980 Census of Population: Persons in Institutions and Other Group Quarters. U.S. Department of Commerce, 1984.

nity plus institutionalized population of 25,493,248, 10.7% of the older U.S. population are estimated to need mental health services. The community elderly needing care comprise 69.2% of the total needing services and the institutionalized elderly the remaining 30.8%. Although institutionalized elderly use a larger share of total health care dollars, twice as many persons in the community need some form of treatment.

The extent to which elderly people either in the community or in institutions receive the care they need is influenced by the prevalent philosophy of health care and by policies regulating the provision and financing of care, as well as by the specifics of the service system. A brief discussion of these issues offers the context for understanding data on the present use of mental health services by the elderly.

Philosophic and Policy Considerations

Widely held premises regarding the mental health care of the elderly underlie policies for the provision of that care. These include: 1) a preference for providing care in the community instead of institutions, 2) a belief in the value of managed care approaches (case managers, primary care physicians as gatekeepers, or organizations such as health maintenance organizations and preferred provider organizations), 3) a preference for service provision by generalist providers instead of specialists when feasible, and 4) a belief that care should be comprehensive, continuous, coordinated, and of high quality.

These premises represent a compromise between concerns about individuals' quality of life and the interests of society as a whole. The latter reflects the value placed by society on the welfare of older persons and the costs to society both of treatment and of its absence. Promoting access, containing costs, and assuring quality are the (sometimes incompatible) goals.

Concern about costs gives rise to efforts to substitute less costly care in the community, at home, or in a nursing home, for more costly hospital services. Community care is likely to be managed by primary care physicians or nurse clinicians. Access to specialized psychiatric care is likely to be constrained by limited private and public insurance coverage and by the limited availability of public sector services, restricted today in many areas to state and county mental hospitals or to Medicaid-funded nursing homes.

Table 4–3. Continuum of care for the mentally ill elderly

Type of care	Type of service organization
Community Services	
1. Evaluation—detection, diagnosis, referral	Primary care (general practitioners health plan), mental health clinic or private practice, social services
2. Outpatient treatment—case management, psychotherapy, drug management, support groups	Mental health, health organization, with mental health consultation
3. Day care—supervision, stimulation, maintenance	Social services (e.g., area agency on aging) with mental health consultation
4. Partial hospitalization—crisis intervention, treatment of symptoms, social skills training, maintenance	Mental health
5. Emergency—crisis intervention, behavioral management, or medical intervention	Home-based mental health mobile team, hospital emergency room, mental health center
6. Home care—assistance with activities of daily living (ADL) or occupational therapy	Home health care

7. Respite care—relief for family care givers for time-limited periods — Home health care agency, mental health agency, nursing home

8. Inpatient—medical treatment to stabilize acute psychiatric problems — General hospital, psychiatric hospital

9. Housing—supervised housing to assist with ADL or independent activities of daily living — Local housing organization, mental health agency

10. Hospice—supervised setting for terminally ill patients (likely to be limited to dementia) — Health organization with mental health consultation

Long-Term Care Institutions

1. Nursing home—fully supervised nursing care, mental health evaluation, and limited treatment — Health organization with mental health consultation

2. Psychiatric hospital—long-term treatment for severe mental illness that cannot be treated in an acute setting — Mental health

3. Prisons—mental health consultation or treatment — Other human services with mental health consultation

4. Other (chronic disease hospitals, mental retardation facilities) — Health organization with mental health consultation

A Continuum of Care

Before proceeding to the realities of the current system of mental health services for the elderly, an ideal continuum of services is outlined. The principles of community-based care, significant reliance on the general health care system and use of existing elderly services are respected in this approach, but in the ideal case greater attention is given to quality and comprehensiveness. In addition to ensuring that a comprehensive array of services is available, an ideal system must assure that services are coordinated within and across service delivery organizations and sectors. The relationships between general health providers and mental health professionals (Schulberg and Burns 1988) are critical, as are the relationships between social service agencies, such as Area Agencies on Aging (Lebowitz et al. 1987; Light et al. 1986), and the health care providers. Since the point of entry into the system can occur in the health or social services sectors, mental health professionals must be accessible to health and social service providers to provide consultation or treatment for their clients.

The services listed in Table 4-3 exist at least partially in most communities. However, the capacity of any given service may not be sufficient, providers may not consider referring elderly people to them, or those services designed for a range of age groups may not be staffed with personnel who have expertise in treating the elderly. Most of the services listed are traditional mental health services. Some, such as home health care and hospice, have not generally been available to psychiatric patients. Other services, like respite care, have become more available as recognition about the burden of dementia on family members has increased.

The proposed continuum of care is largely a theoretical concept. In most communities this continuum has many holes in it. Even when the services do exist, clients may not receive what they need. Availability of services does not insure accessibility which is influenced by insurance coverage, transportation, judgments by providers and families regarding need, and the ability of service providers under different organizational auspices to work together.

Use of the Current Service System

Several studies over the past decade have shown the elderly are underserved in outpatient mental health settings (Taube and Redick 1980; White House Conference on Aging 1981), and that mental health services received in long-term care settings are also inadequate (Burns et al. 1988; Shadish and Bootzin 1981). Following is an attempt, using ECA data, to provide a contemporary estimate of unmet need for mental health services.

Use of mental health services by older Americans can be assessed for those traditional mental health services on which data are available. Evaluation, emergency services, and therapy are grouped under outpatient care categories; partial hospitalization, acute- and long-term inpatient care are reported separately. For the general health sector, limited data are available on outpatient, inpatient, and nursing home care. Certain categories of services are excluded entirely including day care, respite care, home care, housing, and hospice.

In this estimate, a person is counted as receiving care if any mental health care is provided, with certain qualifications. For mental health providers this includes a visit for any reason. For general medical providers, mental health treatment is defined by the prescription of a psychotropic drug in the presence of a mental disorder diagnosis or the provision of counseling or psychotherapy regardless of diagnosis. When information showed that no treatment was provided, as in the NIMH hospital surveys, patients were not counted as receiving care. In nursing homes, treatment is counted if a patient was seen at least once by any type of mental health professional. Receipt of services is without regard to the extent, quality or appropriateness of the care given.[3]

Mental Health Services Use in the Community

Table 4-4 presents national statistics on the use of mental health services in the specialty mental health sector (SMH) and the general health (GH) sector by persons 65 years of age and older who do not reside in institutions. Outpatient services are subdivided into clinics, community mental health centers, Veterans Administration Medical Center clinics, the private practice of psychiatrists and psychologists, and partial hospitalization. Persons in mental institutions are included subsequently under institutional settings.

The specialty sector treated 617,025 persons or 2.5% of this older population. Thus, based on an estimated community need of 7.8%, *about one-third of those who need care receive it from mental health specialists.* Persons who receive care in specialty mental health facilities are likely to receive more care than those who obtain their mental health care in the general health sector (described below). The recorded mental disorder diagnoses of persons treated by nonpsychiatric physicians tend to be somewhat less serious (Schurman et al. 1985).

Table 4–4. Use of mental health services in the community by persons 65 +

Sector and service type	No. of persons	Percentage of total	Percentage of U.S. elderly noninstitutionalized population
Mental Health Special Sector			
Outpatient clinics[1]	79,630		
Community mental health centers[2]	75,545		
VAMC clinics[3]	9,733		
Private practice psychiatrists[4]	368,165		
Private practice psychologists[5]	60,831		
Partial Hospitalization[6]	23,121		
Subtotal	617,025	51.0	2.5
General Health Sector			
Outpatient medical settings[7] (excluding psychiatrists)	482,141		
Nonfederal general hospitals[8] without psychiatric units	110,400		
Subtotal	592,541	49.0	2.4
Unduplicated health sector total[9]	1,209,839	100.0	4.9

[1]Based on National Institute of Mental Health, Division of Biometry and Applied Sciences, Survey and Reports Branch, 1975 survey of admissions to outpatient clinics. Admissions (53,087) were multiplied by a factor of 1.5 to obtain persons under care in a year (personal communication, Carl A. Taube, Ph.D., Johns Hopkins University, October 1, 1988).

[2]Based on National Institute of Mental Health (NIMH), Division of Biometry and Applied Sciences (DBAS), Survey and Reports Branch (SRB), 1978 survey of community mental health centers. Admissions (50,363) were multiplied by 1.5 to obtain persons under care (see note 1).

[3]Based on NIMH, DBAS, SRB, 1975 survey of admissions to VAMC clinics. Admissions (6,489) were multiplied by 1.5 to obtain persons under care (see note 1).

[4]Based on estimates from the 1980 Medical Care Utilization and Expenditure Survey (NMCUES), psychiatrists saw 2,345,000 persons in office-based practice (Bonham GS, Procedures and Questionnaires of the National Medical Care Utilization and Expenditure Survey. National Medical Care Utilization and Expenditure Survey [Series A, Methodological Report No. 1. DHHS Pub. No. ADM 83-2001, National Center for Health Statistics, Public Health Service. Washington, DC, U.S. Government Printing Office, 1983]). Further analysis revealed that 15.7% of the patients of psychiatrists were 55 years or older (Taube CA, Burns BJ, Kessler L: patients of psychiatrists or psychologists, 1980. *American Psychologist* 39:1433-1447, 1984). Although a slight overestimation of the elderly, this percentage was applied to the total number of patients of psychiatrists to obtain the number of older persons treated.

[5]Based on the NMCUES, psychologists were estimated to have seen 2,253,000 patients (see Bonham reference above) and 2% were older than 55 (see Taube et al. reference above). Although a slight overestimate of the elderly, this percentage was applied to the total number of patients of psychologists to obtain the number of older persons treated.

[6]Based on NIMH, DBAS, SRB, 1983, survey of partial hospitalization. Admissions (15,414) were multiplied by 1.5 to obtain persons under care (see note 1 above).

[7]Estimate derived from unpublished data from the 1985 National Ambulatory Medical Care Survey conducted by the National Center for Health Statistics (personal communication, Ann Hohman, Ph.D., M.P.H., National Institute of Mental Health, October 1988). Visits for mental health treatment to nonpsychiatric physicians incuded 7,841,944 for psychotropic drugs and 202,495 for counseling/psychotherapy. To correct for visits in which a psychotropic drug was prescribed without a mental disorder diagnosis, 66% of these visits were eliminated (based on Larson et al. presentation at APHA, November 1989, Psychotropics Prescribed to the U.S. Elderly in 1980 and 1981); to unduplicate visits, the first number was divided by 7 to obtain an estimate of persons (personal communication, Robert Beardsley, Ph.D., School of Pharmacy, University of Maryland, October 1, 1988); counseling/psychotherapy visits were divided by 2 to obtain an estimate of persons served.

[8]Based on the National Center for Health Statistics ["Utilization of Short Stay Hospitals, United States, 1985, Annual Survey," Vital and Health Statistics Series 13, No. 91 (May 1987)] first-listed diagnoses for mental disorders occurred in 250,000 discharges. To split these discharges between psychiatry units and scatterbeds, the proportion of scatterbeds (46%), based on 1984 Medicare data, was applied to total discharges (personal communication, Carl A. Taube, Ph.D., October 1, 1988).

[9]Since persons admitted for a general hospital inpatient stay for a mental condition see a physician in an outpatient visit, these admissions were eliminated from the general health sector total.

Table 4–5. Use of mental health services in institutional settings by persons aged 65 or over

Sector	Number needing services (see Table 4–2)	Number receiving services	Percentage of unmet need
Mental Hospitals[1]	51,105	48,550	5%
Nursing Homes[2]	789,093	32,113	95.9%
Total	840,198	80,663	91.4%

[1]Based on Mental Health Statistical Note 181 (Use of Inpatient Services by the Elderly Age 65 and Over, April 1987), the rate of no psychiatric treatment for persons 65+ ranged from 1.7% in general hospitals to 7.0% in state and county hospitals. A value in between, 5%, was adopted as the no treatment rate; thus, 95% received mental health treatment. This was multiplied by the 1980 psychiatric hospital census figure (see Table 4–2).

[2]This estimate, derived from the National Center for Health Statistics 1985 National Nursing Home Survey (NNHS), is based on unpublished data. The rate of mental health treatment (2.45%) was applied to the 1980 nursing home population ages 65 and over (see Table 4–2). The rate is based on any contact with a mental health professional in the past month.

According to the data presented in Table 4-4, about half of elderly persons receiving treatment get it in the general health sector.[4] The mental health outpatient care received by this population in the general health sector consists primarily of psychotropic medications: the ratio is 4:1 of drugs to counseling/psychotherapy.

The overall rate of mental health service use is 4.9%. When contrasted with a 7.8% estimate of need for services presented earlier, the gap between need and use is 2.9% of the population, or 37% of those needing services.

Mental Health Service Use in Institutions

The institutional picture for the mentally ill elderly is similar to the community picture: the critical treatment role belongs to the general health sector. Although older persons with mental disorders are more likely to receive treatment if they reside in a mental hospital than if they reside in a nursing home, the size of the population needing mental health treatment in nursing homes is about 16 times larger (Table 4-5). Unmet need is 91.4%. An estimated 840,198 persons needed mental health care, and an estimated 80,663 persons received it. This figure could be reduced somewhat if the prescription of psychotropic drugs by nonpsychiatric physicians in nursing homes were counted as treatment. Based on the 1984 National Nursing Home Survey pretest, approximately 30% of residents received psychotropic drugs (Burns et al. 1988). However, psychotropic prescribing was judged to be inappropriate on the basis of lack of a mental disorder diagnosis, a dosage problem or an inappropriate drug in 51% of the cases (Burns and Kamerow 1988). Thus, if *correct* prescribing were used as the criterion for mental health treatment, 15% of the unmet need figure would be eliminated, reducing this amount to around 76%. However, to do this with confidence, it would be important to know that diagnoses were valid and that treatment needs had been adequately assessed and provided for.

Service System Problems and Options for Change in the General Sector

The preceding section documented significant gaps in the provision of mental health services to the mentally ill elderly in institutional settings relative to the need for services and raised questions about the adequacy of mental health care for this population in the community. Among the 7.8% of older persons who need some mental health treatment in the community, 2.5% appear to receive it from mental health professionals, while another 2.4% obtain care from general medical providers. The total is 4.9% in contrast to an estimated need of 7.8%. In institutional settings the rate of unmet need, 91.4%, is especially striking due to the large nursing home population with mental illness who virtually receive no mental health treatment. However, the number of older persons in the community who need care is significantly greater than the number in institutional settings.

The observation of limited mental health specialist care in the community and negligible care in nursing homes reflects a general lack of capacity in the mental health service system. Because the general population, particularly older persons, has regular contact with the general health sector (85% see a physician during any year) (National Center for Health Statistics 1987), the most important place to begin altering practice patterns is there. The data presented indicate high rates of treatment with psychotropic drugs. Although it appears that over 60% of the community elderly with mental disorders are receiving some therapeutic attention, there is no information about whether those persons who need it are the ones who receive it, or, if they are the right people, whether they are diagnosed correctly and whether the amount and type of treatment provided is appropriate. Referrals to mental health professionals are likely to be low unless cases are properly identified by general health service providers. Thus, very basic steps to increase accurate case identification need to be taken including:

1. Increased training of primary care nurses and physicians in the differential diagnosis of frequently occurring mental disorders in the elderly population (especially dementia, depression, and anxiety disorders).
2. The development and use of screening tools in primary care settings as an aid to improve detection. There is some evidence of the effectiveness of mental health screening for older persons (German et al. 1987).

Along with training in the evaluation of mental disorders in older persons, further efforts need to be directed toward treatment and/or referral of patients with mental disorders. Recommendations include:

3. Training of primary care physicians regarding the appropriate use of psychotropic medications for older persons with mental illness.
4. The development and use of structured criteria for referral by primary care providers to mental health specialists of older patients with mental illness.
5. Training for psychiatrists and other mental health professionals to work in primary care settings—assisting primary care physicians in differential diagnosis, consulting on use of psychotropic medications, or providing psychotherapy services.

There are problems with paying for the training proposed above (e.g., caps on subsidies for medical education) and further problems when it comes to physicians' employing mental health knowledge in practice. Better reimbursement by Medicare for cognitive services (see Chapters 6 and 7) may be a start. However, it is not certain that reimbursement alone will offer a sufficient incentive for general health practitioners to invest the time required to evaluate and treat psychiatric disorders in the elderly.

The preceding two sets of recommendations regarding screening, referral, and training of primary care providers are as applicable to general hospitals as to outpatient settings. A further issue for general hospitals is that the availability of separate psychiatric units in general hospitals remains limited despite significant growth. Only 14% of general hospitals have such units (Redick and Witkin 1982) and a slightly, but not significantly larger proportion (17%) have a psychiatric service (Manderscheid et al. 1985) which provides consultation to a subset of medical beds known as scatterbeds. The limited availability of psychiatric inpatient services in general hospitals represents a particular problem for the elderly who may have a comorbid physical illness that would require that psychiatric treatment be received in a general medical setting. Recommendations for improving mental health treatment in general hospitals would add the following:

6. Increasing the number of hospitals with psychiatric consultation services and assuring that consultation services have special geriatric expertise.
7. Increasing the number of psychiatric-medical units in general hospitals which specialize in treating combined medical and psychiatric illness (Burns and Schulberg 1986). This would require sufficient Medicare reimbursement to cover the comprehensive care provided on such units.

Other health services in the community which could improve the care of older persons with mental illness, such as home health care, respite care or hospice services, would also benefit from improved availability of mental health specialist consultation. As the emphasis on community, versus institutional care, is progressively implemented, such service organizations will provide care for a larger number of mentally ill older persons. It is essential that consultation and education are made available to such providers so that they can more effectively manage mentally ill patients.

Nursing homes, the major health sector institutional settings for older persons, present the greatest service delivery challenge when the gap between the diagnosis of mental disorder and the provision of treatment is assessed. The OBRA 1987 Nursing Home Reform legislation should facilitate the identification of persons needing mental health treatment, but it does not provide funds for rendering the treatment required.[5] Coverage of partial hospitalization and mental health services in nursing homes by Medicaid and by other third-party payers is critically needed.

OBRA 1987 also mandates the monitoring of psychotropic medications, historically a problem of substantial magnitude (Ray et al. 1980; Gurland et al. 1979). Again, better funding of mental health services in nursing homes probably will be needed to translate monitoring into better care.

While efforts to upgrade the mental health knowledge and skills of physicians and nurses will help mentally ill patients in nursing homes, homes of substantial size should be required to employ a mental health professional, at least part time. In addition, consideration might be given to the following:

8. Addition of psychogeriatric units in larger nursing homes for intensive treatment of acute psychiatric episodes without discharging the patient.
9. Addition of a rehabilitation component to provide social skills training to patients with dementia or other chronic psychiatric conditions whose quality of life could be improved, possibly increasing the potential for some patients to return to the community.

Research Priorities

Data presented on the use of mental health services in the general health sector point to major needs for research on the appropriateness, adequacy, quality, and effectiveness of the care provided. Questions such as the following need attention:

1. To what extent are the psychotropic drugs being adequately prescribed for specific psychiatric conditions?
2. To what extent is prescribing for symptoms in the absence of a diagnosis appropriate?
3. Are dosages adequate and are important drug or illness interactions being given sufficient consideration?
4. Are such drug prescriptions being monitored with sufficient frequency?

ECA data from New Haven indicate that over 16% of older persons receive psychotropic medications (Tischler et al., unpublished document), and research by Wells et al. (1988) point out problems of limited treatment plans and infrequent drug monitoring for all age groups. The need for research concerning the prescribing of psychotropic medications applies equally to the general medical outpatient settings and to nursing homes.

5. What is the role of the psychosocial therapies for older mentally ill persons in the general health sector?
6. What types of services are most critically needed, which are effective, and what types of providers can be prepared to provide them?
7. Given limited attention to psychosocial treatments by non-psychiatric physicians, how can mental health professionals be effectively integrated into general medical settings for the purpose of teaching, consultation, or treatment? Various models for achieving these aims need to be designed and tested.

Conclusion

This chapter has identified a number of problems relevant to providing mental health services to older persons in the general health sector. With an increased emphasis on curtailing the use of specialty health services through managed approaches to health care (or simply by inadequate reimbursement), the mental health role of the general health providers will only increase over time. While the data presented provide some evidence of recognition of mental health problems by general health providers, their almost exclusive focus on use of psychotropic drugs for intervention is problematic. Based on national survey data, drugs are their primary mental health treatment modality, and relatively little non-pharmacologic therapy is provided to treat the mental disorders of general medical patients whether in the community or in nursing homes. Approaches to address this problem include training, consultation by mental health specialists to general health providers, and adding mental health specialists to treatment teams in general medical settings and in larger nursing homes. Further research is needed to develop more effective approaches to improving the quality of mental health care in the general health sector.

The author would like to recognize critical assistance in the preparation of this chapter. Sam Shapiro, Johns Hopkins University, and Ann Hohman, Ph.D., M.P.H. of the National Institute of Mental Health and Robert S. Beardsley, Ph.D., School of Pharmacy, University of Maryland, contributed by providing data and/or deriving estimates. Lenna Babigian Janick and John Taube, University of Maryland School of Medicine, and Elizabeth Anne Gwaltney, Frederick Community College, assisted with editing and presentation of data. Finally, special appreciation goes to Bonita Chandler for carefully typing multiple drafts of the manuscript.

References

American Psychiatric Association: Diagnostic and Statistical Manual of Mental Disorders, 3rd ed. Washington, American Psychiatric Association, 1980

Bureau of Census: 1980 Census of Population: General Population Characteristics, United States Summary. Washington, DC, U.S. Department of Commerce, 1983

Burns BJ, Kamerow DB: Psychotropic drug prescriptions for nursing home residents. Journal of Family Practice 26:155-160, 1988

Burns BJ, Schulberg HC: Organizing psychiatric care in general hospitals to meet medical and psychiatric needs. Administration in Mental Health 13:180-188, 1986

Burns BJ, Larson DB, Goldstrom ID, et al: Mental disorders among nursing home patients: preliminary findings from the national nursing home survey pretest. International Journal of Geriatric Psychiatry 3:27-35, 1988

Butler RN, Lewis MI: Aging and Mental Health. St. Louis, Mosby, 1982

Cohen GD: Mental health services and the elderly: needs and options. American Journal of Psychiatry 133:65-68, 1976

Cohen-Cole S, Harpe C: Diagnostic assessment of depression in the medically ill, in Principles of Medical Psychiatry. Edited by Stoudemire A, Fogel B. Orlando, Grune and Stratton, 1987

Crook T: Pharmacotherapy of cognitive deficits in Alzheimer's disease and age-associated memory impairment. Psychopharmacology Bulletin 24:31-38, 1988

George LK, Blazer DG, Winfield-Laird I, et al: Psychiatric disorders and mental health service use in later life: evidence from the Epidemiologic Catchment Area Program, in Epidemiology and Aging. Edited by Brody J, Maddox G. New York, Springer, 1988

German PS, Shapiro S, Skinner EA, et al: Detection and management of mental health problems of older patients by primary care providers. Journal of the American Medical Association 257:489-493, 1987

Goldstrom ID, Burns BJ, Larson DB, et al: Mental health services use by elderly adults in a primary care setting. Journal of Gerontology 42:147-153, 1987

Gurland B, Cross P, Defiguerido J, et al: A cross-national comparison of the institutionalized elderly in the cities of New York and London. Psychological Medicine 9:781-788, 1979

Lebowitz BD, Light E, Bailey F: Mental health center services for the elderly: the impact of coordination with area agencies on aging. The Gerontologist 27:699-702, 1987

Light E, Lebowitz BD, Bailey F: CMHCs and elderly services: an analysis of direct and indirect services and service delivery sites. Community Mental Health Journal 22:294-302, 1986

Manderscheid RW, Witkin MJ, Rosenstein MJ, et al: Specialty mental health services: system and patient characteristics—United States, in Mental Health, United States 1985. Edited by Taube CA, Barrett SA. Rockville, National Institute of Mental Health, 1985

National Center for Health Statistics: Current Estimates from the National Health Interview Survey, United States 1986. Vital and Health Statistics Series 10, No. 164, October 1987

Ray WA, Federspiel CF, Schaffner W: A study of antipsychotic drugs in nursing homes: epidemiological evidence suggesting misuse. American Journal of Public Health 70:485-491, 1980

Redick R, Witkin M: Separate Psychiatric Settings in Non-Federal General Hospitals, United States 1977-78. Series CN No. 4, DHHS publication no. (ADM)82-1140. Washington, DC, U.S. Government Printing Office, 1982

Regier DA, Boyd JH, Burke JC, et al: One-month prevalence of psychiatric disorders in the U.S.: based on five epidemiological catchment area sites. Archives of General Psychiatry 45:977-986, 1988

Regier DA, Goldberg ID, Taube CA: The de facto U.S. mental health services system. Archives of General Psychiatry 35:685-693, 1978

Robins LN, Helzer JE, Croughan J, et al: National Institute of Mental Health Diagnostic Interview Schedule. Archives of General Psychiatry 38:381-389, 1981

Rosenstein MJ, Milazzo-Sayre LJ, MacAskill RL, et al: Use of Inpatient Psychiatric Services by Special Populations, in Mental Health United States. Edited by Manderscheid RW, Barrett SA. DHHS Pub. No. (ADM) 87-1518. Washington, DC, Department of Health and Human Services, 1987

Salzman C: Treatment of agitation, anxiety, and depression in dementia. Psychopharmacology Bulletin 24:39-42, 1988

Schulberg HC, Burns BJ: Mental disorders in primary care: epidemiologic, diagnostic, and treatment research directions. General Hospital Psychiatry 10:79-87, 1988

Schurman RA, Kramer PD, Mitchell JB: The Hidden Mental Health Network. Archives of General Psychiatry 42:89-94, 1985

Shadish WE, Bootzin RR: Nursing homes and chronic mental patients. Schizophrenia Bulletin 7:478-488, 1981

Shapiro S, Skinner EA, Kramer M, et al: Measuring Need for Mental Health Services in a General Population. Medical Care 23:1033-1043, 1985

Shapiro S, Skinner EA, German PS, et al: Need and demand for mental health services in an urban community: an exploration based on household interviews, in Mental Disorders in the Community: Progress and Challenge. Edited by Barrett J, Rose RM. New York, The Guilford Press, 1986

Taube CA, Redick RW: Demography and mental health care of the aged, in Handbook of Mental Health and Aging. Edited by Birren JE, Sloane RB. Englewood Cliffs, NJ, Prentice Hall, 1980

Thompson JW, Burns BJ, Bartko J, et al: The use of ambulatory services by persons with and without phobias. Medical Care 26:183-198, 1988

Tischler GL, Leaf PJ, Holzer CE, et al: Mental Health Care and the Elderly, I: Age, Psychiatric Status and Expressed Demand. Unpublished document

U.S. Department of Health and Human Services: The International Classification of Diseases, 9th rev–Clinical Modification, 2nd ed. Publication no (PHS) 80-1260, Washington, DC, Department of Health and Human Services, 1980

U.S. Department of Health, Education and Welfare: Mental Health and the Elderly. Washington, DC, U.S. Government Printing Office, 1979

Wells KB, Goldberg G, Brook R, et al: Management of patients on psychotropic drugs in primary care clinics. Medical Care 26:645-656, 1988

White House Conference on Aging: Report on the Mini-Conference on the Mental Health of Older Americans. Washington, DC, U.S. Government Printing Office, 1981

Zung WWK: Affective disorders, in Handbook of Geriatric Psychiatry. Edited by Busse EW, Blazer DG. New York, Van Nostrand Reinhold, 1980

Notes

1. The one-month prevalence data are cited in this paper because rates for other time periods (e.g., 6-month and lifetime) are only available for the elderly by site.

2. The major disadvantage of this estimate is that it is based only on one site. However, the concern about a potentially inflated national rate associated with the high rate of phobia is eliminated.

3. These estimates, if they err, will tend to underestimate unmet need in the community, both because of quality of care issues and inability to unduplicate persons. Although Regier et al. (1978) were able to estimate the overlap between users of general health versus mental health services for all ages of adults, insufficient data exist on patterns of elderly mental health service to do so at this time. Future research with ECA data could address this problem.

4. Analysis of ECA data from four sites by George and colleagues (1988) does not fully agree—they estimate that the rates of older persons with mental illness seeing a general medical provider for a mental health reason are around 1.5 times higher than for such diagnosed persons using outpatient mental health services.

5. Ironically, implementation of this legislation will result in the discharge of mentally ill persons who do not require nursing care back into the public mental health system, or elsewhere. When such patients are discharged they will need outpatient, home-based care and partial hospitalization in the community. These services do not exist in many communities.

5

Division of Responsibility Among Payers

Howard H. Goldman, M.D., Ph.D.
Richard G. Frank, Ph.D.

Historical Perspective

Historically, financing has driven the system of mental health care for the elderly, as it has for the nonelderly. The predominant source of that financing has been the government. Initially a personal and family responsibility in the United States, the care of the elderly became a public responsibility in the early 19th century. The development of public welfare institutions meant then that the indigent and dependent elderly were placed in poorhouses and almshouses operated by local government. Some elderly with mental disorders were admitted to the state-operated asylums established during this period of social reform, but many remained in undifferentiated local welfare institutions. (State resources built the asylums, but local communities were expected to pay for the cost of each episode of care.) Senility was not recognized as a mental disorder (i.e., dementia), and local governments found it less costly to provide for the elderly in their own community institutions, rather than pay for their care in state asylum facilities.

Incarceration in a local almshouse was an alternative to total neglect rather than a form of medical care. Also, it was less costly than the available medical alternative. It was not until the turn of the 20th century that a medical approach was introduced for the care of the indigent, elderly insane, and demented. Again, it was a change in financing that encouraged the move of the mentally ill elderly from local welfare institutions to state mental hospitals. Reacting to the criticism that the mentally ill were neglected in local public welfare institutions, reformers sought the centralization of the responsibility for their care in state government. The State Care

Acts at the turn of the century made state agencies directly responsible for providing and financing the care of the indigent insane. Local governments, relieved of the financial responsibility for the mental care of their poor citizens by state-operated mental hospitals, sent everyone to the asylum, including the elderly. Dementia, already being recognized by the developing field of neuropathology as a disease, became defined fiscally as a mental disorder, and throughout the first half of the 20th century the population of the senile and dependent elderly in the state mental hospital system rose dramatically nationwide (Grob 1983).

Financial incentives sent the elderly mentally ill to the state hospitals. The same incentives kept them there until, in 1965, the Medicare and Medicaid programs shifted the burden of financial responsibility from the states to the federal government. Medicare would fund up to 190 lifetime days of acute care in a psychiatric hospital, pay for the treatment of mental disorders in general hospitals and allow a small benefit for physicians' services in outpatient settings. Medicaid provided at least a 50% match to state funding for the care of the elderly in psychiatric hospitals, general hospitals, and nursing homes. The result was that states incurred 100% of the costs of treating the indigent in state hospitals and between 20% and 50% of the costs of treating them in acute care hospitals under Medicaid. For Medicare, relative prices of settings changed only for long stay and chronic patients. As a result of this dramatic change in funding, the mentally ill elderly began to receive acute psychiatric care in hospitals, especially in general hospitals, while states sought to reduce direct support for long-term care by moving the mentally ill elderly from state hospitals to nursing homes and sharing the fiscal responsibility for their care with the federal government. This process was a significant element of the deinstitutionalization effort made during the 1965–1980 period (Foley and Sharfstein 1983).

During that same time, the expansion of the Medicare and Medicaid programs was accompanied by the growth of private insurance coverage for acute psychiatric treatment and resulted in a dramatic development of private sector resources for the mentally ill. While government financing continued to dominate the care of the elderly, there was a shift from categoric support in public institutions to third-party subsidies for care in private, as well as public, facilities.

These trends led to a system of care that is complex and highly differentiated, serving a multiplicity of functions and financed by many streams of funding. Although the private sector has expanded, the public sector remains the "floor of the system." The private sector has been able to flourish because the public sector continues to serve the most difficult and compromised patients and to absorb the bad financial risks. The complexity of the system has resulted in fragmentation, but also diversification and growth. Responsibility for the care of the mentally ill elderly is now diffused between the private and public sectors, among many levels of government and their bureaus and agencies (Goldman et al. 1987 [reprinted as Appendix II to this volume]).

Further details of the current, complex system of care for the elderly mentally ill can be found in Chapters 4, 9, 10, and 14. Details of the inpatient care system, based on data of Manderscheid and Barrett (1987), are offered in Appendix II to this volume.

Financial Perspective

In 1980 nearly 100,000 Americans over the age of 65 years were admitted to specialty mental health inpatient settings, accounting for 7% of all admissions. Among these admissions, 59% were to general hospitals, 14% to private psychiatric hospitals, 20% to state and county mental hospitals, and 7% to Veterans Administration hospitals. Third parties paid for almost all of the care in general hospitals and private psychiatric hospitals, 58% of care in state facilities and virtually none of the care in the VA. (Although the state hospitals are public facilities, they are eligible for third-party reimbursement. Typically, however, state hospitals do not retain the payments, and they revert to the state's general treasury. This produces little direct incentive for state hospital administrators to optimize third-party revenues.)

Regarding outpatient care for the elderly, data are scarce because institutional services are few and third-party reimbursement is limited. Medicare is presumed to be the principal source of third-party payment for individuals over the age of 65 years. For the indigent elderly, Medicaid is a secondary pay source. Most private insurance policies for the elderly (e.g., Medigap) do not augment psychiatric benefits. Since Medicare benefits have been severely limited (until 1988 covering only $500 of services with a 50% copayment), it is presumed that most of the care, beyond the approximately $100–200 million of Medicare expenditures and an unknown amount of Medicaid expenditures, has been an out-of-pocket expense incurred by the elderly and their families. Recent increases in the outpatient Medicare mental health care benefit (introduced by the Budget Reconciliation Acts of 1987 and 1989) are likely to expand Medicare expenditures considerably, shifting costs from other payers and perhaps increasing demand to meet previously unmet mental health care needs (see Chapter 4 for an estimate of unmet need). Over the past two years, the 1987 legislation increased the coverage of most services up to $2,200 annually with a 50% copayment. Services for the medical management of psychotropic drugs were exempted from the $2,200 limit and are subject to the same 20% copayment as other Medicare outpatient services. In addition, a partial hospitalization benefit has been offered. The 1989 legislation eliminated the dollar limit for outpatient services entirely. Building on a precedent established for Medicare beneficiaries with Alzheimer's Disease and related disorders (Goldman et al. 1985), these benefit changes were the first statutory expansions of Medicare mental health coverage since 1965 and may serve as a model for other outpatient coverage (Goldman and Taube 1989).

The hope is that increases in outpatient coverage will not only increase access but also increase the efficiency of the health care system by providing alternatives to extended hospitalization. Partial hospital services have been shown to substitute effectively for certain full hospital services and outpatient care may substitute for some inpatient care even if it cannot routinely substitute for a hospitalization. The emphasis is on parity of coverage for those neuropsychiatric services that most resemble general medical services in terms of "medical necessity," practice style (i.e., brief biomedical or cognitively oriented office visits, often involving the use of medication) and economic behavior (i.e., relatively low responsiveness of patients' demand to changes in visit fees).

Financing of long-term care, not a Medicare benefit, is primarily the responsibility of Medicaid and state health care resources that are otherwise used mainly by the poor. These systems also serve those who have been impoverished because of chronic disability or the expense of their long-term care needs. Patients pay for their care out of pocket until they "spend down" to Medicaid eligibility.

The emphasis of these funding mechanisms has been on long-term hospital and nursing home care yet, most mentally ill elderly do not need to be institutionalized. They do, however, require community-based long-term care services and the financing of that care varies considerably from state to state. Case management and psychosocial rehabilitative services appropriate for the elderly are available in some state Medicaid plans and mental health systems, but not in others (though federal Medicaid regulations provide for federal matching funds if states cover these services). Respite care services to relieve families when 24-hour care and supervision of the elderly person is required, are virtually never covered by Medicaid. Private insurance coverage for long-term care is developing slowly, but policies often exclude care for beneficiaries with "nonorganic" mental disorders (see Chapter 15). Many long-term care policies have very limited home health benefits, favoring nursing home care over its alternatives or over those services required prior to admission to long-term institutional care.

The total cost of care of those who have been institutionalized is difficult to determine with precision, but we know that it places an enormous burden on families and on Medicaid and state mental health resources. Recent attempts to improve the long-term care coverage of all Americans (e.g., through a part C benefit in Medicare) marked a major shift in policy. While the benefits initially were favored by the elderly, their concern about bearing the costs imposed in the form of new taxes and premiums led to the repeal of the Catastrophic Coverage Act. In the area of long-term care financing there is a large gap between need and available resources.

Current Policy Issues

During the past 150 years, financial responsibility for the mentally ill has been shifted from one level of government to another. With the advent of "new federalism" in the 1980s, an effort has been made to shift the burden and responsibility of federal health care financing back to the states. The preadmission screening requirement of the 1987 Omnibus Budget Reconciliation Act (see Chapter 15) is an excellent example of such a cost-shifting policy. Also, the major problems being addressed have been those of cost-containment and efficiency, not equity and access. Such a shift in policy may be justified by resource scarcity and the consequent need for austerity, but it disregards the fact that mental health needs for the elderly are growing as the population of elderly Americans grows. Few policy makers are asking the basic question of what resources are needed to effectively address the mental health care needs of our elderly population. Historically, mental health services have been underfunded, especially for the mentally ill elderly. And, while determining the optimal allocation of resources is the central task of formulating a mental health care financing policy, it is not the principal criterion currently used to determine the role of government in financing the care of the elderly. During this era of cost-containment, the focus has been on efficiency and, when possible, on avoiding the direct provision of care. For mental health, an added emphasis has been placed on streamlining the administration of care to reduce fragmentation in a highly differentiated system of services.

The Policy-Making Framework

The overriding question about the role of government remains that of whether the government should provide adequate mental health services to the elderly as a right or a privilege. In other words, should adequate services be expected from our government or should the government be a provider of last resort? Answers are ambivalent. While the Medicare program is regarded as an "earned entitlement," as are Social Security retirement benefits, the Medicaid program may be considered a payer of last resort.

This basic question has been ignored in recent years. On the assumption that there are no resources to pay for universal programs, the debate (and this discussion) focuses on the more mundane, but practical, question of who will pay, and how. Therefore, let us begin with the assumption that the role of government is to finance an array of needed services not paid for privately from out-of-pocket outlays or through various risk-pooling mechanisms.

Which Level of Government?

First, one might consider the traditional question: Which level of government (local, state, or federal) should take responsibility for the mental needs of the elderly? Local government, the first governmental level involved in the care of the mentally ill, presently pays only a few percent of the total direct costs of mental health care for the elderly (Frank and Kamlet 1985). In 1985, state governments with the longest and largest capital-intensive investment in this area of health care accounted for 40% of direct expenditures (the larger share) while the federal government contributed only 6% of the total.

The federal government is best suited to compensate for inequities among states in the quantity and quality of care provided, to protect citizens from possible abuses by state political majorities, and to offer financing, technical assistance and regulatory oversight for state and regional systems of care. Although the federal government's direct funding role diminished in the 1980s, its influence has much greater impact than its financial investment. Recently, federal efforts have been focusing on promoting cost containment and efficiency; but they could be equally well placed to promote equity and access.

The states have historically accepted public responsibility for the care of the indigent mentally ill. State government, being closer to regional needs, can respond more rapidly to local initiatives for change and innovation. On the other hand, when local needs are not well articulated and promoted, few services may be provided. In fact, state government seems, at worst, to have inherited some of the shortcomings of both local and federal agencies. States may lack the centralized control of the federal government and at the same time be too far from the "real communities" being served. In the 1960s, the federal government, believing that most state mental health agencies would not sponsor comprehensive community-based care, went directly to the local communities for implementing the Community Mental Health Centers Program. Therefore, many state governments did not contribute to the growth of community mental health resources until the late 1970s and 1980s. Then it was realized that deinstitutionalization could not be accomplished humanely without supporting the development of community mental health services. Presently, many states are promoting community services and divesting themselves of some or all of direct care responsibilities through new financial arrangements with local communities, particularly counties and municipal governments (Taube and Goldman 1988).

Cities and counties are the closest to the mental health needs of the communities they serve but, historically, they have neglected the responsibility of addressing them. Throughout the 19th century, and since the passage of the State Care Acts at the turn of the century, cities have played a very small role in the mental health care delivery system. In the 1960s the Community Mental Health Centers Program gave local governments and private providers an investment in mental health services. In 1975 the elderly were included explicitly with the amendments to the Community Mental Health Centers Act. As noted earlier, very few local governments raise more than a token amount of resources for the mentally ill. Since the 1960s, some states have shared responsibility with local government, giving them an annual budgetary allocation including, in some cases, the responsibility for the use of beds in state hospitals.

The current trend, being modelled by the Robert Wood Johnson Program for the Chronically Mentally Ill, is to centralize responsibility for the mentally ill in an established or newly created "mental health authority" at the local level (Aiken et al. 1986). This approach requires the cooperation of the state in providing a large share of the resources needed by the new health authority. Also, it may require changes in federal regulations to give local authorities greater control over the allocation of federal resources. The difficult balance among the sources of funds for mental health services has encouraged the diversification of the health care delivery system. At the same time, however, it has diffused responsibility for implementing adequate services, resulting in neglect of the mentally ill. The challenge of finding the best methods to organize and finance the care of the mentally ill elderly is discussed in the next section.

Direct Versus Indirect Service Providers

Originally, public responsibility for the care of the mentally ill meant providing services directly—in hospitals, and later, in clinics and other organized care settings. In the 19th century there were few cases of foster care for the elderly mentally ill financed through subsidies to private individuals, but the approach was never used in a sizable program. Until the 1960s, public financing was almost exclusively for direct service provision through categoric support from budgetary allocations.

The advent of community mental health services and centers promoted some of the first forms of indirect provision, through grants and contracts from federal and state budgets to local providers. And, of course, the Medicare and Medicaid programs initiated a major trend toward the use of mainstream health care providers. A few small demonstration programs, such as the National Institute of Mental Health Community Support Program, used federal grant mechanisms to support local efforts. The Mental Health Systems Act of 1980 made state government the fiscal intermediary and agent of the federal government in allocating funds to community-based projects (Foley and Sharfstein 1983). None of these programs developed into large federal programs, but served as models that state governments began to imitate. In 1981, with the Reagan Administration emphasis on fiscal austerity for human service programs, the Mental Health Systems Act became a block grant program to the states, and the mainstream resources of Medicare and Medicaid gained new importance, in spite of their limited mental health benefits (Mechanic and Aiken 1987).

The advantages and disadvantages of government agencies providing health care directly are still debated. Direct provision of services allows the greatest degree of control over quality assurance, but requires a costly capital investment and a bureaucratic infrastructure that may work better for building schools and roads than for running health care services. Direct provision of services means complicated rules about procurement, rigid personnel regulations and total dependency on annual budget allocations resulting from a highly politicized process rarely under the direct influence of mental health care providers or even the mental health authority.

On the other hand, when government provides the care directly, it has the powerful incentive of fulfilling its public obligation and it is likely to be responsive to public preferences. There is no economic incentive to undertreat patients. However, there may also be tolerance for inadequate resources, generalized neglect, inefficiency, and substandard quality of services.

Indirect provision of services through grants, contracts, and other third-party mechanisms is receiving increased attention in discussions about health care financing. Advantages, such as flexibility and efficiency, and the main disadvantage, lack of control, vary with the type of indirect mechanisms used. They are discussed in the next section.

Alternatives for Indirect Service Provision

Grants were the most common mechanism used in the early years of indirect service provision. Through grants, resources are transferred from the government to a service provider for an array of services specified somewhat loosely in a grant agreement. Usually, there are no specific contractual obligations to perform the services in order to receive payment, but renewal of funding usually depends on fulfilling the intent of the granting agency. The grant gives the provider the greatest flexibility to innovate and offers the least degree of control to the government.

To establish tighter controls and performance specificity over the direct providers of care, grants were replaced by contracts which specify the delivery of specific services within a specific framework. Compared to grants, contracts offer more control but may retard innovation. Also, if services are described simultaneously in great detail, it may be difficult to specify outcomes or build in meaningful incentives for desired outcomes (see also Chapter 11).

Third-party payments may take the form of fee-for-service, retrospective reimbursements, or a variety of prospective payment mechanisms, including capitation and per-service predetermined rates. (Fee-for-service and retrospective reimbursement finance services at prices set by providers, and therefore these are financing mechanisms that encourage utilization. In contrast, prospective mechanisms pay providers predetermined amounts to encourage efficiency by reducing utilization and allowing providers revenues that exceed costs.) The advantage of third-party payments for the neuropsychiatric care of the mentally ill elderly rests on its linkages with other third-party mechanisms in health care. Medicare and Medicaid, in particular, as mainstream programs, are less likely to suffer special budgetary reductions than categoric programs for the mentally ill. Medicare is a true insurance program, and Medicaid is an open-ended voucher program. Although the mentally ill have suffered from benefit limitations in these programs, there is now an opportunity to achieve financing parity for those mental health services that conform most closely to the pattern of general medical practice. Third-party payments provide the greatest flexibility to patients and providers and the least control to government. They often stimulate the development of services by the private sector and hold promise for the elimination of a two-class system of care, provided that the buying power of government-funded third-party benefits is comparable to that of third-party benefits funded by private sector mechanisms.

Conclusion

The elderly population grows each year. The mental health problems of the elderly and their lack of care has been documented (Shapiro et al. 1984). Congressional interest in this problem seems to be increasing. However, there is no consensus on the role of government and only an awareness that more needs to be done. There is concern about the duplication of services, the fragmentation of care, the use of inappropriate levels of care, the high cost of individual cases, and inefficiency (Goldman et al. 1987; Mechanic and Aiken 1987). There is also concern about problems of equity and access. Not only do we seem to spend too little, but we spend too much of it on the wrong kinds of care. Some of the elderly are drowning in too many of the wrong services, while others have limited access to any care at all.

The differentiation of the mental health service system may serve many functions, but it has also created additional dysfunctions. The complexity of the system makes it very sensitive to disruption by changes in policy. Sensitivity is attractive to those who would alter the system, but should serve as a warning to those who make changes whose effects cannot be predicted or would be likely to be untoward. (Preadmission screening, a provision of OBRA 1987, offers a good example of a policy with unpredictable effects. It is discussed further in Chapter 15.)

Almost everyone acknowledges the need for change, but there is little agreement on what to do. In another analysis, we have reviewed the pros and cons of various mechanisms for financing the care of the severely mentally ill (Frank and Goldman, 1989). We conclude that selecting the proper mechanism depends entirely on the conditions within a specific circumstance. Market-based approaches, using indirect mechanisms, work best when an adequate supply of providers and informed consumers exist. Prospective mechanisms depend heavily on consumers being able to distinguish efficiency from undertreatment and on providers being able to balance advocacy on behalf of patients with their incentive to derive profits from care. Direct financing mechanisms work best with adequate resources and uniformly high quality providers. Determining the optimal financing approach requires a keen awareness of strengths and limitations of each mechanism and careful study of the market conditions to which they will be applied. Increasingly, empirical evidence and analysis will be essential to the policy debate. Those concerned about the neuropsychiatric care of the elderly need an extended, thoughtful forum for discussing the fundamental issues. The elderly depend on the outcome of the policy debate. With any luck, all of us could be the beneficiaries of that outcome.

References

Aiken LH, Somers SA, Shore MF: Private foundations in health affairs: a case study of the development of a national initiative for the chronically mentally ill. American Psychologist 41:1290-1295, 1986

Foley H, Sharfstein SS: Madness and Government: Who Cares for the Mentally Ill? Washington, DC, American Psychiatric Press, 1983

Frank RG, Goldman HH: Financing care of the severely mentally ill: incentives, contracts, and public responsibility. Journal of Social Issues 45:131-144, 1989

Frank RG, Kamlet MA: Direct Costs and Expenditures for Mental Health Care in the United States in 1980. Hospital and Community Psychiatry 36:165-168, 1985

Goldman HH, Cohen GD, Davis M: Economic grand rounds: change in Medicare outpatient coverage for Alzheimer's disease and related disorders. Hospital and Community Psychiatry 36:909-942, 1985

Goldman HH, Taube CA: State strategies to restructure state psychiatric hospitals—a selective review. Inquiry 26:146-156, 1989

Goldman HH, Taube CA, Jencks S: The organization of the psychiatric inpatient services system. Medical Care Supplement 25:S6-S21, 1987

Grob GN: Mental Illness and American Society, 1875-1940. Princeton, Princeton University Press, 1983

Manderscheid R, Barrett S (eds): Mental Health, United States 1987. National Institute of Mental Health. DHHS Pub. No. (ADM) 87-11518. Washington, DC, U.S. Government Printing Office, 1987

Mechanic D, Aiken L: Improving the care of patients with chronic mental illness. New England Journal of Medicine 317:1634-1638, 1987

Shapiro S, Skinner EA, Kessler LG: Utilization of health and mental health services: three epidemiological catchment area sites. Archives of General Psychiatry 41:971-978, 1984

6

Payment for Services: A Provider's Perspective

Steven S. Sharfstein, M.D.

Any impairment of brain function creates an adaptational challenge for the affected individual, the family, and the community which provides the support for treatment and care. Modern medicine, with its capacity to cure or ameliorate most acute medical illness, has contributed to the challenge of an aging population that must at times face chronic maladies, both physical and mental. Paying for the psychiatric component of health care to the elderly is a substantial and unresolved problem of our affluent society. Including psychiatric care in the mainstream of medical care financing, and using in diagnosis and treatment a "neuropsychiatric" rather than a "psychiatric" approach (see Chapter 1) may be one way to introduce needed improvements in elderly health care.

This chapter addresses the major problems in financing psychiatric care for the elderly, places the problems in historical perspective and then concludes with a discussion of a recent breakthrough in Medicare coverage permitting the "medical management" of psychiatric illness in a nondiscriminatory manner similar to that of all other illnesses.

As psychiatrists begin defining or redefining their work more in the medical context than has traditionally been the case, reimbursement opportunities will expand and access by the elderly to specialty psychiatric care will increase. Research and clinical applications of geropsychiatry will continue to expand well into the 21st century as the mature population continues to grow faster relative to younger population groups.

Paying for Psychiatric Care: The Role of Government, the Private Sector, and Third-Party Insurance

Since President Franklin Pierce vetoed the Indigent Insane Act of 1854, the treatment of mental illness has largely been the responsibility of state governments (Foley and Sharfstein 1983). After a citizen-led movement petitioned state legislature after state legislature for asylum care of the mentally ill, Dorothea Dix and her allies managed to initiate during the 1855–1875 period the establishment of 32 state mental hospitals. As the passage of state health care acts during the late 19th century led to the admission and transfer of senile elderly from local institutions to state hospitals, large numbers of immigrants with a high prevalence of psychiatric disorders contributed to fill the hospitals to capacity and helped to justify the increase in the number of state mental hospital beds. By the early 20th century one out of two hospital beds in this country was occupied by a psychiatric patient.

The Depression of the 1930s created a health care crisis, and health insurance was introduced primarily to consolidate hospital resources and to develop a risk pool that would pay for care that had become inaccessible to most individuals and families.

Private health insurance, from the time of its origins, excluded psychiatric care, together with the treatment of tuberculosis, because a large system of government-supported hospitals was available for the clinical support of these conditions (Sharfstein et al. 1984). The peak of public asylum for psychiatric patients was reached by 1954, when 560,000 Americans resided in state and county mental institutions (Talbott 1980). In that same year Blue Cross/Blue Shield adopted a major policy change that allowed the treatment of psychiatric conditions in general hospitals on the same basis as all other medical illness (Sharfstein et al. 1984). This began a shift of the main site for care of psychiatric illness and the reorientation of psychotic care from long-term custodial to active acute care. The shift began even before the widespread use of prescription drugs which, over the following twenty years, transformed the treatment of severe psychiatric illness. Also, it provided an ever-growing number of individuals suffering from treatable but relapsing psychiatric conditions, with general hospital care in small psychiatric units. In 1965, Medicare eventually adopted the Blue Cross and Blue Shield model but limited the treatment of Medicare patients in psychiatric hospitals to 190 days and outpatient benefits to $250. The advent of Medicare and Medicaid in 1965 transformed the overall health system—including the mental health services delivery system—and fueled the rapid expansion of the nursing home industry and the growth of health care settings beyond hospitals. Community mental health centers, halfway houses, day treatment programs, psychiatric consultations in nursing homes, consultation liaison psychiatry in general hospitals, and office practice psychiatry grew because of these changes in method of payment, and the availability of private as well as public third-party dollars in lieu of the tax-supported funding of state hospitals (National Institute of Mental Health 1987).

Gaps and shortfalls became obvious as many patients discharged from hospitals required, but did not obtain, ongoing treatment and support. Deinstitutionalization and homelessness have gone hand in hand among the elderly who increasingly were deprived of access to treatment for neuropsychiatric illness.

Insurance Shortfalls, Inside Limits, Adverse Selection, Moral Hazard, Demand, and Supply-Side Cost Sharing

Before looking at the problems with the Medicare program and the financing of neuropsychiatric care for the elderly, it is useful to discuss the difficulties that are likely to be found when health insurance is used to pay for psychiatric treatment. As mentioned earlier, when, in the mid-1950s, Blue Cross/Blue Shield and other insurance carriers began to pay for the psychiatric care provided in general hospitals over the next few decades, more than 1200 psychiatric units were added to hospitals. However, most health insurance in the private sector, as well as Medicare, had "inside limits" (high deductibles, greater copayment, lower lifetime limits) for both inpatient and outpatient psychiatric care. A recent survey showed that over half of private health insurance plans had dollar limits for inpatient care and over 90% of them had dollar limits for outpatient care, as well as higher deductibles and copayments (Brady et al. 1986).

Health insurers justify these inside limits on the basis of cost considerations. In particular, they are concerned about "moral hazard" and "adverse selection."

"Moral hazard" is a health insurance term denoting the risk of financial loss because of certain behavioral "propensities" of the insured. They include dishonesty, carelessness, lack of judgment, and the innate desire of people to utilize to a maximum what is believed to be advantageous to personal welfare. The term "moral hazard" therefore is used to illustrate the fact that certain needs are created or stimulated by the availability of what is capable to satisfy them. Health insurers believe that psychiatric treatment, especially psychotherapy, has a high degree of "moral hazard" type of risk. This observation is reinforced by studies that indicate that the utilization of psychiatric treatment is on average more price sensitive than general medical care (Frank and McGuire 1986).

The term "adverse selection" refers to an insurance company's excessive assumption of bad risks (such as in the case of enrolling in the insurance plan too many persons who are likely to suffer more losses or make more claims than the estimated average for that population group). Since all health insurance is based on risk sharing among those who are ill and those who are well, if only one insurance company covers the treatment of a certain illness, over time it may enroll a disproportionate number of persons at risk, incur excessive losses, be forced to increase premiums, and lose customers to less expensive and limited programs. This indeed is what happened with the Federal Employees Health Benefits Program of the early 1980s. The High Option Blue Cross/Blue Shield Program was the only program with acceptable psychiatric benefits but eventually lost enrollees to less expensive plans void of psychiatric coverage but including other benefits such as dental coverage. The BC/BS plan had been adversely selected and suffered serious financial setbacks.

The phenomenon of the "dental/mental trade-off," as it was called, led to a concern about "market failure" in supporting psychiatric care and the need for government regulation to insure minimum benefits through the mandated insurance laws (McGuire 1981).

To guard against phenomena such as "moral hazard" and "adverse selection," cost-containment strategies are employed. One kind of cost-containment strategy, known as demand-side cost sharing, emphasizes the relationship between the fiscal third party and the patient. The objective here is that of making the consumer more price conscious through larger copayments and deductibles. The approach takes advantage of the price sensitivity of psychiatric care to decrease health care utilization (Wells et al. 1982). However, this approach is unfair to the poor and it is usually unpopular because of the adverse emotional reactions of insured patients to out-of-pocket payments.

The lack of popularity of demand-side cost sharing makes supply-side cost sharing, the second major form of cost-containment strategy, more prevalent. This approach induces providers to be cost conscious by placing them at economic risk when more services are utilized by users. Examples of supply-side cost sharing are prepaid medical care, contract medicine, diagnostic-related groups (DRGs), health maintenance organizations (HMOs), and preferred provider organizations (PPOs).

In trying to promote access to quality care at a reasonable cost, a mix of demand- and supply-side cost sharing that addresses fundamental human needs is necessary.

The Shortfalls of Medicare

Neuropsychiatric disease can develop into very costly and catastrophic illnesses. The progressive deterioration of the patient's ability to function occurring over months and years creates difficulties of adaptation and growing economic dependency. Dealing with the emotional trauma of seeing a loved one undergoing personality changes and deteriorating intellectually imposes a large emotional and economic burden on families. There is a close correlation between deteriorating mental status as a result of neuropsychiatric illness and the fiscal status of families in Medicare and other related pooled financing arrangements.

Although Medicare is designed to cover the acute care needs of the elderly and the disabled, it provides a limited range of medical benefits and little support for long-term care. Therefore, a large portion of medical expenditures incurred by the elderly is outside the scope of Medicare. For example, Medicare pays almost 70% of the hospital and medical expenses of the elderly, but less than 50% of their total health care bill. And, because of especially restrictive provisions for the diagnosis and treatment of neuropsychiatric illness, Medicare pays less than 50% of total hospital and physician psychiatric care expenses. Even with the improvement of psychiatric benefits in 1987 and 1989, Medicare remains an acute care benefit. For instance, one-quarter of the elderly's total health care expenditures occurs in nursing homes, yet, since skilled nursing benefits are restricted to acute illness, Medicare pays for only 3% of all the elderly's nursing home expenses (Congress of the United States 1983).

These glaring gaps in supporting the diagnosis and treatment of neuropsychiatric and long-term care services must be addressed in a thoughtful reform of Medicare.

The Stigma of Neuropsychiatric Illness in the Elderly

While prevalence of neuropsychiatric disorders in the elderly is high, the use of psychiatric, diagnostic, and treatment services is low. The apparent contradiction results from the threat that neuropsychiatric conditions pose to individual self-image and self-sufficiency. People tend to cover up lapses in mental functioning and resist suggestions to seek professional help fearing incipient senility and loss of faculties as the forerunners of a decline inevitably leading to recovery in a nursing home. Misdiagnoses of depression and lack of treatment of reversible deterioration in mental functioning is a major problem among the elderly and their families.

Recently, I examined an 84-year-old woman whose children, both in their 60s, surprised by her sudden decision to move permanently into a nursing home, had asked for my advice. A widow for 20 years, she had been living independently and, with the aid of a walker, was able to get around well, do her own grocery shopping, cook, and attend to her own total care. In consultation, she complained of a deteriorating memory and general mental functioning, as well as the perceived humiliation of having to seek the services of a psychiatrist. In short, she felt that her survival was compromised and improbable. The consultation uncovered all the symptoms of depression, including change in sleep patterns, decreased eating, low energy, and frequent crying spells. Yet, a recent complete physical exam had been entirely negative with the exception of some long-standing osteoarthritis. Finally, it was discovered that the symptoms had begun on the 20th anniversary of her husband's death. Treated with an antidepressant and short-term psychotherapy, she recovered her cognitive function within a two-month period and was able to remain in her apartment and live independently. If it were not for her enlightened and concerned children, she might have been misdiagnosed and inappropriately sent to a nursing home.

The stigma of mental illness, keenly felt among the elderly, is also commonly affecting judgment among third-party payers.

Medicare and the Medical Management of Neuropsychiatric Illness

The fact that mental illness may be produced by conditions not directly related to an easily recognized and consistent set of causes (the so-called "functional" or nonetiologic basis of mental illness) is often used to justify the limits imposed on health insurance for the diagnosis and treatment of psychiatric disorders. The onset of a psychiatric problem, its course and ultimate outcome are not as likely to be precisely diagnosed as rheumatoid arthritis, hyperthyroidism, or other well-known ailments. Because of the clinical uncertainty, these cases bring potentially greater financial risks for third-party payers than would be true for cases involving nonmental disorders.

This financial uncertainty is underscored by the findings of studies which examined the impact of the Medicare DRG system for psychiatric patients. Since the DRGs (a supply-side cost-sharing approach) are based on accurate predictions of the cost of treatment and of the length of hospital stay, and since it is extremely difficult to predict accurately causes and outcomes of neuropsychiatric illness, the coverage of neuropsychiatric care by Medicare is grossly lacking (English et al. 1986).

The progress made in understanding the neuropsychiatric basis for Alzheimer's disease and other types of dementia, the improvements in the treatment of depression, the greater sophistication in laboratory techniques for diagnosis, and the enhanced capacity to medically treat, are all contributing in breaking down barriers to a more effective financial coverage of neuropsychiatric care. Indeed, it is the recognition of these advances in psychiatry that, as part of the Omnibus Budget Reconciliation Act (OBRA) of 1987, the limits and special copayments for the "medical management of psychopharmacologic agents" (prescription drugs) for Medicare beneficiaries were eliminated. (This type of medical management is now covered on a par with all other medical illnesses, that is with a 20% copayment and no visit or dollar limits, in contrast to a psychotherapy benefit that involves a 50% copayment. While OBRA 1989 eliminated dollar limits on outpatient care, it retained the 50% copayment.)

This change in Medicare is an expansion of the regulatory change that occurred in 1984 when the Department of Health and Human Services redefined appropriate physician services provided outside of a hospital. For Alzheimer's disease, physician treatment services for patients were not to be subject to the then-prevailing $250 Medicare outpatient benefit limitation, except if the treatment was psychotherapy. The removal of limitations on Medicare coverage for patients with Alzheimer's disease promoted greater access to appropriate medical and psychiatric care. Also, the broader coverage was a first step for Medicare toward recognizing the scientific basis of neuropsychiatry.

The policy change in Medicare separating medical management from psychotherapy implies that medical treatment of patients with mental disorders will not be limited by concerns about excessive or uncontrolled use of psychotherapy.

Medicaid policy, the program for the poor and disabled, follows the improvements in Medicare coverage by no longer considering organic mental disorders "mental diseases" for the purpose of limiting Medicaid payments to certain patients or nursing homes.

When this author was asked at a hearing of the House Health Finance Subcommittee of the Ways and Means Committee to define medical management of mental disorders, the answer was that it did not differ from the management of diabetes or arthritis. For psychiatric care, reimbursement that is treatment-specific and not disorder specific, such as that regulated by the DRGs makes sense both clinically and fiscally. However, DRGs poorly predict the use of inpatient psychiatric care and a pricing strategy focused on the type of treatment received by the patient is likely to be easier to implement and more beneficial to the public.

There is, of course, the danger that once economic incentives favor medical management, the use of biomedical treatments, especially prescription drugs, will be increased at the expense of the time spent talking to patients. For patients with severe neuropsychiatric illness, the use of prescription drugs is critical and access to treatments and to effective medications should not be restricted by the effort to control the possible excessive use of psychotherapy. On the other hand, if the reimbursement system favors the reduction of time spent with patients, additional problems will be created for psychiatry and for those patients and families who deal with the more severe types of mental illness. Time-intensive activities with patients and families include taking detailed histories of the cases, medical counseling with the patient and the family for coping with chronic illness and multiple medications. It includes promoting better medication compliance, and, finally, dealing with their specific anxieties about the illness and its outcome.

The reimbursement of medical management is presently defined more like a typical office visit with an internal medicine specialist averaging about 15 minutes. In the case of neuropsychiatric care it is often necessary to spend a half hour or more per visit to effectively assist the patient and his family. These medical management services dealing with the personal interaction of physicians and patients have been traditionally under-reimbursed and have been a source of complaint from conscientious family practitioners and internists over the past several years.

Perhaps a useful distinction for reimbursement purposes could be that short-term psychotherapy is aimed at specific clinical outcomes while long-term psychotherapy is aimed at personality restructuring. In the elderly, however, these distinctions may not be warranted.

Resource-Based Relative Value Scale and Current Procedural Terminology

Changes included in the Omnibus Budget Reconciliation Act of 1987 (PL100-203) increase access by the elderly to appropriate psychiatric services. Additional changes are being anticipated and are likely to focus on physician payment reform and perhaps adopt the recommendations of the Physician Payment Reform Commission established by Congress in 1986. This has led to a re-thinking of the procedural terminology currently in use for psychiatric services. The Resource-Based Relative Value Scale (RBRVS) developed at Harvard to provide guidelines for physician charges had one segment devoted to psychiatric care through a special study funded by the National Institute of Mental Health (NIMH). The Harvard RBRVS emphasizes cognitive assessment as well as patient management and caring activities by physicians. These activities are quite congruent to the tasks performed by psychiatrists. However, the preliminary report submitted by Harvard to the Health Care Financing Administration contains significant problems. The American Psychiatric Association (APA) noted difficulties with the measurement of the clinical work performed, with the Current Procedural Terminology (CPT—the American Medical Association system of terms and codes for reporting medical services and procedures) codes for psychiatric services, and with the measurement of practice costs.

The RBRVS system attempts to develop a fee schedule based on the intensity and quality of work provided to patients. They rely on assessment of case vignettes and assign values to these as a principal step in developing the fee schedule. For psychiatry, the vignettes were not representative of practice. Severe cases such as the management of a psychotic or suicidal patient were not included among the vignettes. Hospital cases were under-represented and the standard vignette was toward the simpler end of the scale of case complexity.

In addition, the psychiatry CPT codes are very broadly defined and the ability to map the codes in relation to the vignettes is impaired. The American Psychiatric Association met with the AMA CPT Advisory Board and has proposed changes in the psychiatric codes to make them more specific and accurate. It was clear that the current CPT-4 had definitions which neglected crucial activities in areas of inpatient care, medical management, partial hospitalization, and drug monitoring. There was no differentiation between medical management and medical psychotherapy and the number of codes for both inpatient and outpatient services was inadequate.

The APA recommended to the AMA additional codes—six for inpatient care including psychiatric admission and evaluation activity, initial psychiatric care, multidisciplinary treatment planning, physician supervision, subsequent psychiatric care, and discharge planning. Partial hospitalization received a separate set of codes. As for psychiatric medical management, new codes were assigned to office and home medical services, diagnostic evaluation of the patient's general medical and psychiatric status, and when appropriate, drug management. These changes incorporated a broader approach to defining medical management in contrast to the recent changes in Medicare. The AMA adopted only two additions, medical psychoanalysis and family therapy without the patient present. They also wrote a note to carriers asking to make certain that psychiatrists could bill under medical codes. Psychiatry will participate in an AMA consensus conference that will review methods of more accurate billing through generic visit codes.

These changes in service definitions and fee schedules will have an impact on the services provided by psychiatrists to Medicare beneficiaries. The process of study continues even as Congress moves ahead with its recommendations. An extensive discussion of the issues related to physician payment reform can be found in Chapter 7.

Long-Term Care Shortfalls

Even as access to effective diagnosis and treatment of neuropsychiatric conditions improves, the problem of long-term care support for patients with chronic illness remains. The success of modern medicine has contributed to the aging of the population, the diffusion of chronic illness, and the increased prevalence of neuropsychiatric conditions. Paying for the necessary long-term care support has eluded our affluent society. An effort to finance adequate nursing home care benefits recently failed in the House of Representatives. Presently most Americans must divest themselves from everything they own in order to receive public support (Medicaid) for nursing home recovery.

The problems of prolonged economic dependency and unending care constitutes the ultimate frontier in area health and social insurance: a challenge not only to the government and to the market but to all of us since we are all are at risk of developing neuropsychiatric illness in our later years, and with few exceptions, needing care that we will not be able to afford. It is a moral test for our society and its value system as we move into the 21st century.

References

Brady J, Sharfstein SS, Muszynski IL: Trends in private insurance coverage for mental illness. American Journal of Psychiatry 143:1276-1279, 1986

Congress of the United States, Congressional Budget Office: Changing the Structure of Medicare Benefits: Issues and Options, March 1983

English JT, Sharfstein SS, Scherl DJ, et al: Diagnosis-related groups and general hospital psychiatry: the APA study. The American Journal of Psychiatry 143:131-139, 1986

Foley HA, Sharfstein SS: Madness and Government: Who Cares for the Mentally Ill? Washington, DC, American Psychiatric Press, 1983

Frank RG, McGuire TG: A Review of Studies of the Impact of Insurance on the Demand and Utilization of Specialty Mental Health Services. Health Services Research, June 1986

McGuire T: Financing Psychotherapy: Costs, Effects, and Public Policy. Cambridge, MA, Ballinger Publishing Company, 1981

National Institute of Mental Health: Mental Health, United States 1987. Edited by Manderscheid RW, Barrett SA. DHHS Pub. No. (ADM) 87-1518. Washington, DC, U.S. Government Printing Office, 1987

Sharfstein SS, Muszynski IL, Myers EJ: Health Insurance and Psychiatric Care: Update and Appraisal. Washington, DC, American Psychiatric Press, 1984

Talbott JA (ed): State Mental Hospitals: Problems and Potentials. New York, Human Sciences Press, 1980

Wells KB, Manning WG Jr, Duan N, et al: Cost Sharing and the Demand for Ambulatory Mental Health Services. Santa Monica, CA, Rand Corporation, September 1982

7

Physician Payment Reform

Barry S. Fogel, M.D.

In a system of medical care increasingly driven by reimbursement, Medicare policies have a profound effect on the supply of services available to the elderly. In earlier chapters, several authors have linked the shortfall in mental health services for the elderly to inadequate and discriminatory reimbursement of these services by Medicare (see Chapters 4, 5, and 6). Medicare policies affect not only specialty mental health providers, but also general health care providers, who provide a majority of outpatient mental health services to the elderly. To date, reimbursement of primary care physicians for office visits has been too low to compensate them for relatively time-consuming mental health interventions, such as making a psychiatric diagnosis, counseling families, educating patients in detail about psychotropic drugs, or offering brief psychotherapy. Thus, even those primary care physicians whose talent, training, and inclination would permit them to perform optimal mental health interventions for the elderly face financial disincentives for doing anything more than prescribing medications at brief office visits.

Concerns about escalating costs of medical care, increasing specialization of physicians, and an excessive focus on high-cost high-technology procedures led Congress to establish the Physician Payment Reform Commission (PPRC) in 1986. It was hoped that a new methodology could be developed for reimbursing physicians that would provide incentives for primary physicians to provide high-quality general medical care, and for specialists to render cognitive services and perhaps rely less upon the performance of separately reimbursed technical procedures. An additional hope was that the Commission could find a way of containing the overall escalation of physician payment without undue adverse effects on care quality. As the PPRC approached its task, it reached consensus on the general principle that physician payments should be based on resource inputs, the latter comprising time, effort, assumption of risk, operating overhead, and the investment in human capital represented by specialty training.

The implementation of Medicare physician payment based on resource inputs was subsequently mandated by Congress as part of OBRA 1989. Under the provisions of that bill, a new fee schedule, derived from a resource-based relative value scale (RBRVS) for physician services, will be phased in over five years from 1992 to 1996. By 1993, charges to Medicare beneficiaries by nonparticipating physicians (i.e., those not agreeing to accept the Medicare fee schedule as payment in full) will be limited to 115% of the Medicare payment. Thus, all physicians, regardless of Medicare participation status, will be significantly affected by the new incentives of the RBRVS.

The adoption of a new physician payment scheme might offer an unusual opportunity to incorporate mental health concerns into the description and reimbursement of evaluation and management (EM) service performed by physicians in general. Ideally, the identification and treatment of mental health problems in general medical practice would be sufficiently reimbursed so that physicians would have financial incentives to do it. This chapter will report on the ongoing development of physician payment methodology for psychiatric services, noting important limitations of work to date, and suggesting improvements. Much of the discussion will focus on the Harvard Resource-Based Relative Value Scale study, carried out by William Hsiao and his colleagues, under the auspices of the PPRC (Hsaio et al. 1988). The RBRVS developed by the Harvard study represents a first approximation to the RBRVS the PPRC is working to develop and implement. Further studies, including some specifically focusing on psychiatric care (with NIMH participation), are under way at the time of this writing.

In the Harvard study, which will be described further below, values for services were assigned on the basis of clinical vignettes that briefly described typical patients and services rendered to those patients. It is salient that no vignette in the Harvard study dealt with the diagnosis and treatment of a mental health problem in an elderly person by an internist or a family practitioner, although these providers are the usual source of mental health treatment for the elderly. Further, the vignettes on psychiatric services devoted limited attention to the elderly, and did not substantially address the problem of combined medical and psychiatric diagnoses, although this is a usual occurrence in geriatric psychiatry. Geriatrics was not represented as a separate specialty in the Harvard study, so nowhere was specific attention given to the problems of medical/psychiatric comorbidity.

While this chapter will deal specifically with the limitations of the Current Procedural Terminology (CPT) and the Harvard RBRVS study for psychiatric services, the issues raised here apply not only to services rendered by psychiatrists, but to the services of all medical specialists who undertake the effortful and time-consuming task of integrating the care of mind and body in elderly patients. (In particular, when cross-linkages between psychiatrists' and internists' services are criticized below, the emphasis is on the nature of the services provided, and not on the identity of the providers.)

The CPT

Two kinds of psychiatric services are coded by the CPT (American Medical Association 1986): Brief office visits, consultations, etc. are considered to be equivalent to services rendered by other medical specialties, and they share common codes. Other services, such as medical psychotherapy, use codes that are unique to psychiatry. In OBRA 1989, Congress directed the Secretary of HHS to establish a single rate of payment for each CPT code regardless of provider specialty. Therefore, the issue of unique versus shared codes is relevant to payment: If a consultation rendered by a psychiatrist is more time-consuming than a consultation rendered by an internist, a common code would be to the psychiatrist's disadvantage.

CPT codes unique to psychiatry are displayed in Table 7-1. Codes shared with other specialties for some services are displayed in Table 7-2.

A *psychiatric* admission requires not only a comprehensive history and mental status examination, but also the interviewing of collateral sources, the initial organization of efforts by a multidisciplinary team, communication with family caretakers, and, especially in the case of elderly patients, a complete assessment of physical health status. For this reason, it usually takes longer than a medical admission. The American Psychiatric Association (APA) therefore has recommended to the American Medical Association that an additional CPT code be added for psychiatric inpatient admissions, to distinguish them from medical admissions. For similar reasons, five other psychiatric inpatient codes were recommended to the AMA by the APA. These include initial psychiatric care, multidisciplinary treatment planning, physician supervision, subsequent psychiatric care, and discharge planning.

A specific code for psychiatric medical management was also recommended. This would permit recognition of the time-consuming nature of psychiatric medical management, which often involves more detailed mental status assessment, as well as patient and family

Table 7–1. CPT codes for services unique to psychiatry

CLINICAL PSYCHIATRIC DIAGNOSTIC OR EVALUATIVE PROCEDURES

90825 Psychiatric evaluation of hospital records, other psychiatric reports, psychometric and/or projective tests, and other accumulated data for medical diagnostic purposes

90830 Psychological testing by physician, with written report, per hour

90831 Telephone consultation with or about patient for psychiatric therapeutic or diagnostic purposes

90835 Narcosynthesis for psychiatric diagnostic and therapeutic purposes, eg, sodium amobarbital (Amytal) interview

PSYCHIATRIC THERAPEUTIC PROCEDURES

MEDICAL PSYCHOTHERAPY

90841 Individual medical psychotherapy with continuing medical diagnostic evaluation, and drug management when indicated, including psychoanalysis, insight oriented, behavior modifying or supportive psychotherapy; time unspecified

90843   approximately 20 to 30 minutes

90844   approximately 45 to 50 minutes

90847 Family medical psychotherapy (conjoint psychotherapy) by a physician
(90848 has been deleted. To report, use 90847)

90849 Multiple-family group medical psychotherapy by a physician

90853 Group medical psychotherapy (other than of a multiple-family group)

PSYCHIATRIC SOMATOTHERAPY

90862 Chemotherapy management, including prescription, use, and review of medication with no more than minimal medical psychotherapy

90870 Electroconvulsive therapy (includes necessary monitoring); single seizure

90871   multiple seizures, per day
(90872 has been deleted. To report use 90899)

Table 7–1. CPT codes for services unique to psychiatry (*continued*)

OTHER PSYCHIATRIC THERAPY

90880 Medical hypnotherapy

90882 Environmental intervention for medical management purposes on a psychiatric patient's behalf with agencies, employers, or institutions

90887 Interpretation or explanation of results of psychiatric, other medical examinations and procedures, or other accumulated data to family or other responsible persons, or advising them how to assist patient

90889 Preparation of report of patient's psychiatric status, history, treatment, or progress (other than for legal or consultative purposes) for other physicians, agencies, or insurance carriers

OTHER PROCEDURES

90899 Unlisted psychiatric service or procedure

Biofeedback

90900 Biofeedback training; by electromyogram application (eg, in tension headache, muscle spasm)

90902 in conduction disorder (eg, arrhythmia)

90904 regulation of blood pressure (eg, in essential hypertension)

90906 regulation of skin temperature or peripheral blood flow

90908 by electroencephalogram application (eg, in anxiety, insomnia)

90910 by electro-oculogram application (eg, in blepharospasm)

90915 other

Source. CPT only is copyright 1988 American Medical Association. Reproduced with permission from American Medical Association: Physicians' Current Procedural Terminology (CPT). Chicago, American Medical Association, 1989.

Table 7–2. CPT codes for services rendered both by psychiatrists and by other physicians

(see Introduction for definitions and examples of levels of service)

Office Medical Services

NEW PATIENT

90000	Office medical service, new patient; brief service
90010	limited service
90015	intermediate service
90017	extended service
90020	comprehensive service

ESTABLISHED PATIENT

90030	Office medical service, established patient; minimal service
90040	brief service
90050	limited service
90060	intermediate service
90070	extended service
90080	comprehensive service

Home Medical Services

NEW PATIENT

90100	Home medical service, new patient; brief service
90110	limited service
90115	intermediate service
90117	extended service

ESTABLISHED PATIENT

90130	Home medical service, established patient; minimal service
90140	brief service

Table 7–2. CPT codes for services rendered both by psychiatrists and by other physicians (*continued*)

90150	limited service
90160	intermediate service
90170	extended service

Hospital Medical Services

NEW AND ESTABLISHED PATIENT

INITIAL HOSPITAL CARE

90200	Initial hospital care; brief history and examination, initiation of diagnostic and treatment programs, and preparation of hospital records
90215	intermediate history and examination, initiation of diagnostic and treatment programs, and preparation of hospital records
90220	comprehensive history and examination, initiation of diagnostic and treatment programs, and preparation of hospital records

SUBSEQUENT HOSPITAL CARE

90240	Subsequent hospital care; each day, hospital subsequent care requiring; brief services
90250	limited services
90260	intermediate services
90270	extended services
90280	comprehensive services

HOSPITAL DISCHARGE SERVICES

(Final day of a multiple day stay)
(For a single day hospital care, use appropriate Initial Hospital care 90200-90220)

Final Hospital Care for discharge of a patient when it includes final examination of the patient, discussion of the hospital stay, instructions for continuing care, and preparation of discharge records.

90292	Hospital discharge day management

Table 7–2. CPT codes for services rendered both by psychiatrists and by other physicians *(continued)*

Consultations

A consultant is expected to render an opinion only. If he also assumes responsibility for patient management, he is rendering concurrent care or has had the case referred to him.

(For descriptions of levels of consultation, see page xvii)
(For concurrent care, see Modifier-75 or 09975)

INITIAL CONSULTATION

90600	Initial consultation; limited
90605	intermediate
90610	extended
90620	comprehensive
90630	complex

FOLLOW-UP CONSULTATION

90640	Follow-up consultation; brief visit
90641	limited visit
90642	intermediate visit, evaluation, and/or treatment
90643	extended visit requiring re-examination or re-evaluation and/or treatment, same or new illness

CONFIRMATORY (ADDITIONAL OPINION) CONSULTATION

This section should be used when the consulting physician is aware of the comtirmatory nature of the opinion that is sought, e.g., when a patient requests a second/third opinion on the necessity or appropriateness of a (previously) recommended medical treatment or surgical procedure.

90650	Confirmatory consultation; limited
90651	intermediate
90652	extended
90653	comprehensive
90654	complex

Source.   CPT only is copyright 1988 American Medical Association. Reproduced with permission from American Medical Association: Physicians' Current Procedural Terminology (CPT). Chicago, American Medical Association, 1989.

Table 7–3. Harvard RBRVS study vignettes concerning elderly patients

A4d.	Hospital consultation for psychiatric evaluation of a 68-year-old cardiac surgical patient with severe post-operative depression.
A7g.	Office visit for termination of a 66-year-old business executive from twice weekly in-office psychotherapy sessions after three years of psychotherapy. Patient had initial complaint of marital problems and "ulcers."
A12l.	Hospital emergency room evaluation of a 78-year-old woman who ingested alcohol and Valium in an apparent suicide attempt.
A14n.	Office consultation for psychiatric evaluation of 65-year-old man with intellectual deterioration and behavior problems, including verbal and physical abuse of coworkers.
A16p.	Electroconvulsive therapy, single seizure, in an 82-year-old widowed man hospitalized with severe depression. Anesthesiologist present.
A19s.	Office visit for diagnostic reevaluation of a 68-year-old woman with chronic depression, unresponsive to treatment.

education, than a typical brief office visit in internal medicine or family practice (Sharfstein and Goldman 1989; Anonymous 1989). However, as this book goes to press, the AMA has not adopted any of these proposed changes.

The Harvard RBRVS Study

The Harvard RBRVS assigned relative values to medical and surgical activities by obtaining a consensus from a large panel of physicians regarding intensity of services rendered. These were adjusted mathematically for practice costs and opportunity costs of training. The consensus on time and effort was based on clinical vignettes deemed typical of services rendered by each of the specialties studied; services not described in the vignettes were assigned values based on the ratio of their current prevailing charges to the charges for services covered by the consensus items.

Relative values for psychiatric services were based on 25 vignettes, comprising 15 different CPT codes. Six of the vignettes described patients over 65 (see Table 7-3). Only one of the six vignettes described a definite physical comorbidity.

In the Harvard study, internal medicine evaluations receive substantially higher relative values than psychiatric evaluations. For example, an emergency hospital consultation by an internist on a 73-year-old new patient with a possible bowel obstruction is given a CPT code of 90630, for a complex consultation, and is assigned a relative value of 361. A hospital consultation for diagnosis and management of fever following abdominal surgery is assigned a code of 90610 for an extended consultation, and a relative value of 250. By contrast, hospital consultation for psychiatric evaluation of a 68-year-old cardiac surgical patient with a severe post-operative depression, and an office consultation for psychiatric evaluation of a 65-year-old man with intellectual deterioration and behavior problems, including verbal and physical abuse of coworkers, are both assigned codes of 90620, for a comprehensive consultation, and given a relative value of 204. The comprehensive evaluation of depression in a patient who has recently had cardiac surgery will require a detailed psychiatric history, behavioral observations from nurses, a complete review of the medication list, a cognitive evaluation to screen for neurologic complications of the surgery and anesthesia, and a complete mental status examination with evaluation of suicidal risk. The evaluation of the 66-year-old man with behavior change will likewise include cognitive evaluation, neurologic screening, a psychiatric history, observations from collateral sources, and an assessment of risk of danger to others. These highly time-consuming procedures contrast with what is often a fairly straightforward and routine evaluation of a post-operative fever. The latter is nonetheless accorded a higher relative value.

These observations suggest that the Hsaio et al. study assigns a higher value to evaluation and management of common problems seen by internists than to the evaluation and management of often more subtle and complex problems seen by psychiatrists. Part of the reason for this is the assignment of a higher weight to internists' practice costs. Additionally, however, the psychiatric vignettes fail to convey the common occurrence of medical comorbidity in elderly psychiatric patients. For example, in the cardiac surgery vignette, if it were mentioned that the patient were on seven medications, including several with potential central nervous system side effects, the raters' perception of the effort and time involved, and risk assumed, might have been different. While there were no vignettes specifically dealing with the prescription of medication in the elderly, it is likely, for example, that a higher value would be assigned to the prescription of an antidepressant drug to a 75-year-old man with a history of cardiac arrhythmia and several falls than to the prescription of the same drug to a 35-year-old who was totally healthy apart from depression.

Before a resource-based relative value scale is adopted as a standard for Medicare reimbursement, the limitations of CPT codes for psychiatry, and the problem of medical comorbidity, should be addressed. If not, the system will build in disincentives for psychiatric treatment of the frail or multi-problem elderly. Even without revision of CPT, existing modifiers for severity exist within the CPT coding system, so operationally defined criteria for using the modifiers would permit the development of increased relative values for psychiatric services to more complex and compromised patients.

Internists and geriatricians also are concerned that their services are covered by a very limited number of codes, whereas the services of procedure-oriented specialties are described by a wide range of codes. In a personal communication, a member of the Physicians Payment Reform Commission shared with this writer his concern that a limited number of codes for internists' services would create financial incentives for them to avoid the sickest and most complex patients, while reliable and valid codes for severity and complexity could help remove these disincentives (John Eisenberg, M.D., personal communication). Further studies of relative values, based on an expanded range of vignettes mapped onto a larger set of codes, offer the best hope of developing an RVS that is equitable in its evaluation of EM services (Ginsburg 1989).

Cross-Links and Further Implications of Inter-Specialty Differentials

In the RBRVS study, comparisons of service intensity across specialties were arrived at by consensus, relying in part upon estimates by experts within each specialty of the time involved to perform the service. Comparisons between services not explicitly cross-linked were made by extrapolation, using within-specialty relative values and starting from explicitly cross-linked services. Seven psychiatric services were cross-linked with medical services—three in general internal medicine and four in rheumatology. Four of the psychiatric services were rendered to elderly patients (see Table 7-4). For example, a hospital emergency room evaluation of a 78-year-old woman who ingested alcohol and Valium in an apparent suicide attempt, is deemed equivalent to an emergency hospital consultation on a 72-year-old new patient with a possible bowel obstruction. The assumption of equivalency is questionable. The internist evaluating the potential bowel obstruction does not need to obtain extensive information from collateral sources regarding the patient's behavior, while this would be essential in a recent suicide attempter. The internist does not need to conduct a detailed mental status examination, while the psychiatrist must do a detailed mental status examination evaluating both suicidal intent and cognitive status. Both the psychiatrist and the internist must review patients' medication lists, medical histories, and laboratory data. The only service uniquely provided by the internist might be the physical examination, and this would not be extremely time-consuming, as

Table 7–4.   Cross specialty links: Harvard RBRVS study

Psychiatric service	"Equivalent" medical service
1. Hospital emergency room evaluation of a 78-year-old woman who ingested alcohol and Valium in an apparent suicide attempt.	Emergency hospital consultation of a 72-year-old new patient with possible bowel obstruction.
2. Office visit for diagnostic reevaluation of a 68-year-old woman with chronic depression, unresponsive to treatment.	Initial office evaluation of a patient with negative lab and x-ray studies, with question of fibrositis.
3. Office consultation for psychiatric evaluation of a 65-year-old man with intellectual deterioration and behavior problems, including verbal and physical abuse of coworkers.	Initial office evaluation of a 70-year-old woman with polyarthralgia.
4. Hospital consultation for psychiatric evaluation of a 68-year-old cardiac surgical patient with severe postoperative depression.	Hospital consultation of a 35-year-old woman with fever, swelling joints, and rash of one week duration.

Source.   Adapted from Table 48 (Hsaio et al. 1988).

some time-consuming parts of the general physical examination (such as a detailed neurological and sensory assessment) usually would be omitted in the setting of a possible acute bowel obstruction.

The examples in Table 7-4 suggest that the cross-links between psychiatry and internal medicine are questionable. Further, the estimates of time involved in rendering a psychiatric service may be influenced by traditions of payment for a 50- to 60-minute therapy hour, and not accurately estimate the actual time a psychiatrist would choose to take to properly address the case.

Faulty cross-specialty linkages in a revised payment scale have several possible implications for access to neuropsychiatric care: If psychiatric services are under-reimbursed relative to the time, stress, and intensity of the work involved, physicians will have an incentive to avoid psychiatry, psychiatrists will have an incentive to avoid Medicare recipients, and psychiatrists treating Medicare recipients will have an incentive to avoid patients who might require more stressful or complex services. Training programs in teaching hospitals, the likely locus of care for complex cases, which rely upon Medicare Part B revenues to partially fund faculty, will find it disadvantageous to focus their services on the most complex and severely ill patients. Consequently, training for the next generation of physicians in the management of complex neuropsychiatric problems would suffer.

The potential adverse consequences of "locking in" inappropriate relative values, as might occur if the current RBRVS were adopted, are described in a recent article by Holahan and Zuckerman (1989). At worst, physician payment reform could gain cost control at the price of diminished access to care (Sammons 1989). Patients would lose their option to directly express their demand for services they wanted and needed, but were poorly reimbursed by the Medicare system. Recognizing this potential problem, OBRA 1989 requires the Secretary of HHS to monitor utilization and access to care as physician payment reform is implemented. While the major focus of monitoring appears to be the detection of overutilization or decreased Medicare assignment rates, advocates could press for monitoring to also address concerns regarding *underutilization* of mental health services by Medicare beneficiaries.

Complexity: Addressed or Finessed?

The comprehensive evaluation of the many dimensions of an elderly patient's physical, mental, and functional status is obviously a time-consuming task. Nonetheless, it is quite possible to treat specific illnesses, disabilities, and medical problems in elderly patients without getting involved in the complexities of a holistic approach. For example, an ophthalmologist can perform a lens implant without evaluating the patient's cognitive function or family environment. A cardiologist can prescribe treatment for angina pectoris without intervening to change the patient's lifestyle, or assessing the effect of the diagnosis or prescription on the patient's mood. In these cases, the evaluation performed by the specialist can nonetheless be labeled "comprehensive" because the requisite history and general physical examination are performed. Likewise, a psychiatrist can prescribe antidepressant medication without fully considering the effects of the patient's medical diagnosis on drug metabolism, or evaluating family and environmental factors that might be relevant to the patient's mood. As long as a psychiatric history is taken and a formal mental status examination is performed, that consultation also can be labeled "comprehensive." Thus, issues can be finessed, rather than addressed.

It is tempting to speculate that some of patients' dissatisfaction with medical care may lie in the frustration of seeing multiple specialists, each of whom perform an adequate or even excellent within-specialty examination, but choose not to address the total picture. Part of the clamor for more primary care physicians may be motivated by these frustrations. However, primary care physicians are not immune from finessing complex issues. They may choose to treat less serious problems symptomatically and superficially, while referring more complex problems to specialists, who then may initiate intensive and invasive procedures according to the customs of their specialties, without involving the primary care physician in an integrative role. Further, primary care physicians are known to underrecognize and undertreat the psychiatric disorders that are ubiquitous in primary care practice, whether as principal diagnoses or as comorbidities.

Within a course of treatment by an individual provider, services may be more or less complex. The emergency room evaluation of a suicidal patient may involve extraordinary complexity, which can decline rapidly if a prompt decision is made to admit the patient to a psychiatric hospital. As long as that decision is pending, the psychiatrist must not only evaluate mental status and history in detail, but also obtain collateral information about the patient's social supports, behavior, and environment (Marson et al. 1988). Once the decision to admit is made, much of this information-gathering can be deferred. Similarly, the decision to discharge a patient to a nursing home may be less complex than the decision to send the patient to his/her own home, which might involve family education, arrangement of supportive services, patient education for treatment adherence, and evaluation of safety risks if the patient is functionally impaired or intermittently dangerous to self. In each of these cases, the physician decision that leads to a less complex physician service is likely to result in greater costs for the health care system. Since physician payment should not indirectly encourage institutional treatment when there are satisfactory alternatives, a system of relative values for EM services ideally would take into account not only the severity and complexity of a patient's illness, but also whether the complexity of illness was actually addressed by the physician's service. The PPRC is committed to addressing this issue, at least to the extent of providing some additional payment to physicians when services require an unusually long time. However, the PPRC is unlikely to make the supplement very great, because of fears of encouraging inefficiency or overutilization (Paul Ginsburg, Ph.D., personal communication).

Research Priorities

Establishing reliable, valid, and operationally defined measures of complexity and severity is of evident importance. In developing such measures, neuropsychiatric comorbidities deserve attention, as they have been shown to correlate with greater mortality, poorer rehabilitative outcome, and higher utilization of services (see Chapter 1). Consideration might be given to further exploration of the model of Cromwell et al. (1989) for incorporating a measure of complexity into a relative value scale. According to their system, which appeared reliable for a number of medical and surgical procedures, the value of a service is expressed by the equation

$$F = AT^\alpha C^\beta,$$

where F is the relative value of the service, A is a constant, T the time taken, C a measure of complexity, and α and β are exponents chosen to permit nonlinear relationships of time and complexity with service value. The exponent for case complexity could be adjusted according to whether or not the complexity was addressed by the consultation. Service to a more compromised or multi-problem patient would receive a somewhat greater relative value even if complexity were not addressed, because medical judgments involved would be more difficult, and might involve the assumption of greater risk of adverse outcome. However, a system ought to build in incentives for addressing complexity, or at least eliminate disincentives for addressing complexity.

It might be argued that simply adjusting for time spent with a patient would suffice. This would be satisfactory only if it did not require greater effort, judgment, and skill to integrate a complex set of data and set priorities for one patient, compared with delivering more limited and narrowly defined services to several patients in the same stretch of time. This question is perhaps more philosophical than empirical. However, if there is a widespread desire for more holistic and less fragmented medical care for elderly people, incentives should be biased to encourage integrative cognitive activity by physicians.

References

American Medical Association: Physicians' Current Procedural Terminology, 4th ed. Chicago, American Medical Association, 1986

Anonymous: APA Proposes 15 New Codes for Fourth CPT Edition. Psychiatric News, April 7, 1989

Cromwell J, Mitchell JB, Rosenbach ML, et al: Using physician time and complexity to identify mispriced procedures. Inquiry 26:7-23, 1989

Ginsburg P: Physician payment policy in 101st congress. Health Affairs 8:6-20, 1989

Holahan J, Zuckerman S: Medicare mandatory assignment—an unnecessary risk. Health Affairs 8:66-79, 1989

Hsaio WC, Braun P, Becker E, et al: A National Study of Resource-Based Relative Value Scales for Physician Services: Final report. Boston, Harvard School of Public Health, 1988

Marson DC, McGovern MP, Pomp HC: Psychiatric decision making in the emergency room: a research overview. American Journal of Psychiatry 145:918-925, 1988

Sammons JH: Physician payment reform: don't forget the patient. Health Affairs 8:132-138, 1989

Sharfstein SS, Goldman H: Financing the medical management of psychiatric disorders. American Journal of Psychiatry 146:345-349, 1989

8

The Cost-Offset Effect

Judith R. Lave, Ph.D.

People with diagnosable mental disorders use more general health care services than those without such disorders. The association between diagnosable mental disorders and the use of general health care services holds for the general population as well as for the population aged 65 and over (Hankin and Oaktay 1979; Shapiro et al. 1984; Goldstrom et al. 1987). There is a general hypothesis, the offset hypothesis, that the treatment of mental illness results in a subsequent reduction in the utilization of other health care services. If such a decrease takes place, then the cost of mental health services will be "offset," in whole or in part, by the reduction in the cost of other services. The offset issue is explored here as it relates to neuropsychiatric care for people over 65 years of age.

After a discussion on the use of health care services by elderly persons with mental disorders, relevant findings from the literature on treatment offsets are summarized. Then, the reasons why the treatment for mental disorders may be accompanied by a reduction in the use of other medical services are examined, limitations of our present knowledge are identified, and the offset issue reassessed in a broader context.

Treatment of Mental Disorders in the Elderly Population

The issue of offsets usually arises in the context of arguments favoring the increase in services or payment for the treatment of mental disorders. Therefore, it may be useful to ascertain whether or not mental health services are underutilized by the elderly.

There is some evidence that the elderly are much less likely to visit physicians for the treatment of mental disorders than are the nonelderly (Shapiro et al. 1984) and that they are less likely to obtain care from specialty mental health providers (Leaf et al. 1985; Shapiro et al. 1984).

These utilization data and other studies of clinical practice have led to the general conclusion that mental disorders in the elderly are likely to remain under treated (German et al. 1985). The elderly may not seek treatment because they are unaware of being ill or because of denial employed to avoid the stigma associated with mental disorders. Other barriers to treatment are low expectations about treatment outcome and the restricted coverage for mental health available under Medicare (Gottlieb 1986). Finally, many physicians do not recognize mental disorders and, therefore, fail to prescribe appropriate treatment or to refer their patients to specialists. And, when illnesses such as dementia, depression, and anxiety are diagnosed, they are often ascribed to the normal aging process and left untreated. These issues are discussed in greater detail in Chapter 4.

Evidence on the Offset Effect

The offset hypothesis states that appropriate and timely treatment of mental disorders is conducive to subsequent decreases in the utilization of other health care resources. The hypothesis emerges from observing a reduction in the use of other health care services following treatment for mental illness. This observation alone may not be evidence of a cause and effect relationship since the use of general health services often peaks just before the onset of mental health care and the decrease in their use may be resulting from a natural return to the average level of utilization. Such regression to the mean is a phenomenon likely to occur even without a neuropsychiatric intervention.

Many studies have examined the offset effect, and two among them are based on a comprehensive review and analysis (meta-analysis) of the published evidence on the topic (Johns and Vishi 1979; Mumford et al. 1984). The studies report on the effects of initiating psychotherapy and similar types of interventions (Budman et al. 1984), on the introduction of a psychiatric liaison program in hospitals (Levitan and Kornfeld 1981; Strain et al. 1989), and on the utilization patterns among the enrollees of HMOs by those who received mental health services versus those who did not (Hankin et al. 1983). Although a few studies found that general health care utilization increased after the initiation of mental health treatments (Budman et al. 1984), the general conclusion of both meta-analyses is that the treatment for mental disorders is accompanied by about a 20% overall decrease in the use of general health care services.

The "offset effect" is more likely to occur in the case of inpatient than outpatient services. However, the studies examined in the meta-analyses did not compare the estimated dollar savings from the decreased utilization of services with the cost of the mental health interventions.

Only one study in the published literature specifically focuses on the offset effect for the population over the age of 65 (Levitan and Kornfeld 1981). In the study, a liaison psychiatrist participated in the post-operative care of 24 patients who had received surgery for fractured femurs. Compared to a group of comparable patients admitted to the hospital in the 6 months prior to the study period, these patients had a significantly shorter average hospital stay (30 days compared to 42 days) and were much less likely to be admitted to a nursing home (30% compared to 65%). Of the 24 study patients, 17 suffered from psychopathological disorders. In this case, the dollar amount saved from the decreased utilization of other health care services more than offset the cost of the liaison psychiatrist. A possible reason why the addition of psychiatric liaison made such a difference is that neuropsychiatric problems of patients in the comparison group were not identified and treated in the course of their hospitalization. This observation is consistent with the findings of another study on the use of psychiatric consultations: Wallen et al. (1987), in an analysis of hospital discharge data from over 300 hospitals in the 1970s, found that very few discharged patients had psychiatric consultations and that proportionately fewer patients over 65 received one.

The replication by Strain et al. (1989) of the Levitan and Kornfield study was conducted at two sites: Mt. Sinai Hospital in New York and Northwestern Memorial Hospital in Chicago. The total N was 356: 208 intervention subjects and 148 controls. A psychiatric liaison intervention involving structure screening of all hip fracture patients over 65 for depression, anxiety, cognitive deficits, and functional impairment was instituted on two orthopedic services; when psychiatric comorbidities were identified they were addressed by the liaison psychiatrist according to the psychiatrist's judgment. Baseline data were collected for a full year on both services prior to institution of the liaison program; acute care costs were directly determined. While only 10% of elderly hip fracture patients received psychiatric consultation during the baseline year, more than 50% of patients during the experimental year were identified as having significant comorbid psychiatric disorders, such as major depression or delirium. Both hospital length of stay and acute care costs fell during the intervention year at both sites. In New York, average length of stay dropped from 21.7 days to 19.6 days, with a total cost savings of $136,800 for 114 patients, compared with the expected costs projected from the baseline year. In Chicago, length of stay dropped from 15.5 days to 14.1 days, with a calculated cost savings of $56,400 for 94 patients. In contrast to the Levitan and Kornfield study, Strain et al. did not find a significant change in post-discharge dispositions between the control year and the intervention year, so the cost savings they found were due to a reduction in acute care costs rather than to a reduction in institutional long-term care placements.

The study of Strain et al. illustrated the effectiveness of standardized structured instruments for screening an elderly inpatient group for psychiatric comorbidities relevant to their health services utilization. The instruments used in the Strain et al. study can all be administered by nonphysicians, showing that the initial case-finding stage of psychiatric liaison need not require direct physician involvement.

Although only one publication reports on interventions targeted to older patients, other studies do examine the relationship between the offset effect and age. Mumford et al. (1984) conclude in their meta-analysis that the offset effect increases with age in the study populations. However, the oldest patients in these investigations were usually between 45 and 65 years old. Very few patients were over 65 years old.

In spite of the attractive "common sense" appeal of the offset effect, estimates of the effects must be viewed with some caution. Only in a few cases did researchers use a randomized controlled design and many methodological flaws are associated with the more frequent "before and after" and case control studies. For example, several studies examined the relative service utilization of people with diagnosed mental illness who did or did not seek treatment from specialty mental health providers (Hankin et al. 1983; Schlesinger et al. 1983). However, there are fundamental differences among these two groups: one group sought treatment and therefore was self-selected, while the comparison group might not have changed utilization patterns even with treatment.

Why Should the Treatment of Mental Disorders Lead to a Decrease in the Use of Other Services?

Some reasons why the treatment of mental disorders may lead to a decrease in the use of other health care resources (Morlock 1987; Hankin et al. 1983) are described here.

First, mental disorders are associated with the amplification of minor symptoms of physical illness or a heightened concern about such symptoms. These responses may increase the demand for treatment of physical illness while at the same time diminishing the patient response to treatment. The problem is likely to be more common among older persons since, for example, psychiatric co-morbidities are higher among people with chronic medical conditions (Wells et al. 1988), which, in turn, are more prevalent among the elderly. Consistent with these speculations are the findings from a previously mentioned study that reported longer hospital stays for Medicare patients with psychiatric comorbidity (Fulop et al. 1987). In those cases, treating the mental disorder possibly led to a decrease in the use of health services.

Second, mental disorder may be accompanied by somatization—"the conversion of mental experience or states into bodily symptoms" (Dorland 1988) which is associated with a coping style of increased health care utilization. People may move from doctor to doctor while seeking an explanation for what bothers them. The result is an increase not only in the number of doctor visits, but also in the use of ancillary services such as the diagnostic tests undertaken to determine the origin of the symptoms. Therefore, linking certain perceived physical symptoms to treatable mental disorders could shorten the search for physical pathology and, after the successful treatment of the mental condition, eliminate the physical distress and the need for related medical services.

Third, mental disorders, in particular depression, may affect the functional status of older people more than that of younger persons. Depressed older people may be less able to carry out activities of daily living and, therefore, be more in need of services provided by friends, family, or community providers. The effective treatment of depression would then lead to a decrease in the utilization of support services.

Fourth, the early identification and treatment of mental disorders may avert institutionalization. For example, depression can cause social withdrawal, at times mimicking dementia. The cases reviewed in the Levitan and Kornfeld study emphasize the importance of identifying and treating depression early and, consequently, keeping some patients from being discharged to nursing homes. In the same vein, Sharfstein (in Chapter 6) reports the case of a woman successfully retained within her community because of the diagnosis and the successful treatment of depression.

Fifth, mental disorders may produce physical illness. An obvious example is liver disease due to alcoholism. In this case, a decrease in drinking could ameliorate a decrease in the physical illness and its related costs. Among the elderly, depression, by disrupting sleep, diminishing morbidity and decreasing appetite, may lead to blatant physical problems such as malnutrition, disturbed gait, and infectious disease without the mediation of exogenous toxins.

Finally, treatment by the specialty mental health provider could substitute for the treatment by the general medical practitioner.

Discussion

With this background, the offset effect can be viewed in a broader context. The arguments above suggest that, in some circumstances, the treatment of mental disorders may lead to a decrease in the use of general medical services, and that this decrease will offset some of the costs of the mental health interventions. This statement does not imply that total costs of care will be lower if mental health services were expanded. It does, however, suggest that there might be targets of opportunity, where specific interventions could have significant offsets. Any intervention will have associated with it some costs and some benefits (Warner and Luce 1982). The costs of the mental health intervention depend upon the type of service provided (screening, drug therapy, short-term counseling), the qualifications of the providers (family practitioner, psychologist, psychiatrist) and the intensity of services (the number of services offered plus the time period over which the services are offered). The benefits of the intervention are associated with the utility derived from the appropriate diagnosis of the disease, the decrease in morbidity, and the increase in the patient's ability to function. These benefits are realized both by the patient and the patient's family. As discussed earlier, other benefits may be derived from decreases in the use of other health care services. However, intervention could produce an increase in the use of other services. For example, a screening program which diagnoses a patient as having Alzheimer's disease may trigger the use of several community services. Or, the decision to administer antidepressant drugs may lead to a cardiological evaluation to assess the safety of those medications.

Costs and benefits may have differing time frames. For example, the costs of treating depression might be incurred over months, while the benefits of preserved function and decreased utilization of supportive services might be recovered over years. Finally, benefits may accrue to parties other than those that incur the cost of treatment. More Medicare dollars spent for acute psychiatric treatment, if correctly applied, could reduce Medicaid dollars that would otherwise be spent on nursing home care.

While it is possible to identify the nature of the costs and benefits of clinical interventions, it is often quite difficult to quantify them (Warner and Luce 1982; Pincus 1984). A way of approaching the measuring task would be that of conducting randomized clinical trials with one group of patients receiving specialty neuropsychiatric treatment and another group receiving general health care. In the best case, investigators would collect information on health status, mental health status, the quality of life and the use of services by the two groups. Having the groups selected at random, those observed differences that were statistically valid could be ascribed to the treatment.

The magnitude of the differences, however, would depend on the costs, the efficiency, the quality, and the effectiveness of the intervention. Overall results might also depend on how the efforts of informal care providers were accounted for.

There is considerable evidence that the neuropsychiatric problems of the aged are underdiagnosed (see Chapter 4). Also, there is evidence that the signs of depression or prescription drug side effects may be misinterpreted as indicating the presence of dementia. Further, as a result of clinical trials, it is known that many neuropsychiatric conditions are responsive to treatment (see Chapter 3). Given the evidence of undertreatment and the potential for cost offsets, the need for obtaining more definitive information on the economic implications of treating neuropsychiatric disorders is evident.

Four areas of research are likely to produce scientifically sound and policy relevant results:

1. Studies of psychiatric liaison programs in hospitals, such as those by Levitan and Kornfeld (1981), should be replicated in other sites and under different conditions. During the past few years, progress has been made in geriatric medical training, the number of geriatric assessment units has grown, and the diagnosis and treatment of neuropsychiatric disorders may have improved for the older hospitalized population. Yet, many cases of neuropsychiatric disorders are likely to remain undiagnosed. In the present era of cost-containment strategies, hospitals have incentives to cut back rather than to expand programs, and hospital administrators need good information for adequately allocating their scarce resources. Hospital administrators may be reluctant to fund psychiatric liaison programs if their goals are seen as merely educational. However, they may be willing to fund targeted neuropsychiatric programs empirically shown to reduce the cost of care for specific populations. In an era of prospective payment,

behaviorally disturbed medical patients awaiting placement are money losers. Levitan and Kornfeld's study suggests that some patients' need for nursing home placement would be obviated by timely psychiatric intervention.

2. More detailed analysis is needed of patients referred for nursing home placement, to identify those whose functional impairments may be aggravated by reversible neuropsychiatric disorders such as depression or prescription drug toxicity. Analysis must be based on actual direct evaluation of patients, rather than based on recorded diagnoses, since it is known that neuropsychiatric diagnoses are under-recorded, when they are made at all. The identification of specific groups at risk for this aggravation of functional deficit could be followed by controlled studies of groups at risk. Utilization of nursing home services would be the measured outcome, with one group receiving neuropsychiatric intervention, and a control group receiving conventional care.

3. Studies of clinical effectiveness should, if possible, include a health services research component. For example, Robinson (1987) has recently published the results of a study in which he examined the prevalence of depression among people who have suffered a stroke and then studied the effectiveness of treating these patients for depression. Over 40% of the depressed patients were found to respond to treatment. It would be interesting to know whether there were any differences in the utilization of health services between the treated and the untreated groups.

4. There should be some investigation of the treatment patterns of older people who are enrolled in capitated systems. In capitated health plans there are strong incentives to increase the efficiency with which care is provided. Consequently, the potential for offset should be exploited by the organization. For example, are the physicians in these settings who care for older people more likely to have formal training in geriatrics? Do they use more psychiatric consultations?

In conclusion, it is possible for the treatment of neuropsychiatric disorders to be accompanied by a decrease in the use of other health services, but it is likely to not be true in all cases, or perhaps even in the majority of cases. Even when there is a decrease in utilization of other health care services, the proportion of the costs offset may be small. Therefore, given the present state of our knowledge on the offset effect, it is unwise to base an increase in services for neuropsychiatric disorders in the elderly on the basis of the costs offsets alone. The purpose of neuropsychiatric care is to decrease psychiatric morbidity and to increase function. It should be evaluated largely on how effectively it achieves those treatment goals.

References

Budman SH, Demby AB, Feldstein ML: A controlled study of the impact of mental health treatment of medical care utilization. Medical Care 22:216-222, 1984

Dorland's Illustrated Medical Dictionary, 27th ed. Philadelphia, W. B. Saunders, 1988

Fulop G, Strain J, Vita J, et al: Impact of psychiatric comorbidity on length of hospital stay for medical/surgical patients: a preliminary report. American Journal of Psychiatry 144:878-882, 1987

German PS, Shapiro S, Skinner EA: Mental health of the elderly: use of health and mental health services. Journal of the American Geriatric Society 33:246-252, 1985

German PS, Shapiro S, Skinner EA, et al: Detection and management of mental health problems of older patients by primary care providers. Journal of the American Medical Association 257:489-493, 1987

Goldstrom ID, Burns BJ, Kessler LG, et al: Mental health services use by elderly adults in a primary care setting. Journal of Gerontology 42:147-143, 1987

Gottlieb GL: Contemporary psychiatry: providing psychiatric care for medicare patients. Psychiatric Annals 16:660-662, 1986

Hankin J, Oaktay JS: Mental Disorders and Primary Care: An Analytical Review of the Literature. (ADM) 78-661. Series D. No 5. Rockville, MD, U.S. Department of Health and Human Services, 1979

Hankin JR, Kessler LG, Goldberg ID, et al: A longitudinal study of offset in the use of nonpsychiatric services following specialized mental health care. Medical Care 21:1099-1110, 1983

Johns KR, Vishi TR: Impact of alcohol, drug abuse and mental health treatment on medical care utilization: a review of the research literature. Medical Care 17(Suppl):1-82, 1979

Leaf PJ, Livingston MM, Tischler GL, et al: Contact with health professionals for the treatment of psychiatric and emotional problems. Medical Care 23:1322-1337, 1985

Levitan SJ, Kornfield DS: Clinical and cost benefits of liaison psychiatry. American Journal of Psychiatry 138:790-793, 1981

Morlock LL: Recognition and treatment of mental health problems in the general health care sector. Paper presented at the Conference on the future of Mental Health Services Research, Tampa, Florida, February 1987

Mumford E, Schlesinger HJ, Glass GV, et al: A new look at evidence about reduced cost of medical utilization following mental health treatment. American Journal of Psychiatry 141:1145-1158, 1984

Pincus HA: Making the case for consultation-liaison psychiatry: issues in cost effectiveness analysis. General Hospital Psychiatry 6:173-179, 1984

Robinson RG: Depression and stroke. Psychiatric Annals 17:731-739, 1987

Schlesinger H, Mumford E, Glass GV: Mental health treatment and medical care utilization in a fee-for-service system: outpatient mental health treatment following the onset of a chronic disease. American Journal of Public Health 73:422-429, 1983

Shapiro S, Skinner EA, Kessler LG, et al: Utilization of health and mental health services: three epidemiological catchment area sites. Archives of General Psychiatry 41:971-978, 1984

Strain JJ, Hammer JS, Lyons JS, et al: Cost offset from the psychiatric liaison intervention for elderly hip fracture patients (abstract). Psychosomatic Medicine 51:261, 1989

Wallen J, Pincus H, Goldman H, et al: Psychiatric consultations in short-term general hospitals. American General Psychiatry 44:163-168, 1987

Warner KE, Luce BR: Cost-Benefit and Cost-Effectiveness Analysis in Health Care: Principles, Practice and Potential. Ann Arbor, MI, Health Administration Press, 1982

Wells KB, Golding JM, Burnam MA: Psychiatric disorder in a sample of the general population with and without chronic medical conditions. American Journal of Psychiatry 145:976-981, 1988

9

Market Segmentation

Gary L. Gottlieb, M.D., M.B.A.

The diverse group of professionals and paraprofessionals who administer mental health services to the elderly participate in a fragmented system with limited commonality in training, philosophy, therapeutic methods, and objectives. Additionally, geriatric mental health care delivery is tainted by factors that have been associated with psychiatric care in younger populations: controversial definitions of illness, poor standardization of triage and clinical decision making, a large variety of intervention strategies, and few gold standards of outcome.

A number of inspiring and innovative programs deliver care and comprehensive services to a relatively small number of older adults. However, the general organization and availability of resources have evolved in response to the mandates of the Older Americans Act and to the evolving design of Medicare benefits (Gottlieb 1988). Solo and group private practice continue to dominate the marketplace (Beigel and Sharfstein 1984). Because of individual tastes and reimbursement exclusions, most private practitioners choose not to care for elderly patients (Mitchell and Schurman 1983; Mitchell et al. 1986). As a result, while the overall supply of mental health providers has grown in parallel with the elderly population, the elderly have little access to mental health specialty services (Mumford and Siblinger 1985; Borson et al. 1987; Gottlieb and Bloom 1988).

Many studies and proposals have addressed style of practice, practice patterns and provider behaviors in general health care (Hornbrook and Berki 1985; Eisenberg 1985, 1986). These efforts assume that rational economic behavior, training, incentives, and feedback mechanisms will allow some manipulation of provider function, thereby enhancing uniformity in decision making and in resource utilization. However, these factors may be difficult to control.

Eddy (1984) and Wennberg et al. (1982) have addressed the importance of uncertainty in diagnosis, treatment, and practice styles. Wennberg et al. identified three characteristic sources of clinical uncertainty:

> [(1)] ...difficulties in classifying a particular patient so that the probabilities of existence of disease, extent of disease, prognosis and treatment outcomes are reasonably ascertained. [(2)] ...information on the probabilities of treatment outcome under controlled circumstances does not exist. [(3)] ...the utility of the physician—who makes vicarious decisions—may not correspond to the patient's utility. (Wennberg et al. 1982, p. 812)

These sources of uncertainty are pervasive in the delivery of neuropsychiatric care to the elderly. Strategies for the delivery of high quality, efficient services for complex problems cannot succeed unless they adapt discipline-specific solutions that exploit the assets of each provider discipline and address the differences in training, diagnostic ability, treatment dogma, and outcome objectives among provider types.

Provider Profile

Beitman (1983) estimates that there are at least 100,000 independently practicing psychotherapists in the United States. However, estimates of the size of institutional provider categories indicate a much larger supply of potential providers of neuropsychiatric care. The specialty mental health sector provides some kind of care to about 21% of people with a known diagnosable mental disorder who receive formal treatment each year; the remainder receive treatment from primary care medical providers (NIMH 1987). The specialty sector provides an even smaller proportion of total mental health care for older adults (Mumford and Siblinger 1985; see Chapter 4).

There are four major clusters of professionals in the specialty sector: psychiatric nurses, psychiatric (or clinical) social workers, psychologists, and psychiatrists. The roles of each of these provider groups have evolved remarkably over the past 25 years. However, the diagnoses, the types of patients, and the problems treated by individual provider groups are unknown. Similarly, the patients treated in the specialty mental health sector have never been compared directly to those treated in the nonspecialty sector.

Nurses

Of the roughly one million employed registered nurses in the United States, about 60,000 are engaged in some form of neuropsychiatric care (Taintor 1984; Lewis 1984). Sixty-five percent of this group are graduates of two-year programs, 22% have bachelor's degrees, and 13% are at the masters, specialist, or doctorate level. Psychiatric nurses are licensed and have a minimum of two years of experience in a "psychiatric" setting (Lewis 1984). Their functions include triage, intake screening, home visits, psychotherapy, "counseling," medication monitoring, implementation of medical regimens, etc. They function in Community Mental Health Centers (CMHCs), inpatient settings, HMOs, public and private agencies, hospitals, nursing homes, and, in small number, in private practice. Standards of practice, certification, and licensure have been established (American Nurses' Association 1982). Masters programs for geriatric nurses and geriatric nurse practitioners have grown remarkably over the past decade. In addition to an extensive didactic curriculum, these programs generally require substantial supervised clinical experience in specialty geriatric settings. Approximately 1200 geriatric nurse practitioners have been certified (Mezey and Lynaugh 1989).

Social Workers

There are about 130,000 professionally qualified social workers in the United States. Most of these providers have masters level training from accredited programs (Lee 1984). However, it is estimated that about half of the graduates of bachelors' granting social work programs do not pursue graduate education. Positions in social work may be occupied by as many as 300,000 individuals who function as social workers, with or without professional qualification (Taintor 1984). The philosophy of social work "emphasizes the life processes of adaptation and reciprocal interactions between individuals and their social and physical environments" (Lee 1984). Geriatric social worker practice is represented in community mental health, general health facilities, family service agencies, nursing homes, and area agencies on aging (AAA) (Waldfogel and Rosenblatt 1983). Approximately 70,000 social workers are thought to be engaged as psychiatric social workers and about 20,000 are involved in some form of private clinical practice (Klerman 1985). Specialized training in psychiatric social work at the masters level includes concentrated coursework and clinical practice in psychiatric settings. Specific requirements vary among programs. About half of the states have licensure requirements for social workers (Lee 1984).

Psychologists

Training in psychology is a combination of curricula in psychological assessment and treatment, in clinical modification of behavior and in research methods and evaluation (American Psychological Association 1983). Psychologists who pursue the Ph.D. are required to complete an original research dissertation. Those in programs offering a professional degree, the Psy.D., have similar clinical programs with less rigid research requirements. The American Psychological Association has established standards for accreditation of trainees. Accreditation requires a broad, general curriculum in general psychology with competence demonstrated in biological, social, and cognitive-affective bases of behavior and in individual behavior (APA 1983). There are more than 100,000 masters and doctorate-level psychologists. Probably a quarter of these are doctoral-level psychologists who provide clinical services (Taintor 1984). A substantial and growing proportion of all psychologists provide care in office-based practices. Licensure requirements vary substantially by state (Vanden Bos et al. 1981). Many third-party carriers require that an independent vendor have an APA approved internship and supervised predoctoral and postdoctoral experience in health care settings. An independent group, the National Register of Health Service Providers in Psychology, has attempted to codify these requirements (Council for the NRHSPP 1987). Specialty training in neuropsychology and in geriatric psychology has grown steadily over the past decade. A separate division, division 20, of the American Psychological Association is responsible for practice and policy issues related to aging.

Psychiatrists

Four years of training beyond medical school is required for eligibility for certification by the American Board of Psychiatry and Neurology. Some 33,000 psychiatrists are trained in psychiatric theories and treatments including growth and development, psychopathology, biological psychiatry, drug treatment, psychotherapy, and diagnostic procedures. Diagnostic training includes an emphasis on identifying medical conditions that may cause or contribute to mental symptoms (American Board of Psychiatry and Neurology 1985). Licensure requirements are those required by individual states for all physicians. While general requirements for clinical and didactic experiences in psychiatric residency are established nationally (Accreditation Council for Graduate Medical Education 1988), there is substantive variability in specific training experiences and controversy about what training is ideal (American Psychiatric Association 1986). About two-thirds of psychiatrists do some private practice (Klerman 1985) and evidence of increasing participation in office-based practice has been reported (Knesper and Carlson 1981; Fenton 1987).

The nature and intensity of training in the neuropsychiatric care of older adults vary considerably among residency programs. Subspecialty training in geriatric psychiatry has increasingly become available, but the content of post-residency fellowships in the clinical and research elements of the mental health of the elderly is not well standardized. Formalization of certification for added qualifications in Geriatric Psychiatry by the ABPN should provide a framework for subspecialty curricula. The American Association for Geriatric Psychiatry (AAGP) is comprised of psychiatrists with a reported interest in care of the elderly. There is considerable variability in geriatric specialty training and experience among the AAGP's more than nine hundred members.

The Nonspecialty Sector

The majority of patients with a psychiatric disorder who receive treatment obtain their care from providers who are not mental health specialists (NIMH 1987). Several studies suggest that an even greater percentage of psychiatrically ill older people are treated by general health care providers (Waxman et al. 1984; also see Chapter 4). Six percent of visits to the nearly 500,000 nonpsychiatric physicians in the United States are related to a diagnosis of a mental disorder (NIMH 1987). The majority of these visits are to primary care providers in general and family practice, internal medicine, and obstetrics and gynecology (Taintor 1984). However, there is evidence that primary care providers diagnose, appropriately treat, or refer only a small proportion of patients with mental disorders with whom they have contact (German et al. 1987). Comprehensive efforts to screen for mental disorders in primary care practices confirm a substantial prevalence of untreated psychiatric disorders in these settings (Zung et al. 1983; Wilkinson 1986; Von Korff et al. 1987). Diagnosis and treatment of cognitive impairment and of depression in older patients by primary care providers are generally inadequate (Waxman and Carner 1984). Attempts to remedy this situation have included teaching to improve primary care physicians' interviewing skills (Caroll and Monroe 1979; Linn et al.

1980; Cope et al. 1986). However, general improvement in interviewing skill does not substitute for specific knowledge of mental disorders. Systematic diagnostic protocols may be useful in improving the ability of primary care providers in assessing psychopathology in the elderly (Von Korff et al. 1987).

The growth of geriatric internal medicine and geriatric family practice may improve neuropsychiatric outcomes for older adults in primary care settings. The standard curriculum for subspecialty training and added qualifications in geriatric medicine includes a considerable emphasis on geriatric psychiatry (American Board of Family Practice and American Board of Internal Medicine 1987; American Geriatrics Society 1987).

Feedback programs established to influence the abilities of primary care providers to deliver mental health care have been undertaken (Hoeper et al. 1984; Moore et al. 1978; German et al. 1987; Shapiro et al. 1987). Hoeper et al. (1984) found that feedback from screening had no measurable effects on the rate of detection of mental disorder by physicians in a primary care clinic. In contrast, Moore et al. (1978) demonstrated that feedback from depression screening significantly improved the ability of family practice residents to recognize the disorder. Recently, German et al. (1987) and Shapiro et al. (1987) evaluated the effects of feedback from mental health screening data on the practice behaviors of primary care providers. German et al. showed that feedback significantly increased the likelihood of detection of mental disorders in elderly patients. Management of mental disorders improved also, but the trend was statistically insignificant (German et al. 1987).

Other Providers

Mental health care may be provided also by "counselors and therapists" who are only beginning to be accounted for by regulatory agencies (e.g., California developed the title of "marriage and family counselors" in an effort to license therapists who were not trained in an identified discipline). There are also about 130,000 other mental health professionals (bachelors degree and above) and mental health workers (no bachelors degree) providing services in organized mental health care facilities. Pastoral counseling, provided in some form by the close to 500,000 identified ministers, is perhaps the most widely available, stigma-free, mental health care resource. While specific qualifications have been established for certification by the American Association of Pastoral Counseling, only a fraction of the ministry has pursued membership (Taintor

1984). While the elderly are served extensively by the clergy, there are no universal geriatric curricula required for pastoral counselors.

This extraordinary conglomeration of providers delivers diverse services and procedures: 1) Diagnostic abilities and nomenclature are not consistent among these groups (Hoeper et al. 1979); 2) A large number of treatments exist. There are probably about 400 different psychotherapies (Karasu 1986) and few have established outcome probabilities (Guillette 1984); 3) The individual utilities (motives) of these providers necessarily agree neither with one another nor with patient utility.

Each of the disciplines has a unique ethos. Training standards have been linked to the philosophy and identified tasks that have become associated with each provider group. The growth of private practice in an environment of limited resources and uncertain demand has driven interdisciplinary competition. Research to date has failed to identify unique discipline-specific talents. However,tradition and regulation have created monopolies for specific disciplines for the provision of some services. The medical profession has long claimed a unique ability to provide certain procedures. For example, psychiatry maintains that medical training is necessary for adequate differential diagnosis, especially in complicated populations like the elderly. Similarly, the prescription of medication and other somatic interventions has been the exclusive domain of physicians. Recent state and federal legislation has expanded the practice horizons of nonphysician providers in traditionally medical areas: Nurse practitioners, nurse anesthetists, nurse midwives, physicians' assistants, and optometrists can now provide many services previously delivered only by physicians. Turf battles between psychiatrists and psychologists regarding so-called medical aspects of care including hospital privileges have intensified (Schindler et al. 1981; Sharfstein 1982a). However, neither discipline offers scientific evidence supporting its peculiar ability to provide better care or more favorable outcomes. Instead, prevention and treatment methods are applied generally to any consumer (i.e., client or patient) who demands them. Collaborative efforts specifically exploiting the assets of specific providers for different aspects of a given problem are only beginning to emerge (Coordinated Care Management Corp. 1988).

Determinants of Provider Behavior

Attempts to develop guidelines for clinical care are difficult even within identified mental health specialties. Formal algorithms for diagnosis and treatment of common conditions are poorly established, if they exist at all. Each of the major mental health professions has developed requirements for licensure. However, licensure does not create uniformity in provider behavior. Even in psychiatry, where medical licensure and residency requirements are reinforced by specialty board certification, "schools of thought and treatment modality" are adequately powerful to divide clinicians in determining the specific course of action that should be taken in a given set of circumstances (Smith et al. 1980). Most outcome studies have evaluated very specific diagnostic entities (e.g., depression) and focused intervention strategies (Rush et al. 1977; Klerman et al. 1984; Horowitz et al. 1986). While generic psychotherapy in general has been shown by meta-analysis to be associated significantly with improvements in mental symptoms, the most appropriate length, intensity, and nature of treatment for various conditions has not been established (Smith et al. 1980). Therefore, in many cases, a true "standard of care," the legal system's yardstick for provider performance, may not exist (Curran and Shapiro 1982).

Psychotherapeutic techniques vary considerably in their appropriateness to specific patient populations. They vary in frequency and duration of patient visits, in intensity of the provider-patient relationship and in the amount of provider effort per patient contact. A provider's style of practice is dependent upon personal motives, and is influenced substantially by the provider's discipline and theoretical inclination. In the specialty sector, trainees, influenced by a mentor or a body of knowledge, often pursue and apply the teachings of a specific theoretician. Social workers and psychologists, despite similar, relatively eclectic training, often become affiliated with psychoanalytic institutes, cognitive therapy centers, and/or family therapy programs. The selected practice style might be adaptable to numerous settings including solo private practice. However, the process of clinical work will be affected substantially by the treatment mode selected. Therefore, outcome is only one of many factors likely to influence providers in clinical decision making. The basic training requirements of specialty disciplines include some exposure to many treatment modalities without imposing rules or paradigms for their application. It is reasonable to expect that an ethical clinician, trained extensively in a specific therapeutic technique, is behaving rationally and optimizing his/her own utility when selecting that intervention for most patients (Karasu 1984).

At least one major study indicates that a therapist's allegiance to a specific school or belief system is necessary for the confidence and professional identity of the therapist and is associated with more favorable outcomes (Smith et al. 1980). Style and school of practice can influence numerous factors. These include: process of treatment, cost of treatment, likelihood of using diagnostic tests and inpatient settings, socioeconomic and functional status of a provider's caseload, and productivity (Karasu 1984; Guillette 1984; Craig and Patterson 1981). Similarly, allegiance to a specific therapeutic philosophy is likely to influence acceptance of standardized diagnostic methods, like the DSM-III (Jampala et al. 1986).

In summary, provider diversity affects the following:

1. *The objectives of treatment.* For example, given the same patient, a behaviorist or a psychopharmacologist might initiate treatment with the expectation of acute symptom reduction, while a psychoanalyst might set out to affect a major change in character.
2. *The means of achieving a given set of objectives.* Various psychotherapeutic approaches or somatic interventions might be appropriate to a given set of clinical circumstances and goals.
3. *Potential outcomes.* For many patients, the competence of the therapist, regardless of school, is the most relevant input related to outcome (Karasu 1984). But, there may be some patients who require a specific intervention, regardless of provider. A provider who is unlikely to select the correct intervention will affect potential outcome adversely. Specificity of this nature is most clear in conditions like psychosis, where drug therapies are clearly superior to virtually all other interventions (Richelson 1986).

Patient/client populations can be distinguished by: those who can benefit from rehabilitation and those who cannot; those individuals who require acute rather than chronic treatment; and those who may become the burden of the public sector if not cared for adequately (Beigel and Sharfstein 1984). These patient distinctions influence provider decision making at the point of referral or first contact. Similarly, the patient's demand for services has a complicated impact on mental health care. Patient expectations influence the ordering of medical tests and reactive, "defensive" medical practices in general health care settings (Eisenberg 1985; Garg et al. 1978; Brett and McCollough 1986). Although patients often have limited knowledge about psychotherapeutic techniques, their demands and expectations affect the treatment process (Orne 1984). In the worst case, patient desires influence the provider's treatment plan in a way that affects outcome adversely.

In the general health sector, increased numbers of physicians are associated with higher, rather than lower, prices for care and more abundant use of services (Feldstein 1970; Newhouse 1970; Fuchs 1978). This observation of apparent supplier-induced demand has been a focus of health care policy debate for over 25 years

(Wennberg 1984). The most comprehensive evaluations of the effects of competition on mental health specialty practice patterns and behaviors have examined psychiatrists in private practice settings.

Mitchell et al. (1986) and Frank (1985) studied the effects of competition on psychiatric practice, psychiatrists' fees, and psychiatrists' income. They found that psychiatrists are not immune to market forces. Increases in the number of psychiatrists per capita and direct reimbursement of psychologists (under Freedom of Choice insurance regulations) reduce workloads and hourly earnings for psychiatrists. However, Mitchell et al. (1986) suggest that larger numbers of nonpsychiatric general health care providers may increase referrals and increase fees and real income for psychiatrists.

These studies reflect the overall market for psychiatric services. Procedurally, talking psychotherapies are the modal intervention for all but the most severely ill patients, and only a small fraction of providers have adapted themselves to market niches that exploit their training or discipline specifically (Fenton 1987). However, as the supply of general mental health providers grows larger than the demand for office-based psychotherapy, the roles of specific provider types should become better defined.

In efficient capital markets, the low cost, high quality supplier ultimately captures the greatest market share. However, the market for neuropsychiatric services for the elderly is broad and multifaceted. Numerous distinct services may be required simultaneously and/or in sequence. While the least expensive provider may be readily identifiable, the appropriate resource (i.e., the highest quality) for a given situation may be unknown to the consumer. In fact, the most appropriate response to a given need may, as yet, also be unknown to providers, third-party payers, and regulators.

Each of the specialty mental health disciplines can make important and unique contributions to the neuropsychiatric care of older persons. However, the only guidelines which pair training and specific service delivery are those imposed by reimbursement and practice regulations (Gottlieb 1988). Given the limits of consumers' understanding of the differences between suppliers, providers frequently become direct competitors unnecessarily. While there are many circumstances in which provider substitutability is reasonable, an assumption of provider homogeneity in this complex marketplace is erroneous and potentially dangerous. Although provider organizations tend to advocate expansion of their specialty's role, the market for neuropsychiatric services for the elderly must be analyzed in terms of specific needs.

The efficient employment of the unique skills of each discipline to meet the specific needs of individual patients could be accomplished through the evolution of clearer market segments. All markets are segmented in the sense that different clusters of potential consumers seek to satisfy substantially different bundles of desires. Segmentation is based on a critical analysis of the demand side of the market (Coddington and Moore 1987). Economically, this process disaggregates the demand schedules of individual consumers where only one schedule was recognized before. In the market for geriatric neuropsychiatric services, the assessment of needs and the linkage between needs and disciplines pose many questions that require and deserve comprehensive research.

Comprehensive geriatric care usually requires interdisciplinary collaboration. The contribution of each type of provider will depend on diagnosis, disease stage and severity, and the availability of patient and caregiver resources. Alzheimer's disease allows an illustration of the value of demand analysis (patient and family needs assessment) and a potential "segmented" response: At initial presentation, individuals with cognitive impairment require extensive medical, psychiatric, neuropsychological, and functional assessment. Interdisciplinary team approaches to this task may facilitate data collection from various sources (Larson et al. 1986). However, discipline-specific assessments must be outlined carefully to prevent redundancy. Once a diagnosis has been made, overall case management, support of family care, and access to necessary legal and community resources could be carried out by a social worker. Ongoing medical, psychiatric, and functional needs could be monitored by a nurse clinician and referred to a physician or a psychologist when necessary. As the illness progresses, acute management of behavioral excess disability and periodic reassessment of cognitive function could be provided by a psychiatrist while acute medical problems would require input from a primary care physician or medical specialist. Changes in environment could require more intensive intervention and management. However, efficient use of manpower would be facilitated by teamwork, based on the principle of assigning work to the provider most specifically able to do the job, or to the least costly provider if more than one is able to meet the need. Teamwork offers an alternative to "turf battles."

While comprehensive interdisciplinary geriatric assessment programs have been shown in some demonstrations to improve some quality of care and quality of life indices, (Rubenstein et al. 1984; Allen et al. 1986) they would appear to be very expensive. Therefore, proper assessment of discipline-specific evaluation and management programs for neuropsychiatric disorders will require cost-related information as well as analysis of patient and family outcome data. Study of provider satisfaction would also be relevant to the goal of inducing providers to focus their efforts where they are most efficient.

Organizational structure and payment schemes have been used frequently to provide incentives for efficient and/or specific service delivery. Sharfstein (1982b) proposes that organized, prepaid "mental health HMOs" could provide comprehensive care while avoiding the massive expenditures imposed by frequent hospitalizations. His innovative formulation is dependent on relatively uniform provider responses to HMO-like incentives to reduce inpatient utilization. These effects have been demonstrated even in the care of the chronically mentally ill (CMI) (Meier 1981; Christianson 1988). The On Lok project in San Francisco has successfully maintained very impaired disabled older adults while reducing utilization of expensive institutional services (see Chapter 9). However, the importance of specific provider function and efficacy in that program have not been studied rigorously. A number of other capitated models of service delivery are emerging as the public sector attempts to provide comprehensive, cost-contained services for CMI populations (see Chapter 12). However, the emphasis on cost outcomes in most managed care systems limits our ability to measure quality and to assess the adequacy of response of providers to specific patient needs.

In lieu of analyzing the demand schedules of specific clients, most capitated providers mandate the use of professionals and procedures that are least costly per unit of service (not necessarily least costly per episode of illness!) (Wells et al. 1986). As a result of provisions for the development of "at-risk" Medicare contracts by the Health Care Financing Administration (HCFA), a number of managed health care providers have undertaken to provide comprehensive medical care for older adults. The quality of care provided and the economic feasibility of these arrangements have been controversial (Gottlieb 1988). However, these models could provide important data regarding the effects of organizational structure and specific provider roles on clinical neuropsychiatric outcomes in well and infirm elderly.

Studies that compare the nature of services rendered and the associated costs in a centralized, managed prepaid program and in the "open market" of the fee-for-service (FFS) system are important (Luft 1983; Luft 1981; Wells et al. 1986). Unfortunately, descriptions of the organizational structures, incentive systems, and triage mechanisms of managed care programs are rarely detailed. However, substantial data regarding utilization were analyzed in the Health

Insurance Experiment (HIE) (Wells et al. 1986): Mental health service users in FFS plans are about 50% more likely to be treated by more expensive providers than are HMO enrollees in studied programs. Patients in prepaid plans are about three times as likely as FFS users to see nonmedical therapists, usually social workers. Similarly, FFS patients are about 60% more likely to receive individual psychotherapy while HMO members are more than twice as likely to be treated with family or group treatments. It is not known if these differences result from an organized set of treatment paradigms, and what their relevance is to patient outcomes.

Manning et al. (1984) have documented that specific patterns of organization of care are associated with substantial cost savings. Their interpretation of HIE data led them to conclude that physicians in the prepaid group practices that they studied were "practicing a different style of medicine from that of fee-for-service physicians." However, the relative importance of management, reporting system, and group ethos versus payment method per se is not known.

Feedback and group participation in the division of labor among neuropsychiatric providers can be useful in reinforcing identified roles and in improving economic outcomes and morale. Craig and Patterson (1981) evaluated the productivity of clinicians in the psychiatry department of a prepaid health program. They defined productivity as the proportion of available staff time actually spent in direct service. All staff participated in the development of productivity standards for each of the provider categories represented in the program. The standards employed were subject to continuing review and actual performance was reported to the staff monthly. Staff members met periodically to evaluate the appropriateness of expectations. Data obtained encouraged therapists to alter traditional scheduling practices to optimize efficiency. Feedback allowed staff members from diverse disciplines to develop "realistic expectations of staff service and . . . to monitor their own fulfillment of these expectations." Notably, the clinical leadership, administrative psychiatrists in this case, was subject to the same system of evaluation and feedback as other team members.

An Agenda for Research

Integrated Clinical Trials

Brook and Lohr (1985) suggest that health services research would benefit from the development of a "macro" model that integrates a focus on issues of efficacy, effectiveness, variations in use, and quality of care. They define efficacy as the probability of benefit from an intervention applied for a specific problem under ideal conditions. Effectiveness is identical to efficacy, except that it describes "performance under ordinary conditions by the average practitioner for the typical patient" (Brook and Lohr 1985). Variations in use refers to differences in the consumption of services specifically related to the style of practice of the individual provider. Finally, "quality of care" is that part of the difference between effectiveness and efficacy that can be attributed to the provider and the setting of care.

Psychiatric research has only begun to address these essential areas. The adaptation of the randomized clinical trial (RCT) as the gold standard of therapeutic efficacy was an enormous step. The development of reliable and valid diagnostic and outcome criteria has contributed to the generalizability of treatments. However, clinical trials have been limited to testing new drugs or psychotherapeutic techniques in relatively small populations, recruited specifically for study. They have established the efficacy of interventions, not their *effectiveness*. For example, in an NIMH multicenter collaborative study, treatment of depression *under average conditions* in academic medical centers fell short of the standards set by a consensus of researchers (Keller et al. 1986). Brook and Lohr (1985) suggest that clinical trials must be designed so that outcome measures can be monitored on a long-term basis. Further, the dissemination of new interventions, including drug therapies and new psychotherapeutic techniques, deserves specific study.

Clinical trials should be integrated with evaluations of effectiveness, quality of care and variations in care. In addition to isolated RCTs which test only the effects of a new procedure, RCTs must be designed to assess the process of treatment administration and the skills it requires. In that way, provider attributes and their relation to quality of care could be assessed prospectively. Perhaps this would allow better definition of costs and task performance by providers of different disciplines. RCTs can be used also to evaluate the efficacy and effectiveness of assessment, triage, and treatment paradigms in different settings.

Innovative Training

A window of opportunity exists in mental health training. Delivery organizations and third parties are scrambling to produce more efficient systems of care. Educational leaders in the various disciplines can become the architects of future delivery systems. University-based programs can study new training models which integrate and define specific provider functions. Effectiveness of these programs can be evaluated prospectively and longitudinally in various settings where prevention and treatment of geriatric neuropsychiatric disorders are necessary.

While potentially expensive (Eisenberg 1985), education, feedback, and participation programs have been used effectively in changing the utilization and diagnostic behaviors of established providers (Craig and Patterson 1981). These methods can be employed to influence mature providers to collaborate more efficiently in the care of their older adult patients. Clinical leaders in the mental health specialties must envision the future more collaboratively. Better economic understanding of the segmentation of markets could facilitate more efficiency, rather than foster interdisciplinary competition and wasteful redundancy of services. Feedback programs aimed at quality and productivity developed and implemented by interdisciplinary clinical leadership are particularly worthy of study.

Organized settings of care, especially community mental health centers and prepaid group practices must study innovative models of organization, provider role identification and quality assurance. Well-studied demonstration projects can determine the optimal roles for providers while quantifying the impact of quality and cost imperatives on provider behavior.

Standardization of Care

Health service research methods that evaluate the process of care may be especially useful in standardizing neuropsychiatric care of the elderly. Diagnosis or symptom-specific sets of criteria have been developed for some medical conditions (Brook and Lohr 1985). These sets of criteria and other types of problem-specific tracers can be applied to treatment records relatively easily. This process allows auditors, supervisors, or peers to assess "what is done to or for a patient with respect to his or her particular . . . complaint" (Brook and Lohr 1985). It has been suggested that this kind of review program could be helpful in the establishment of treatment protocols for various illnesses.

General health care researchers have studied decision analytic methods extensively to provide models of care. These methods, which use data derived from expert judgments and from treatment research to reduce provider uncertainty, may be useful in providing guidelines for individual providers in clinically complex neuropsychiatric situations (Hamm et al. 1984; Widiger et al. 1984). Prescriptive decision analysis has provided numerous models for optimal practice behavior (Eisenberg 1985; Elstein et al. 1983). Many of these studies have been valuable educationally and as tools in analysis of cost-effectiveness and cost-benefit. Decision models are now an accepted component of the diagnostic system in psychiatry (i.e., DSM-III-R) (American Psychiatric Association 1987).

The talents of mental health providers, their behaviors, and the influences of their training are essential components of utilization that are difficult to describe or to quantify. Descriptive decision models could be useful in improving our knowledge of how psychiatry, psychology, social work, and nursing are practiced (Eisenberg 1985; 1986; Elstein et al. 1978). Different providers evaluate risks, benefits, and costs in different ways. It is essential that researchers begin to assess the cognitive processes of providers to better assess the inputs of practice (Elstein et al. 1983). The influences of patient sociodemographic characteristics on clinical decision making are poorly understood (Mitchell et al. 1986; Wells et al. 1986). Yet, it is clear that many well-qualified providers avoid elderly patients (Mitchell et al. 1983; 1986). Descriptive decision analysis could facilitate the development of programs to influence and/or undermine these barriers and thus increase access to neuropsychiatric care for the elderly.

Demonstration Projects

HCFA and private insurance companies must continue to encourage the development of unique practice models for the delivery of geriatric neuropsychiatric services. These microscopic endeavors should be designed as integrated service, research, and training projects. Assessment tools to evaluate the effects of collaboration, organizational structure, and the effectiveness of individual providers for specific functions are essential. Integration of prospective evaluation of benefit and cost will allow the design of larger, more generalizable service delivery systems. Demonstration projects must in every case be linked to well-designed peer-reviewed evaluation protocols, with incentives for the incorporation of economic measures (see also Chapter 10).

Conclusion

Neuropsychiatric disorders are prevalent in the older adult population. These illnesses and syndromes are complex and multifaceted. No individual provider has all of the skills, knowledge, or perseverance to address these problems holistically. The diverse universe of mental health providers is a vast resource that is, in large part, inaccessible to the elderly. Additionally, services delivered by individual providers often are narrow and inefficient responses to perceived needs. Empirically based segmentation of the market for geriatric neuropsychiatric services would allow more efficient utilization of existing resources while improving patient/client outcomes and provider satisfaction, thereby reducing substantial barriers to quality care. Research and demonstrations are needed to elucidate the unique assets of the mental health provider disciplines, and to develop models for efficient interdisciplinary collaboration.

References

Accreditation Council for Graduate Medical Education: Directory of Residency Training Programs 1988-1989. Chicago, IL, American Medical Association, 1988

Allen CM, Becker PN, McVey LJ, et al: A randomized controlled clinical trial of a geriatric consultation team: compliance with recommendations. JAMA 255:2617-2621, 1986

American Board of Family Practice and American Board of Internal Medicine: Certification for Advanced Training in Geriatrics. Journal of the American Geriatrics Society 35:700-701, 1987

American Board of Psychiatry and Neurology: Description of Written Examination. Evanston, IL, 1985

American Geriatrics Society: Guidelines for fellowship training programs in geriatric medicine. Journal of the American Geriatrics Society 35:769-795 1987

American Nurses' Association: Standards of Psychiatric and Mental Health Nursing Practice. Kansas City, MO, American Nurses' Association, 1982

American Psychiatric Association: Scientific Debate: Are We Training Too Many Psychiatrists? Presented at the American Psychiatric Association Annual Meeting, Washington DC, May 1986

American Psychiatric Association: Diagnostic and Statistical Manual of Mental Disorders, 3rd ed., rev. Washington, DC, American Psychiatric Association, 1987

American Psychological Association: Report on Accreditation: Accreditation Handbook. Washington, DC, American Psychological Association, 1983

Beigel A, Sharfstein SS: Mental health care providers: not the only cause or only care for rising costs. Am J Psychiatry 141:668-672, 1984

Beitman BD: The demographics of American psychotherapists: a pilot study. Am J Psychotherapy 37:37-48, 1983

Borson S, Liptzin B, Nininger J, et al: Psychiatry and the nursing home. Am J Psychiatry 144:1412-1418, 1987

Brett AS, McCollough LB: When patients request specific interventions: defining the limits of the physician's obligation. N Engl J Med 315:1347-1351, 1986

Brook RH, Lohr KN: Efficacy, effectiveness, variations and quality: boundary-crossing research. Medical Care 23:710-722, 1985

Carroll JG, Monroe J: Teaching medical interviewing: a critique of educational research and practice. J Med Educ 54:498-500, 1979

Christianson J: Capitation of mental health care in public programs, in Advances in Health Economics and Health Services Research, vol 8. Edited by Scheffler R, Rossiter L. Greenwich, CT, JAI Press, 1988

Coddington DC, Moore KD: Market Driven Strategies in Health Care. San Francisco, Jossey Bass, 1987, pp 47-50

Coordinated Care Management Corporation: Annual Report 1987. Buffalo, NY, Coordinated Care Management Corporation, 1988

Cope DW, Linn LS, Leake BD, et al: Modification of residents' behavior by preceptor feedback of patient satisfaction. J Gen Int Med 1:394-398, 1986

Council for the National Register of Health Service Providers in Psychology: National Register of Health Service Providers in Psychology. Washington, DC, Council for the National Register of Health Service Providers in Psychology, 1987

Craig TJ, Patterson DY: Productivity of Mental Health Professionals in a Prepaid Health Plan. Am J Psychiatry 138:498-501, 1981

Curran WJ, Shapiro ED: Law, Medicine and Forensic Science, 3rd ed. Boston MA, Little, Brown, 1982

Eddy DM: Variations in physician practice: the role of uncertainty. Health Affairs 3:74-89, 1984

Eisenberg JM: Physician utilization: the state of research about physicians' practice patterns. Med Care 23:461-483, 1985

Eisenberg JM: Doctors' Decisions and the Cost of Medical Care. Ann Arbor, MI, Health Administration Press, 1986

Elstein AS, Holmes MM, Ravitch MM, et al: Medical Decisions in Perspective: Applied Research in Cognitive Psychology. Perspectives in Biol and Med 26:486-501, 1983

Elstein AS, Shulman LS, Sprafka SA: Medical Problem Solving: An Analysis of Clinical Reasoning. Cambridge, MA, Harvard University Press, 1978

Feldstein M: The rising price of physicians' services. Review of Economics and Statistics 11:121-133, 1970

Fenton WS: The professional activities of psychiatrists, in The Nation's Psychiatrists. Edited by Koran L. Washington, DC, The American Psychiatric Association, 1987

Frank RG: Pricing and location of physicians' services in mental health. Economic Inquiry 24:115-133, 1985

Fuchs VR: The supply of surgeons and the demand for operations. J Human Resources 13(Suppl):35-56, 1978

Garg ML, Gliebe WA, Elhatib MB: The extent of defensive medicine: some empirical evidence. Legal Aspects of Medical Practice 6:25-29, 1978

German PS, Shapiro S, Skinner EA, et al: Detection and Management of Mental Health Problems of Older Patients by Primary Care Providers. JAMA 257:489-493, 1987

Gottlieb G: Financial issues affecting geriatric psychiatric care, in Essentials of Geriatric Psychiatry. Edited by Lazarus L, Jarvik L, Foster J, et al. New York, Springer, 1988

Gottlieb GL, Bloom BS: Specialty mental health service utilization by indigent older adults in Philadelphia 1984-1987. Unpublished report prepared for the Philadelphia Office of Mental Health, 1988

Guillette W: Third party payer views on mental health providers, in Cost Considerations in Mental Health Treatment: Settings, Modalities and Providers, Series EN No. 2. Edited by Taintor Z, Widem P, Barrett SA. DHHS Pub. No. (ADM) 84-1295. Washington, DC, U.S. Government Printing Office, 1984

Hamm RM, Clark JA, Bursztajn H: Psychiatrists' thorny judgments: describing and improving decision making process. Med Decis Making 4:425-447, 1984

Hoeper EW, Nycz GR, Cleary PD, et al: Estimated Prevalence of RDC Mental Disorders in Primary Medical Care. Int J Ment Health 8:6-15, 1979

Hoeper EW, Nycz GR, Kessler LG, et al: The usefulness of screening for mental illness. Lancet 1:33-35, 1984

Hornbrook MC, Berki SE: Practice mode and payment method: effects on use, costs, quality and access. Med Care 23:484-511, 1985

Horowitz MJ, Marmur CR, Weiss DS, et al: Comprehensive analysis of change after brief dynamic psychotherapy. Am J Psychiatry 143:582-589, 1986

Jampala VC, Sierles FS, Taylor MA: Consumer views of DSM-III: attitudes and practices of U.S. psychiatrists and 1984 graduating psychiatric residents. Am J Psychiatry 143:148-153, 1986

Karasu TB: Politics, practice and *p* value in psychotherapy, in Psychotherapy Research: Where are We and Where Should We Go? Edited by Williams JBW, Spitzer RL. New York, Guilford Press, 1984

Karasu TB: The specificity versus nonspecificity dilemma: toward identifying therapeutic change agents. Am J Psychiatry 143:687-695, 1986

Keller MB, Lavori PW, Klerman GL, et al: Low levels and lack of predictors of somatotherapy and psychotherapy received by depressed patients. Archives of General Psychiatry 43:458-466, 1986

Klerman GL, Weissman MM, Rounsaville BJ, et al: Interpersonal Psychotherapy of Depression. New York, Basic Books, 1984

Klerman GL: Trends in utilization of mental health services: prospectives for health services research. Med Care 23:584-597, 1985

Knesper DJ, Carlson BW: An analysis of the movement into private psychiatric practice. Arch Gen Psychiatry 38:943-949, 1981

Larson EB, Reifler BV, Sumi SM, et al: Diagnostic tests in the evaluation of dementia: a prospective study of 200 elderly outpatients. Arch Int Med 146:1917-1922, 1986

Lee S: Psychiatric social work, in Cost Considerations in Mental Health Treatment: Settings, Modalities and Providers (Series EN, No. 2). Edited by Taintor Z, Widem P, Barrett SA. DHHS Pub. No. (ADM) 84-1295. Washington, DC, U.S. Government Printing Office, 1984

Lewis RV: Nurse supply and reimbursement, in Cost Considerations in Mental Health Treatment: Settings, Modalities and Providers (Series EN, No. 2). Edited by Taintor Z, Widem P, Barrett SA. DHHS Pub. No. (ADM) 84-1295. Washington, DC, U.S. Government Printing Office, 1984

Linn LS, Heinrich RM, Lewis MA, et al: A behavioral medicine course for postgraduate trainees in internal medicine. J Med Educ 55:133-135, 1980

Luft HS: Health Maintenance Organizations: Dimensions of Performance. New York, John Wiley and Sons, 1981

Luft HS: Variations in clinical practice patterns. Arch Int Med 143:1861-1862, 1983

Manning WG, Leibowitz A, Goldberg GA, et al: A controlled trial of the effects of a prepaid group practice on use of services. N Engl J Med 310:1505-1510, 1984

Meier G: HMO Experiences with mental health services to the long-term emotionally disabled. Inquiry 18:125-138, 1981

Mezey MD, Lynaugh JE: The teaching nursing home program: outcomes of care. Nursing Clinics of North America 24:769-780, 1989

Mitchell JB, Cromwell J, Schurman R, et al: Psychiatric Office Practice Study, Final Report. Needham, MA, Health Economics Research, Inc., 1986

Mitchell JB, Schurman R: Practice Patterns and Earnings of Private Psychiatrists. Needham, MA, Health Economics Research, Inc., 1983

Moore JT, Silimperi DR, Bobula JA: Recognition of depression by family practice residents: the impact of screening. J Family Practice 7:509-513, 1978

Mumford E, Siblinger HJ: Economic discrimination against elderly psychiatric patients under Medicare. Hosp Comm Psychiatry 36:587-589, 1985

National Institute of Mental Health: Mental Health, United States 1987. DHHS Pub. No. (ADM) 87-1518. Washington, DC, U.S. Government Printing Office, 1987

Newhouse JP: A model of physician pricing. Southern Economic Journal 37:174-183, 1970

Orne MT: Psychotherapy: toward an appropriate basis for reimbursal, in Cost Considerations in Mental Health Treatment: Settings, Modalities and Providers (Series EN No. 2). Edited by Taintor Z, Widem P, Barrett SA. DHHS Pub. No. (ADM) 84-1295. Washington, DC, U.S. Government Printing Office, 1984

Richelson E: Schizophrenia: Treatment in Psychoses, Affective Disorders and Dementia. Edited by Carenar JO. New York, Basic Books, 1986

Rubinstein LZ, Josephson KR, Wieland GD, et al: Effectiveness of a Geriatric evaluation unit: a randomized clinical trial. N Engl J Med 311:1664-1670, 1984

Rush AJ, Beck AT, Kovacs M, et al: Comparative efficacy of cognitive therapy and pharmacotherapy in the treatment of depressed outpatients. Cog Ther Res 1:17-37, 1977

Schindler F, Berren M, Beigel A: A Study of the causes of conflict between psychiatrists and psychologists. Hosp Comm Psychiatry 32:263-266, 1981

Shapiro S, German PS, Skinner EA, et al: An experiment to change detection and management of mental morbidity in primary care. Medical Care 25:327-339, 1987

Sharfstein SS: Competition or catastrophe: insurance for psychiatric care. Compr Psychiatry 23:430-435, 1982a

Sharfstein SS: Medical cutbacks and block grants: crisis or opportunity for community mental health? Am J Psychiat 139:446-470, 1982b

Smith ML, Glass GV, Miller TI: The Benefits of Psychotherapy. Baltimore, Johns Hopkins University Press, 1980

Taintor Z: Cost considerations about mental health service providers, in Cost Considerations in Mental Health Treatment: Settings, Modalities and Providers (Series EN No. 2). Edited by Taintor Z, Widem P, Barrett SA. DHHS Pub. No. (ADM) 84-1295. Washington, DC, U.S. Government Printing Office, 1984

Vanden Bos GR, Stapp J, Kilburg RR: Health service providers in psychology. American Psychologist 36:1395-1418, 1981

Von Korff M, Shapiro S, Burke JD, et al: Anxiety and depression in a primary care clinic. Arch Gen Psychiatry 44:152-156, 1987

Waldfogel D, Rosenblatt A: Handbook of clinical social work. San Francisco, Jossey-Bass, 1983

Waxman HM, Carner EA: Physicians' recognition, diagnosis and treatment of mental disorders in elderly medical patients. Gerontologist 24:593-597, 1984

Waxman HM, Carner EA, Klein M: Underutilization of mental health professionals by community elderly. Gerontologist 24:23-30, 1984

Wells KB, Manning WG, Benjamin B: Use of outpatient mental health services in HMO and fee for service plans: results from a randomized controlled trial. Health Services Research 21:452-474, 1986

Wells KB, Manning WG, Duan N, et al: Sociodemographic factors and the use of outpatient mental health services. Med Care 24:75-85, 1986

Wennberg JE, Barnes BA, Zubkoff M: Professional uncertainty and the problem of supplier induced demand. Soc Sci Med 16:811-824, 1982

Wennberg JW: On patient need, supplier induced demand, and the need to assess outcome of common medical practices. Med Care 23:512-520, 1984

Widiger TA, Hurt SW, Frances A, et al: Diagnostic efficiency and DSM-III. Arch Gen Psychiatry 41:1005-1012, 1984

Wilkinson G: Overview of Mental Health Practices in Primary Care Settings, with Recommendations for Future Research. NIMH Series DN No. 7. DHHS Pub No. (ADM) 86-1467. Washington, DC, U.S. Government Printing Office, 1986

Zung WWK, Magill M, Moore JT, et al: Recognition and treatment of depression in a family medicine practice. Journal of Clinical Psychiatry 44:3-6, 1983

10

The Psychiatric Component of Long-Term Care Models

Gail K. Robinson, Ph.D.

In recent years, there has been extraordinary interest in developing alternative models of long-term care as a partial solution to the pressing problems of a fragmented service system and skyrocketing costs of care. Four such models developed in the field of aging to manage care and contain costs are reviewed here. Inferences are drawn concerning the relevance of these models for the comprehensive management of mental illness. A need to incorporate a greater concern for mental status into refinements of these models is identified.

Concern for Long-Term Care

In the field of aging, thinking about long-term care has emphasized a systems approach combining managed care and cost control. In the mental health field, long-term care of the chronically mentally ill has developed as a more individually focused case management approach. The contrasting approaches have responded to differences in the populations served and in the external pressures on the system of care. (These concepts are elaborated in Chapters 12 through 14.)

Before the late 1970s, long-term care meant almost exclusively nursing home care. The National Nursing Home Survey (NNHS) in 1977 found a 21% increase in nursing home residents over the preceding three years, and an increase of 225,100 beds—from 1,177,300 in 1974 to 1,402,400 in 1977. The NNHS also found that the proportion of elderly using nursing home services grew from 2.3% of all elderly in 1960 to 5% in 1977. This is an undercount because the NNHS was a one-day (point prevalence) sample; other experts estimate that closer to 20 to 25% of the elderly population use nursing home care *at some time* (Dunlop 1976).

Policy makers were concerned about this dramatic growth in nursing home utilization. The cost concerns focused on Medicaid, which since its passage in 1965 had become the major payer for nursing home care. In 1979, the General Accounting Office (GAO) was asked by Congress to analyze the impact of Medicaid policies and other factors on the placement of chronically impaired elderly in nursing homes. The statistics on expenditures were staggering. In 1969, only 13% of nursing home residents used Medicaid funds as the primary source of payment, but by 1977, 48% of nursing home residents relied on Medicaid. In 1976, 60% of all nursing home days were paid by Medicaid either totally or in part. In 1978, a total of $7.8 billion or 46% of all Medicaid dollars were spent on nursing home care. In 1978, 37 states (74%) spent 40% or more of their total Medicaid expenditures (federal and state) on nursing home care; in 19 states half or more went for nursing home care (GAO 1979).

The GAO findings were quite critical of Medicaid's long-term care policies. Specifically, the report found that Medicaid's eligibility policies contained financial incentives to use nursing homes instead of community services, that elderly persons and their families were discouraged from using community services, and that assessment procedures for determining needs of the elderly for nursing home care were inadequate.

The GAO recommended establishment of a preadmission screening program that would provide comprehensive needs assessments for all applicants to nursing homes, assistance in planning and obtaining services in the community, coordination and monitoring of community care, payment for community services, and control over costs and utilization. Because the cost of such a proposal was unknown, the GAO suggested that Congress fund "a community-wide long-term demonstration project in several areas to obtain more concrete information on costs, people who could be served, service utilization, and system-wide effects" (GAO 1979).

Responding to the GAO report and other criticisms of long-term care, the Federal government initiated a number of long-term care demonstration projects using Medicare and Medicaid waivers. These demonstrations were aimed at reducing the need for institutionalization and controlling the escalating costs of long-term care.

The Mental Health Concern

Experts in the mental health field also became concerned with the predominant role nursing homes played in the provision of long-term care. They were concerned with two questions. First, were nursing home residents receiving adequate and appropriate mental health services? Second, were individuals with histories of psychiatric hospitalizations inappropriately placed in nursing homes?

Evidence to date suggests that psychiatric problems continue to be frequently undiagnosed or misdiagnosed for residents in nursing homes. The case for widespread under*treatment* is made on an epidemiologic basis in Chapter 4. A superb review of clinical literature by Borson et al. (1987) emphasizes the additional problem that *diagnoses* of mental disorders are frequently overlooked and that mental health concerns are infrequently incorporated into treatment planning. "The majority of diagnostic errors made by admitting physicians involved failure to identify a disabling psychiatric or neurologic disease or to address a potentially treatable behavioral disturbance" (Borson et al. 1987). The situation has improved only slightly since 1976, when a field study suggested that *fewer than 1%* of the patients with a diagnosed mental disorder received explicit mental health intervention (Glasscote et al. 1976).

This issue of mental health treatment in nursing homes was recognized by the National Institute of Mental Health (NIMH) as early as 1975 with the amendments to the Community Mental Health Centers Act (P.L. 94-63). More specifically, P.L. 94-63 stipulated twelve services where only five were required under the original legislation. These additional services were targeted to vulnerable populations, including the elderly. Under this requirement, many community mental health centers (CMHCs) developed linkages with senior centers and nursing homes. However, as direct Federal CMHC funding diminished and CMHCs became increasingly dependent on state and Medicaid monies for support, many of these programs gave way to new requirements and priority areas. Medicaid, for instance, would not reimburse CMHCs for services provided to nursing home residents on site, but only for services provided in the clinic.

Low reimbursement rates and unreasonable regulatory requirements were no more favorable for private psychiatrists working with nursing home residents. Under Medicare, the time and expense of travel to and from the nursing home is not covered in the consultation rate charged by the psychiatrist. Furthermore, unless the nursing home resident maintains Medicare Part B coverage for nonhospital care, private psychiatric consultation is not covered at all.

Therefore, the answer to the question of whether nursing home residents are receiving adequate and appropriate mental health services is, with few exceptions, no. For those in the mental health field, particularly geriatric psychiatrists, there is deep concern for nursing home residents in need of mental health services. Residents' primary problems usually are physical, but they often need psychiatric care in addition to medical and personal care services.

Concern about unnecessary utilization of nursing homes by individuals with severe or chronic mental illness was a direct consequence of a larger policy change taking place in the mental health field. Deinstitutionalization—shifting the primary locus of mental health care from the state mental hospital to a decentralized, community-based system of services—was the stated policy direction of the sixties and seventies. But experts soon observed that state hospital reductions often were being realized by discharging thousands of state mental hospital patients to nursing homes.

In Texas, the state hospital inpatient population was reduced from 15,035 in 1968 to 5,260 in 1978. More than 5,000 patients were discharged to nursing homes between 1971 and 1977 (Dittmar and Franklin 1980). The 1974 National Nursing Home Survey revealed that 22% of skilled nursing home patients 65 and under were diagnosed as mentally ill or mentally retarded. The 1977 National Nursing Home Survey found an estimated 670,000 individuals with mental illness. About 54% of these had a primary or secondary diagnosis of senility and another 5% had a physical disorder as well as a mental disorder (Goldman et al. 1986). Thus, an estimated 274,700 nursing home residents had a primary mental disorder other than dementia.

The 1977 GAO report on deinstitutionalization reported that nursing homes were the largest single place of care for individuals with mental illness. A NIMH study estimated that in 1974, 29.3% or $4.2 billion of the estimated total direct care costs of $14.5 billion for individuals with mental illness was spent for nursing home care (GAO 1977).

One major goal of mental health authorities was to remove people from the traditional place for long-term care (state hospitals) and provide an alternative "in the community." Some experts argued that since nursing homes played an important role in community care of individuals with mental illness, policy should be developed to help nursing homes play a more comprehensive and constructive role (Shadish and Bootzin 1981). However, most experts were critical of the use of nursing homes as community alternatives (Bassuk and Gerson 1978; Carling 1981). At the same time, criticisms of the ability and willingness of Community Mental Health Centers to serve individuals with chronic mental illness were mounting (Bassuk and Gerson 1978).

In 1977 NIMH established the Community Support Program (CSP), based on the idea that only by organizing a comprehensive system of care could a community ensure availability of the wide array of human services required by individuals with severe mental illness. The CSP concept is generally considered to be a desirable long-term care model for individuals with severe mental illness. There are 10 service components:

1. *Client identification and outreach*—including crisis stabilization, assistance in meeting basic needs, and transportation as needed.
2. *Mental health treatment and clinical services*—diagnostic evaluation, supportive counseling and psychotherapeutic intervention, medication management services, and services that address both mental illness and substance abuse as appropriate to the individual's needs.
3. *Crisis response services*—24-hour availability of hotline services, walk-in triage services, mobile outreach for in-home crises, crisis residential beds, and crisis respite services.
4. *Health and dental care*
5. *Housing*—with particular emphasis on permanent housing in as "normal," integrated, and unrestrictive a setting as possible, as well as a range of transitional and more structured/supervised settings for individuals with special needs.
6. *Peer support*—consumer-run services and self-help programs, including peer support groups, drop-in centers and social clubs, independent living programs, housing, businesses, crisis and respite services, and community education programs.
7. *Family and community support*—including education as well as support to families and community members who are in contact with individuals with serious mental illness.
8. *Rehabilitation services*—social rehabilitation services which enhance abilities to live and socialize in the community and vocational rehabilitation services and employment opportunities which enable people to be productive, with emphasis on approaches which are based in natural settings.
9. *Protection and advocacy*—including grievance mechanisms and other procedures in line with the Mental Health Patient Bill of Rights.
10. *Case management services*—with emphasis on case management that is "client directed and client empowering" (Parrish 1987).

Case management became a key component for alternative care models geared to individuals with severe and persistent mental illness, in many ways a replacement for the role hospitals played in the oversight of all aspects of a client's life. Case management was intended to facilitate clients' effective use of formal and informal helping systems by designating a single person or team responsible for helping the client make informed choices about opportunities and services, assuring timely access to medical care and concrete assistance, and coordinating all services to meet the client's goals. Case management emerged as the centralizing force in a decentralized, fragmented, and sometimes redundant community-based system (Robinson and Toff Bergman 1989).

The initiation of CSP represented a clear departure from the aging field's concept of long-term care. In the field of aging, long-term care was defined as facility-based (e.g., nursing homes). By contrast, in the mental health field, long-term care was defined as community-based. The main issue for the aging field was cost containment, whereas the predominant issue for the mental health field was access to and coordination of care. Alternative long-term care models developed by the two fields reflect this difference in emphasis.

Defining Long-Term Care Models

Two general models of long-term care in the community have emerged in the field of aging. As in projects for persons with chronic mental illness, these models see case management as the cornerstone of any community model for long-term care. The *brokerage model* reduces fragmentation by placing a coordinating agent between the client and the various services. The *consolidated model* reduces fragmentation by replacing existing services with a single service delivery agency.

In the brokerage model, the case managing agency assesses the need for care, develops a comprehensive care plan, refers the client for services specified in this plan, and monitors ongoing client status and the need for readjustment of the care plan. The brokerage agency may or may not control payment for services; however, it almost never provides services directly. This model leaves the ongoing service system intact and only adds services where there are gaps. The brokerage model, however, is not completely neutral. The case manager is able, through directing or purchasing services for a client, to alter the market behavior of providers and to shape the character of systems for the delivery of long-term care (Austin 1983).

The key feature in the consolidated model is its integration of all aspects of the health care system—delivery, population, financing, and risk. "The provider entity consolidates all primary, acute and long-term care and support services through one provider agency, which manages the care of each patient across the entire system" (Alpha Center 1984). Cost-containment incentives are built directly into the model. The provider entity receives prospective payment, and funds from different sources are pooled, eliminating incentives for increasing utilization that characterize the cost-based reimbursement systems. Because the provider entity is financially at risk for service costs, there is an incentive to find creative ways to prevent institutionalization of its clients.

Long-Term Care Alternatives

Four community long-term care alternatives have evolved out of these two models: the Channeling Demonstration, Social/Health Maintenance Organizations, On Lok, and Life Care Communities. With the exception of the Channeling Demonstration, these alternatives were not tested by research studies with a randomized controlled design. For this reason, their results are affected by selection biases. Nevertheless, examination of how these alternatives met their clients' mental health needs and how successfully they controlled costs should be useful in developing ideas for managing the care and controlling the cost of care for elderly individuals with mental illness.

The Channeling Demonstration

The National Long-Term Care Demonstration—more commonly known as the Channeling Demonstration—was designed to serve severely impaired elderly at risk of being institutionalized, and to test the effectiveness of two types of case management. Substitution of formal and informal community-based services for nursing home care was intended to reduce costs and improve the quality of life of clients and informal caregivers. The Channeling Demonstration represents the brokerage model.

In September 1980, the Department of Health and Human Services (HHS) awarded contracts to 12 states.[1] The states in turn solicited formal proposals from agencies and programs within the state to provide case management services. Specific sites were selected in January 1981. Each of two types of case management was tested at half of the sites. The first, *basic case management,* tested the premise that access (and not financing) was the major barrier in obtaining appropriate long-term care services. Basic case management sites had an overall fixed budget with project funds paying only for the case management service itself. The second, *financial control case management,* tested the premise that inadequate public financing of community services was the cause of inappropriate use of nursing homes. Additional funding in a lump sum was available to these sites for both case management and services. The sites were fully operational by June 1982 and the demonstration was completed in March 1985.

Client eligibility was predicated upon Medicaid eligibility for nursing home admission. Clients had to have at least moderate disabilities in two or more physical activities of daily living (ADL), three severe impairments in instrumental activities of daily living (IADL), or two severe IADL impairments plus one severe ADL impairment. Cognitive or behavioral impairments affecting activities of daily living were considered a severe IADL impairment. The minimum age for participation was 65. There was no income criterion, but higher income clients were expected to contribute to the cost of care. Finally, clients had to reside in the community or, if institutionalized, be certified as likely to be discharged within three months (Applebaum 1988).

Since cognitive and behavioral impairments were considered one of the criteria for participation in the demonstration, non-psychiatric "screeners" asked questions on the mental status of prospective clients. The screeners would talk to providers or family members of the applicant by phone. They asked: 1) Does the applicant exhibit disorientation or inappropriate behavior at times? and 2) If so, then does the behavior affect the applicant's activities of daily living or is daily supervision necessary to ensure personal safety?

Answers in the affirmative demonstrated need for care, and these applicants were eligible for services. Applicants typically were referred to this program from existing agencies serving the elderly including hospitals, area agencies on aging, senior centers, public social service programs, and home health and homemaker programs. Referrals from mental health agencies and state mental hospitals were not generally requested. Consequently, elderly with chronic mental illness may have been underrepresented.

Once the applicant was accepted, the case manager administered the Short Portable Mental Status Questionnaire (SPMSQ) to him/her (Omer et al. 1983). This ten-item questionnaire was specifically designed to be used by nonprofessionals, such as the case managers. The questionnaire asked clients such questions as their age, day of the week, and name of the U.S. president. The baseline assessment indicated that 32% of the clients were classified as having severe mental impairments (missing more than five questions), and on average clients missed between three and four of the ten items (Mathematica Policy Research 1986).

Channeling clients, whose mean age was 80 years, experienced severe functional, health, social, and financial problems.[2] Channeling clients were more likely than the general population to need post-acute care, to receive formal care from the community care system, and to live alone.

To achieve the objective of managing service use, the following five core functions were included:

1. Needs assessment to determine individual problems, resources, and service needs;
2. Care planning to specify the types and amounts of care to be provided;
3. Service arrangement to implement the plan;
4. Monitoring of the services; and
5. Reassessment to adjust care plans to changing needs (Phillips et al. 1988).

Both models used a brokerage approach to arrange for services.[3]

The channeling demonstration was financed through Medicare and Medicaid waivers, and allowed projects to use Medicaid, Medicare, and other public program funds irrespective of a client's categorical eligibility. Clients did, however, have to be covered by Medicare Part A to be eligible for channeling in the financial control sites. Cost control at the financial control sites was implemented by placing a limit on average service expenditures (averaged across all clients), and on individual service expenditures, and by cost sharing by clients.[4]

Evaluation. Compared to a simulated national population, channeling clients were very frail, but not at differentially high risk of institutionalization. They did have a high use of hospitals and other medical services.

Clients were often referred to the channeling demonstration following an acute care episode. "Over 70% reported experiencing the onset or worsening of a serious health condition in the year prior to channeling, and almost half had been hospitalized in the two months before application to channeling" (Kemper 1988). Despite their frailty, only a very small percentage (13%–14%) of the control group members were in nursing homes after one year.

The evaluation found that the average cost increase from expanding case management and formal community services *was not offset* by reductions in nursing home care. Under the basic model total costs increased by 6% and under the financial model costs increased by 18% (Kemper 1988). *Clients' costs,* however, were reduced by 7%. While it did not save money, channeling improved the quality of life of its clients and caregivers—it increased services, reduced unmet needs, increased satisfaction with care and service arrangements, and improved satisfaction with life in general.

Social/Health Maintenance Organization

A second example of long-term care alternatives is the social/health maintenance organization (S/HMO). A S/HMO is a managed system of health and long-term care. A single provider assumes responsibility for a full range of health and support services for a prospectively determined fixed premium. Elderly persons (healthy and frail) who reside in the service area are enrolled voluntarily through the marketing effort of the S/HMO provider. As with a health maintenance organization (HMO), enrollees must receive all covered services through the S/HMO providers. The S/HMO typifies the consolidated model of managed care.

The S/HMO concept was developed by Brandeis University under a three year grant from the Health Care Finance Administration (HCFA). With support from private foundations and HCFA approval of Medicare waivers, four demonstration sites began operation in early 1985.[5] All four are in urban areas with large elderly populations. The sites had experience in delivering comprehensive, high quality services to a significant share of the local elderly population and were interested in expanding services to this target group. By December 1986, a total of 10,626 elderly were enrolled at the four sites. Kaiser had the most enrollees with 4,305, while the other sites enrolled between 2,000 to 2,500 participants.

S/HMO eligibility requirements are the same as those for Medicare. Data obtained so far have shown S/HMO membership to be generally representative of the overall community, including both disabled and able-bodied individuals. There were a few differences. Compared to the overall Medicare population, S/HMO enrollees were slightly more likely to be "old old" (over age 80). Thirty-five percent lived alone, as compared to 30% of the Medicare population. The data showed that 14.5% of S/HMO clients required "assistance getting places" as compared to 8.9% for Medicare beneficiaries in general. Ability to perform other basic activities of daily living (ADLs) was not otherwise different.

Applicants are required to fill out a written form describing their health status and functional impairment. Functional impairment includes *physical* mobility and activities of daily living. No specific information is obtained on mental status. If an applicant has a functional impairment then he/she is placed on a waiting list to ensure that there is a sufficient mix of healthy and impaired members in the S/HMO. Since cognitive or behavioral problems are not part of this standard screen, it is possible that applicants with mental problems but without physical impairment would not necessarily be placed on the waiting list, but would be accepted immediately. It is not clear whether sites have the option of placing mentally ill applicants in a special queue.

Once the application is received, a case manager will call the applicant or family member and administer a health status questionnaire. Initially, the health status questionnaire did not request information on mental status, but this past year one question has been included. Applicants are asked if, during the past year, they have received psychiatric treatment or have had an emotional or psychiatric problem. Not until the applicant becomes a member and is accepted for the long-term care benefit are more comprehensive assessments made.

The case manager, who usually has social work training, makes a home visit to administer the more comprehensive assessment. The assessment includes the use of the Kahn Mental Status Questionnaire (MSQ) (Montgomery and Costa 1983). S/HMO case managers use the MSQ as a trigger mechanism to alert them to a cognitive or behavioral problem, but not to measure the level of cognitive impairment. The MSQ detects dementia of moderate to severe degree, but does not detect mild or limited cognitive problems (Nelson et al. 1986) and does not explicitly evaluate mood. A severely depressed person, for example, can have a normal MSQ score. In addition to administering this instrument, the case managers assess how much supervision the member will require. The case manager in the S/HMO demonstration sites performs a pivotal function in identifying, referring, and qualifying members for expanded care benefits including hospitalization.

If a member requires specific mental health treatment, the case manager will refer the member to psychiatric outpatient services. S/HMO enrollees are offered a full range of acute medical and ancillary services similar to high option Health Maintenance Organizations (e.g., dentures, prescription drugs, optometry, audiometry, eyeglasses, hearing aids). In addition, a full range of long-term care services is provided to frail enrollees, such as homemaker, personal care aide, respite, adult day health care, and transportation. Nursing home services are provided without Medicare's requirements for prior hospitalization or needed skill level.

The S/HMO is financed on a prepaid capitated basis through premium contributions from Medicare, Medicaid, and individual and group subscribers.[6]

Evaluation. Analysis of hospital use indicated that two of the sites (Elderplan and Scan) were at or very close to their capitation estimates, and two (Kaiser Permanente and Senior Plus) were substantially below their estimates. Although there is no hard evidence, the evaluators believe that lower hospitalization was due to more effective use of case management (Greenberg et al. 1988).

Regarding mental health treatment, the S/HMOs have found that their biggest problem is finding psychiatrists who will treat geriatric patients. This was a problem even at the Kaiser and Minneapolis S/HMOs which have staff psychiatrists. A member requiring any service which is not available at the site is referred out. Overall, the members used few formal mental health services.

S/HMOs have two additional shortcomings with regard to the mental health needs of members. First, in-home services are primarily personal care services and do not include assistance with behavioral management. Thus, if a member requires behavioral management services, there seems to be little option other than to place the member in a nursing facility. Second, there is no systematic collection of information on mental health status apart from the initial screening for dementia. The opportunity for a comprehensive plan to identify particular disorders such as depression, and to treat them early, is not exploited by the existing S/HMO models. Since program designers have found that mental status is critical in predicting nursing home placement, they now plan to collect more information on mental status, if funding is obtained to do so (Greenberg et al. 1988).

On Lok Senior Services Program

A third example of long-term care alternatives is the On Lok Senior Services Program. On Lok Senior Health Services in San Francisco provides medical and support services to about 300 frail elderly, who otherwise would be in a nursing home. Like the S/HMO, On Lok is a consolidated model. Responsibility for assessment and service delivery rests with one organization. All service components available are provided either by staff (primary care doctors) or through contracts (e.g., an all-inclusive daily rate at an acute care hospital).

On Lok grew out of community concern for frail elderly in San Francisco's Chinatown, North Beach, and Polk Gulch neighborhoods in 1971. A day health center was introduced in 1973. Now On Lok operates three adult day health centers, a 54-unit housing facility for low-income elderly, and a multidisciplinary team of physicians, nurse practitioners, social workers, therapists, nutritionists, paraprofessionals, and other support staff. In 1983, On Lok received Medicare and Medicaid waivers for assuming full financial risk for the provision of all services to a high-cost, high-risk elderly population. In 1986, Congress approved continuing the Medicare and Medicaid waivers as long as the program's quality and cost effectiveness are maintained. Moreover, the On Lok comprehensive service model has been replicated in four sites in other parts of the country through support from the Robert Wood Johnson and John A. Hartford Foundations.

On Lok's services are targeted to elderly individuals at risk of institutionalization with each state defining the criteria. In New York State, for example, On Lok participants must meet Medicaid eligibility standards for institutional care, as well as New York State's standards for its Long-Term Care Home Health Program.[7]

On Lok's clients in San Francisco have an average age of 81 years. Their average monthly income is $525 (1986). Three-fourths are of Chinese origin. Most live in their own homes, and 64% live alone. Clients average 5.4 serious medical diagnoses. (Three-fourths are incontinent and three-fourths have extremity impairments.)

The key component in the On Lok Program is its multidisciplinary team. The team in San Francisco is composed of 25 professionals and paraprofessionals with extensive knowledge of each participant's condition. Client assessment, treatment planning, delivery of services, and monitoring of care is done by the team as a whole. There are 11 service components: Intake and Assessment, Day Health Centers, In-Home Services, Housing, Appliances (restorative/supportive), Laboratory, X-ray, Ambulance Service, Medical Specialty Services, Skilled Nursing Care, and Acute Hospital Care. Housing is provided through Department of Housing and Urban Development (HUD) Section 202 grants; On Lok operates one congregate housing setting.

Mental health services are provided in the On Lok projects. At the New York site, a geriatric psychiatrist soon will begin to provide mental health services once a week on site. For more serious mental health conditions requiring inpatient hospitalization, services are referred out.

The On Lok Program is based on a capitation financing model. Revenue from all sources goes into one pool and becomes undifferentiated funds. A capitation rate—a monthly rate negotiated annually—is payment in full for all services. Each of the revenue sources is apportioned its contribution to the capitation rate.[8]

On Lok has been unsuccessful in getting private insurance companies to contribute to the program's cost. The overall cost per person per month is $1,300.[9]

Evaluation. A study comparing the service utilization patterns of 70 On Lok enrollees with 70 similarly impaired persons in the community (1979–1983) indicated that On Lok patients used one-third as many hospital days and one-fifth as many nursing home days as the comparison group. The Beth Abraham Hospital (New York) On Lok program found that when comparing their participants to a control group, the estimated total expenditure per patient per month was 17% less than the control group's.

Mental health utilization by On Lok participants has not been systematically studied, but On Lok's difficulty in finding psychiatrists willing to provide mental health services to the elderly, and in persuading clients to use mental health services, has been similar to the S/HMO experience.

Life Care Communities

The final LTC model to be discussed combines the brokerage and consolidated approaches. Life care communities (continuing care retirement communities [CCRC] and life care at home [LCAH]) are housing-based programs that provide residents with health and social services along with other amenities to meet their continuing care needs late in life. They combine elements of the brokerage and consolidated models, providing some services directly and referring residents for others. While these models have not been systematically evaluated, they are described here because of their increasing popularity among middle- and upper middle-class elderly persons.

The basis of the CCRC operation is a lifetime contract between the CCRC and the resident, stipulating each party's obligations. Currently there are more than 600 CCRCs in the United States, most of which are fiscally sound. CCRCs are relatively expensive, with the entrance fee for a residential unit ranging from $50,000 to $100,000 and a monthly service fee of $400 to $1,500. The typical contract stipulates that upon the death of the resident the CCRC operator will retain the entrance fee, regardless of the value of services received prior to the resident's death (Pies 1984).

A study of CCRCs conducted in 1984 found that most residents are among the "old old" of the elderly population. More than half of the CCRCs surveyed have an average resident age of 80 to 82 years or higher. The more-established CCRCs have a larger share of this cohort. Longer-established CCRCs also tend to have sicker and more disabled residents.[10]

Life Care at Home differs from a CCRC in that the member lives at home rather than moving to a central "campus." LCAH insures enrollees against the catastrophic costs of long-term care and provides a case-managed delivery system to ensure access to needed services. The LCAH is still in the marketing phase and has no operational experience. Marketing and enrollment for the first site began in the fall of 1987 (Tell et al. 1987).

The target population for LCAH is expected to be more representative of the general population than CCRCs. Entrance fees will (when implemented) range from $5,000 to $10,000 and monthly fees from $130 to $200 depending on age at entry, marital status, and benefit package. The designers expect that the majority of entrants will be under 75, with nearly half between 65 and 69. This plan is aimed at 1% of the elderly population with a target enrollment per plan of 1,000 members. All new members must be healthy to join the plan, but can continue membership if they become ill (Tell et al. 1987).

Directly provided services usually include: nursing home care not otherwise covered by Medicare, personal care, home health and homemaker services, home-delivered meals, respite care, social/medical day care, social/recreational activities, medical transportation, and an in-home electronic monitoring/call system. Brokerage services that may or may not be covered include nursing home care (if not directly provided) and medical acute care.

The entrance and monthly fees for both types of Life Care Communities usually cover only long-term care services and not the kind of acute care covered by Medicare and Medigap policies. Applicants may be excluded from joining such communities if they have preexisting conditions. LCAH plans do cover nursing home care, while many CCRCs *do not* guarantee nursing home care for "as long as necessary." There may be an extra charge in CCRCs for the nursing home care itself and charges may increase at any time. LCAH limits the total annual benefit for community-based long-term care services to exceed what it would cost to care for the member in a nursing home. This plan also assumes some cost sharing for both institutional and community-based services as an additional cost control mechanism.

Both the CCRC and the LCAH concepts offer structures in which systematic and periodic screening of clients for treatable mental health problems and neuropsychiatric disorders could be incorporated. If CCRC and LCAH programs are at risk for the costs of managing the adverse functional consequences of untreated mental disorders, they may have an incentive to intervene. On the other hand, if lifecare programs do not assume risk for nursing home placement, they may have perverse incentives to undertreat mental disorders. In the worst case, community members with excess functional disability due to neuropsychiatric disorders would be dumped into nursing homes for which they, their families, or unrelated third parties would be at risk. The lifecare community would thereby save the costs of providing supportive services to keep those patients in the community.

To date, there have been no systematic studies of mental disorders or their treatment among residents of CCRCs or LCAH projects. Research to develop an empirical data base for policy in this area would be of great value.

Policy Considerations

In assessing these approaches to long-term care, policy makers in the mental health field must ask to what extent they meet mental health needs of their current participants, and what the models might have to offer the chronically mentally ill elderly. To answer these questions, the models must be viewed in terms of clients, services, and financial incentives.

The treatment of mental illness is not a priority in any of the long-term care models. Moreover, referral sources (senior centers, hospitals, area agencies on aging) typically underrepresent or screen out individuals with diagnosed mental illnesses. Program evaluations have reported relatively little information on mental status even though most recognized that cognitive impairment is a strong predictor of nursing home placement.

Mental health services available to those participating in the models were those traditionally covered by Medicare. By definition, then, these were acute care services. Obtaining the covered acute services proved difficult for *nonfinancial reasons.* Some of the projects had a great deal of trouble finding psychiatrists and psychologists who would treat geriatric patients; other projects found the elderly's resistance to psychiatric care as a barrier to treatment.

For elderly with chronic mental health conditions, appropriate services were almost unavailable. Long-term care services designed to prevent institutionalization were essentially personal care services provided at the clinic or in the home. Case management and psychosocial services associated with the treatment of chronic mental conditions did not appear in any of the models' service descriptions.

Cost-Containment Mechanisms and Their Service Implications

The models included a variety of financial mechanisms to contain costs. In the Channeling Demonstrations, reimbursement was based on an average service unit cost. For example, the average cost of delivering case management is $35 per visit based on an average time of one hour. If the case manager spends less than the time allotted, the program keeps the difference. If the case management visit costs more, the program has to make up the difference. There is an incentive to keep at or below the average on every client. Clients with behavioral problems are therefore less likely to get the full amount of time they may need.

S/HMOs and On Lok operate under a capitation payment system. The cost of all services is averaged over the participants for the year, and a single annual per person amount is assessed regardless of services actually used. Capitation provides the agency with the greatest flexibility to provide services needed, but a financial incentive to underserve is built in. While On Lok and its replications are primarily publicly funded, the S/HMO has an additional financial pressure to control costs since it must sell policies to healthy elderly people. Its premiums must be low enough to be competitive with other health care policies. Adding a number of mental health services may make the plan too costly to be marketable, unless the services lead to offsetting cost reductions or offer something seen as particularly desirable by potential clients (e.g., memory enhancement services or assistance with insomnia).

The two Life Care Community models are financed under a *fixed fee payment system*. A fairly substantial entrance fee is required in advance and then a large monthly fee (in addition to Medicare and Medigap premiums) must be paid. This model is unlikely to attract individuals with severe mental illness because of their high cost and the *preexisting conditions* exclusion in most contracts. Like S/HMO, Life Care Communities must compete in the private market where they must be competitive with other service vendors. Adding mental health services may be seen as too expensive.

In conclusion, the LTC models currently operating may meet some of the acute care mental health needs of the elderly, but do not fully exploit the potential of their comprehensive structure for case finding and early interventions. They also fall short on longer-term mental health care needs. Psychosocial services and case management that take mental and behavioral problems into account must be included at a minimum if the LTC models are to meet those needs.

Application to the Chronically Mentally Ill

The models do shed some light on alternative ways of managing long-term care for elderly persons with chronic mental illness. Models primarily financed by the public sector may be a more feasible strategy for a patient whose long-term care needs are for mental health services, because these models are less dependent on market forces. For example, a model like On Lok might be adapted to the mental health field. On Lok's population is high risk and requires a variety of acute and supportive services. Clients live on their own as well as in specialized housing. The use of a capitated payment system, where public funds are pooled, provides flexibility for needed individualized treatment plans, while the public sector's accountability to the community reduces the risk of underutilization.

In those demonstrations using a consolidated model, the rate of hospitalization decreased with the use of case management. To improve access to mental health care for the elderly, while simultaneously keeping costs under control, various forms of case management combined with a consolidated model would seem to offer hope, as reductions in hospital care might offset the costs of more comprehensive community-based services and of case management itself.

Research Recommendations

In the future, mental health measures and mental health services utilization measures should be incorporated in all studies of long-term care systems for the elderly. When possible, data from existing demonstrations should be reanalyzed to look at the relationship between the care structure and acute mental health services utilization. Research on mental health and services utilization in managed care models offers one of the best opportunities for establishing cost-offset effects, and for identifying opportunities for prevention of excess disability due to neuropsychiatric disorders.

References

Alpha Center: Social/Health Maintenance Organizations. Alpha Center-piece: A Report on Health Policy Issues, May 1984, pp 3-4

Applebaum R: Recruitment and characteristics of channeling clients. Health Services Research 23:51-66, 1988

Austin C: Case management in long-term care: options and opportunities. Health and Social Work 8:16-30, 1983

Bassuk E, Gerson S: Deinstitutionalization and Mental Health Services. Scientific American 238:46-53, 1978

Borson S, Liptzin B, Nininger J, et al: Psychiatry and the nursing home. American Journal of Psychiatry 144:1412-1418, 1987

Carcagno G, Kemper P: An overview of the channeling demonstration and its evaluation. Health Services Research 23:1-22, 1988

Carling P: Nursing homes and chronic mental patients: a second opinion. Schizophrenia Bulletin 7:574-579, 1981

Dittmar N, Franklin J: State hospital patients discharged to nursing homes: are hospitals dumping their more difficult patients? Hospital and Community Psychiatry 31:251-254, 1980

Dunlop B: Determinants of Long-Term Care Facility Utilization by the Elderly: An Empirical Analysis. Washington DC, Urban Institute, 1976

General Accounting Office: Returning the Mentally Disabled to the Community: Government Needs to Do More. Washington DC, General Accounting Office, January 1977

General Accounting Office: Entering A Nursing Home—Costly Implications For Medicaid and the Elderly. Washington DC, General Accounting Office, November 1979

Glasscote RM, Beigel A, Butterfield A, et al: Old Folks at Homes: A Field Study of Nursing and Board-and-Care Homes. Washington, DC, Joint Information Service of the American Psychiatric Association and the National Association for Mental Health, 1976

Goldman H, Feder J, Scanlon W, et al: Chronic mental patients in nursing homes: reexamining data from the National Nursing Home Survey. Hospital and Community Psychiatry 37:269-272, 1986

Greenberg J, Leutz W, Greenlick M, et al: The social HMO demonstration: early experience. Health Affairs 7:66-79, 1988

Kemper P: Overview of the findings: the evaluation of the national long-term care demonstration. Health Services Research 23:161-174, 1988

Mathematica Policy Research: The Evaluation of the National Long-Term Care Demonstration: The Planning and Operational Experience of the Channeling Projects, Vol 1. Washington, DC, U.S. Department of Health and Human Services, July 1986

Montgomery K, Costa L: Neuropsychological test performance of a normal elderly sample. Paper presented at the International Neuropsychological Society Meeting, Mexico City, 1983

Nelson A, Fogel B, Faust D: Bedside cognitive screening instruments: a critical assessment. Journal of Nervous and Mental Diseases 174:73-83, 1986

Omer H, Foldes J, Toby M, et al: Screening for cognitive deficits in a sample of hospitalized geriatric patients: a reevaluation of a brief mental status questionnaire. Journal of the American Geriatrics Society 31:266-268, 1983

Parrish J: The ideal community-based mental health service system for adults with long-term, disabling mental illness. Bethesda, MD, National Institute of Mental Health, October 1987

Phillips B, Kemper P, Appelbaum P: Case management under channeling. Health Services Research 23:67-81, 1988

Pies H: Life care communities for the aged—an overview, in Long-Term Care Financing and Delivery Systems: Exploring Some Alternatives (Conference Proceedings: Health Care Financing Administration). Publication No. 03174. Washington, DC, U.S. Government Printing Office, June 1984

Robinson G, Toff Bergman G: Choices in case management: a review of current knowledge and practice for mental health programs. Bethesda, MD, National Institute of Mental Health, March 1989

Shadish W, Bootzin R: Nursing homes and chronic mental patients. Schizophrenia Bulletin 7:488-498, 1981

Tell E, Cohen M, Wallack S: Life care at home: a new model for financing and delivering long-term care. Inquiry 24: 253-265, 1987

Winklevoss H, Powell A: Continuing Care Retirement Communities: An Empirical, Financial, and Legal Analysis. Philadelphia, The Wharton School, Pension Research Council, 1984

Notes

1.   Florida, Hawaii, Kentucky, Maine, Maryland, Massachusetts, Missouri, New Jersey, New York, Ohio, Pennsylvania, and Texas (Hawaii and Missouri did not participate in the evaluation).

2.   The data show that 32% were classified as having severe mental impairments; 83% reported their overall health as fair or poor; 52% reported incomes below $500 per month.

3.   Under the basic program caseloads were 45:1 and case managers had no discretion over reimbursement rates. Under the financial model, caseloads were slightly higher (49:1) and case managers could authorize funds up to 85% of prevailing nursing home rates for individual clients and 60% across all clients.

4.   The limits on average and individual service expenditures were set at 60% and 85%, respectively, of prevailing nursing home rates. The cost-sharing provision applied only to those clients with incomes in excess of a certain amount, and only for services that would not otherwise have been available without a charge.

5.   Elderplan, Inc., Brooklyn, New York; Kaiser Permanente's Medicare Plus II, Portland, Oregon; SCAN Health Plan, Inc., Long Beach, California; and Seniors Plus, Minneapolis, Minnesota.

6.   Medicare pays 100% of its expected costs in the locality. A monthly premium of $29 to $49 is charged to all members. Medicaid picks up the premium charge for members who are eligible. S/HMOs are provided a higher capitated rate by Medicare and Medicaid for severely disabled enrollees living in the community. By enrolling the nonimpaired as well as the impaired, the financial risk is spread among a larger pool of enrollees.

7. Applicants' eligibility for institutional care is based on the Patient Review Instrument (PRI). This primarily is a medical assessment administered by a nurse trained on the instrument. Information on mental status includes evaluations for verbal disruption, physical aggression, disruptive and infantile behavior, socially inappropriate behavior, and hallucinations. Applicants must have a serious problem with one or more of the aforementioned behaviors to be eligible for the program on the basis of mental status alone.

Eligibility for the New York Long-Term Care Home Health Program is based on the Medical Assessment Abstract, commonly known as DMS-1 Score. Specific mental status items include impaired judgment, regressive behavior, severe depression, and agitation at night. Information on the participant is systematically collected every four months. Systematic data collection of participants' health status is required by all On Lok sites.

8. The proportions are not evenly distributed. Medicare contributes through a waiver. The rate is based on a single adjustor to the county per capita cost. Medicaid also pays through a waiver. The rate is based on comparative Medicaid costs, using the state Medicaid HMO rate-setting methods. An individual not eligible for Medicaid pays the Medicaid equivalent portion of the capitated rate.

9. The daily cost of the day health center is $45 per person. On Lok's day health center includes transportation, activities, meals, and nursing care.

10. In close to 30% of the CCRCs, more than 21% of the residents require nursing and/or home health care. Communities with higher ratios are located predominantly in the North Central and Western United States, where CCRCs have been well-established. Communities with the lowest ratios of nursing care and home health care utilization (less than 10% of the residents) are located in the Southern region where most of the new communities are being built. In addition, the study found that CCRCs having extensive health care guarantees have lower nursing and health care ratios than communities with limited health care guarantees. The study's authors assert that the lower costs are due to greater financial incentives to tightly monitor nursing care utilization (Winklevoss and Powell 1984).

11

Testing New Models
of Service Delivery

Robert L. Kane, M.D.

The basic approach to addressing the issue of how to develop and test new models of care falls back on fundamental principles. It is important to begin at the end. We must determine what we hope to accomplish if we are to know when we have succeeded and to gain insight into the most fruitful strategies to pursue. Too often service programs begin with an innovative idea in search of an appropriate target. In today's geriatric environment, the answer is almost inevitably "case management," whatever the question. No one seems too perplexed by the failure to define the concept or the difficulty in showing that it makes a substantial difference. We do not want to fall into the same trap as we discuss neuropsychiatric care.

This discussion will begin, then, with an examination of the potential goals for neuropsychiatric care, distinguishing at least the two major themes of such care: those devoted to cognition and those to affect. From the goals we can then proceed to examine strategies for implementing them and constraints to be faced in launching innovative efforts. Finally we will explore issues around the question of how to assess the effectiveness—to say nothing of the cost-effectiveness—of new approaches.

Major points of the discussion are recapitulated in Tables 11-1 and 11-2: one listing desirable features of new service delivery models, and the other listing desirable features of program evaluations.

Defining Goals

As others in this volume have noted, the care goals for dementia and depression in the elderly are different. Although the differential

Table 11–1. Desirable features of new service delivery models

---

1. Well-defined goals.
2. Flexibility in use of care providers, allowing substitution of less costly providers and support of informal caregiving.
3. Emphasis on making diagnoses that lead to treatment, while avoiding expense for early diagnoses of irreversible degenerative diseases.
4. Administrative and legal authority to depart from traditional care patterns, with appropriate safeguards for patients' welfare.
5. Explicit recognition of tradeoffs between safety and autonomy.
6. Ascertainment of consumers' desires and expectations.
7. Recognition of neuropsychiatric comorbidities' effects on the course of physical illnesses and disabilities.
8. Targeting of assessment to specific purposes (e.g., identifying resources needed), rather than applying "generic" assessment.
9. Recognition of cuing and supervision as crucial and labor-intensive components of caregiving to demented individuals.
10. Emphasis on improving health and function, as well as on treating pathology.
11. Practical employment of outcome measures with incentives to providers for attaining better outcomes.
12. Adequate weight to appropriately chosen mental health outcome measures.

---

diagnosis between the two conditions is clinically important, the importance of the distinction for health policy lies in the differences in available treatment and the expectations therefrom. We have reasonable expectations that older persons suffering from depression will improve, often dramatically if properly treated. This expectation justifies large efforts at detecting such persons and correctly diagnosing them.

In contrast, a correct diagnosis of a degenerative dementia such as Alzheimer's disease is essentially a life sentence. The emphasis of the health care system should thus be more on eliminating reversible causes of dementia than on looking for early cases of irreversible degenerative disorders. Especially in light of increased public attention to Alzheimer's disease and related disorders, there is a real possibility that many other conditions, especially acute ones such as adverse drug reactions (Larson 1987), may be misdiagnosed as Alzheimer's disease. Because the implications of misdiagnosis are so severe, careful efforts are indicated to make the correct diagnosis *once overt symptoms of dementia are manifest.*

The issue is how aggressively to search for subtle early symptoms. There seems little reason to seek out a condition for which most would agree there is no effective treatment. Having excluded acute and *reversible* cognitive impairment incorrectly labelled as dementia, only a modest proportion of the dementias are reversible.

Table 11–2.   Desirable features of program evaluations

1. Evaluation design done prospectively and integrated with planning of the program itself.
2. Use of control groups with random assignment if possible.
3. Use of face-valid and robust outcome measures (e.g., ability to walk without assistance).
4. Appropriate choice of outcome measure (e.g., caregiver health status rather than patient function in a study of respite care).
5. Adequate measures of caregiver efforts, with recognition of cuing and supervision.
6. Adequate time for the program to reach steady state, to avoid confounds from enthusiasm or inexperience.
7. Adequate time to evaluate costs and benefits properly, considering experience-related cost reductions and possible delayed benefits.
8. Direct verification that the new program was actually implemented as designed.
9. Consideration of *who* realizes cost savings from interventions.
10. Replication at other sites, *after* initial evaluation of effectiveness at one site.
11. Evaluation of costs, effectiveness, and benefits of programs *after* dissemination to nonexperimental settings.

Truly correctable dementias, where the institution of treatment leads to substantial improvement in cognition, appear to be less frequent than formerly hoped, and probably account for no more than 10% to 15% of all dementias (Larson 1984).

Certainly, every dementia victim deserves a diligent search for correctable causes. The challenging question is how hard one should look. Some families will demand that no stone be left unturned. In sophisticated centers the standard of practice seems to demand the use of the newest technology lest the clinician be labelled as superficial. At the same time, there is a point beyond which it is inefficient to go except under the rubric of allaying anxiety and assuring the family that everything possible was done. Prospective studies have suggested that many of the core components of the standard dementia evaluation may not yield much useful information. For example, Larson and his colleagues (1986) suggest that the only laboratory tests of definite value in evaluating dementia were thyroid function tests, a complete blood count, and a screening blood chemistry panel. They suggest reserving CT scanning for only high risk cases. (*Editors' note:* A dissenting view is offered by Katzman et al. [1988], who recommend routine CT scanning in their report to the Office of Technology Assessment on the diagnosis of dementia.) The key question for payers is: How much should I pay to alleviate your anxiety?

The most common stone over which this debate stumbles is probably the use of CT scans. Whereas most clinicians agree that the probable yield from such a test does not justify the expense, most will quickly capitulate to demands for a "thorough" investigation and justify the procedure on the basis of ruling out possible remediable causes such as tumor and trauma. The more interesting way of posing the cost-effectiveness question is: If the same resources represented by a CT scan were made available to the neuropsychiatric clinician, how might they best be used?

One approach to controlling the costs of dementia assessments without jeopardizing their effectiveness is to subject each part of the process to careful cost-effectiveness evaluation. Such an effort would require the synthesis of large amounts of data to identify the contributions of individual tests and to identify potential indications for such tests. Ideally this type of analysis would yield a set of simple first-line screening items from history, physical examination, and basic laboratory tests that would serve as an indication of the probable diagnostic value of more elaborate testing. This was done for lumbar puncture and cerebrospinal fluid examination by investigators from Duke and Pittsburgh (Becker et al. 1985; Hammerstrom and Zimmer 1985). Their studies contributed significantly to a consensus that a lumbar puncture could be dropped from the routine dementia workup. Central to this analysis is a clarification of how much tolerance there is for a false positive versus a false negative result. What is the penalty for missing a potentially correctable case and how many false leads are we prepared to follow in order not to lose one such case?

Some optimists might argue that if treatment is to work, it will be most effectively directed toward those newly stricken, but there is presently little basis for this position beyond theory. Without treatment that arrests or reverses the dementia, the goals of dementia care are the preservation of maximal function consistent with the level of brain degeneration and preventing disruption by eliminating stressful elements in the environment and treating specific psychiatric complications of dementia, such as depression, agitation, and paranoid behavior. Reducing these latter symptoms can reduce caregiver burden and improve the client's functional performance (see Chapter 3 for details).

In dementia assistance is directed not only at the patient, but also at the informal caregiver when one is available. Indeed, many of the most innovative services are designed to provide indirect care by strengthening or relieving the informal caregiver. Evaluating the effectiveness of such strategies poses special problems. It is hard to define and control the use of respite. Many control members may wind up getting similar assistance and many experimental members may not accept any help (Lawton et al. 1989). Some caregivers are very tightly bonded to their charges and are quite reluctant to cede any responsibility to others. Nor is it clear what to assess as an outcome. Is the goal of respite to maintain the client in the community or to relieve caregiver stress regardless of its immediate or long-term effect on the client? What happens if one goal is achieved at the expense of the other, i.e., less institutional care but worn-out caregivers?

Early diagnosis can sometimes confound efforts to assess treatment. Epidemiological literature makes regular reference to the concept of artificial prolongation of survival by early identification of cases. Identifying a case earlier in its natural course artificially extends the period of observation and hence creates the impression of longer survival by starting the clock earlier. The same effect can be seen in conditions where the endpoint is function rather than survival. One can appear to "prolong" the period of good function by finding cases at an earlier stage. This difficulty is especially subtle for Alzheimer's disease, where the early stage may extend for a long period with few specific features.

Problems of dementia and depression can also complicate the management of physical conditions. Prolonged hospitalization, slowed recovery, or poor compliance may result from the influences of these neuropsychiatric problems. In this case, treatment goals may focus on minimizing complications imposed on the physical illness and its treatment regimen. This may involve adapting the regimen to address the neuropsychiatric context, as when drug treatment of a medical disorder is changed to avoid psychiatric side effects. Active efforts to address the neuropsychiatric components of the patient's difficulties might result in overall improvements in efficiency of care (see Chapter 7 on cost-offsets).

Ironically, to the extent that they are underrecognized, neuropsychiatric diagnoses will not emerge as complicating factors in statistical analyses designed to identify problems associated with worse than expected medical care outcomes. More work is needed to identify such factors in routine studies of the course and treatment of physical problems of the elderly. More systematic incorporation of standard measures for depression and cognitive impairment may help to identify the contribution these conditions make to the course of physical problems and to lay the groundwork for interventions that attend to them.

Intervention Strategies

Assessment

One of the most common contemporary long-term care service components is assessment. A broad consensus that function is the common denominator of long-term care led to the technical response of comprehensive functional assessment. However, assessment now needs to be assessed. It occurs in response to different purposes and includes components that are more applicable in some situations than others. Much "generic" functional assessment may be unproductive (Larson 1986). Further, not every profession must be represented in every assessment, nor must all professions assemble *en masse* to process the information.

In evaluating assessment, it is important to distinguish those elements that are directly associated with improved results from those that are the result of tradition. There is some basis for believing that at least part of the effectiveness of assessments may be attributable to the belief of the assessor (and hence the client) in the feasibility of benefit (Kane 1988).

A different approach to assessment is appropriate for finding persons suffering from a given condition than for verifying the presence of a condition already suspected and exploring its implications. In case-finding the emphasis is on those parameters that rule in or out a specific problem. These tend to be primarily clinical. In addressing a problem already tentatively diagnosed, the assessor usually has a broader set of goals in mind. In addition to confirming the diagnosis, the assessment explores the consequences of the diagnosis, including the service needs and resources available to meet them. This more comprehensive assessment addresses several important areas, including functioning (general, cognitive, and affective), resources available and used, and expectations of care and its consequences by the patient and by informal caretakers.

Measures of functioning play a central role in almost any contemporary geriatric enterprise. The standard measure is built around the assessment of abilities to perform activities of daily living (ADLs), or slightly more expansive performance items that constitute the instrumental activities of daily living (IADLs). Such measures can be collected in a variety of ways, which can create great confusion because essentially different measures may look the same when they are presented.

One distinction among measures is the source of the information. Some measures use data derived from actual performance under specified conditions. Others use observed performance in usual living circumstances; in this case it is necessary to find some way of summing patterns of behavior to come up with a single measure, which may be an approximation to usual performance or alternatively the highest level reached in the period of observation. In some instances, reports of behavior rely on things not readily observed by the reporters. For example, family members may not know how well a relative functions in an institution; and institutional personnel can only guess at how well a patient might do in a noninstitutional setting.

Functional measures of cognition and mood generally collect data directly from the client. In the case of cognition, they are usually based on actual performance. Mood is more likely to be reported than observed. Both must attend to the points on the continuum of greatest relevance. Most of the extant scales are designed to detect pathology but are not necessarily sensitive to higher levels of functioning. (For cognitive scales, this issue is addressed by Nelson et al. [1986].) For many purposes, one may want to encourage something more than just the reduction of bad performance. For example, it may be useful to know when a person shows insight or a sense of humor, or when they feel happy rather than just not sad.

In the case of dementia especially, it is important to appreciate that what you see is not necessarily what you get. We have come a long way in appreciating the value of ADLs as central to long-term care. In fact, they may well become the ticket of eligibility for long-term care benefits and are part of eligibility criteria in all long-term care bills currently pending in Congress. If so, how one measures ADLs may be even more important than *what* one measures. In the case of dementia specifically, much of the need is best expressed in terms of the presence of another person. The service required, however, usually is not physical assistance but cuing and supervision. Ironically, such supervision can take more time than simply doing the task for the patient. However, a standard ADL metric records client needs, in terms of inabilities, to perform specified tasks. Unless the metric is specifically constructed to be sensitive to cuing needs, the real level of disability may go unremarked.

An important and often overlooked component of the assessment process is determining the expectations of the several participants. Conflicting expectations may explain the varying levels of satisfaction with the outcomes of a given course of therapy. It is all too easy to assume that the professional has conveyed an adequate picture to the client and his family, when the latter harbor their own independent concepts of what lies ahead. On the other hand, the professional can have a subtle, but profound effect on the outcome itself by communicating deliberately or inadvertently a sense of discouragement about the likelihood of improvement (Siegler 1975; Eisenberg 1986). Because motivation is an important component of function, this sort of negative prophecy can be self-fulfilling.

Therefore, any effort to assess or influence the outcomes of care should include some documentation of the expectations held by patients and family members as well as the prognosis of the responsible clinician.

Treatment

Assessment, per se, like a medical diagnosis will not improve an individual's health unless it leads to meaningful treatment. The translation of functional deficits into care plans is a difficult business. The large body of information inevitably collected must be synthesized and prioritized. For each significant problem, separately and in combination, a goal must be established and resources identified to achieve that goal.

It is important to assess not only the need for resources but also their availability. Care strategies must take into consideration the limitations of the community. Especially when achievements are measured in terms of process, it is important to recognize the constraints on reasonable choice. Further, not all resources that are available are accessible. Eligibility criteria, including financial barriers, may exclude some clients.

In the case of long-term care, many relevant resources come from outside the formal care system. The strategy to provide assistance may be indirect, through supporting the informal caregivers. It is thus necessary to ascertain the burden felt by the caregivers and to estimate their ability to sustain further efforts.

In some cases, an overwhelming number of problems are identifiable. In these cases, priorities must be set on the basis of clear criteria. Accountability will be reasonably directed toward those areas targeted for effort, but the choice of targets cannot rest solely on the likelihood of success.

Assistance

The most effective strategy to affect function is the provision of direct assistance. This seems so straightforward as to need no comment, but there are a few subtle twists to consider. Mention has already been made of the role of indirect assistance to support caregivers. Despite the appeal of the concept, neither respite care nor caregiver support groups have been utilized to anywhere near the extent anticipated (Lawton et al. 1989; Montgomery 1988).

Help, like any therapy, has its side effects. In the case of services, this side effect is best described as dependency breeding. The combination of risk aversion and the general tendency to want to help people can produce problems. Fostering autonomy requires an environment in which the individual is challenged (Lawton 1989), but not put at great danger. At the same time, autonomy does involve risk. Professional caregivers, worried about lawsuits, and family members, worried about catastrophes, can each limit the client's autonomy by restricting activities in the name of safety and prudence. It is important to document the extent to which the client's (and family's) preferences about the trade-off between safety and autonomy were discussed and incorporated into the treatment plan, in order to distinguish from negligence the assumption by the patient, family, and care providers of an acceptable risk of possible bad outcomes.

Much of the help a person may require to function may not require a high level of professional skill. Even in areas of direct therapy, there is good reason to assume that downward substitution may have no untoward consequences. In instances where following a prescribed regimen is deemed an asset, there may even be demonstrable benefits to using less professionally prepared therapists who are more willing to take direction and more eager (and able) to spend time with the client.

Incentives

Especially in this country, incentives are important influences on behavior. Both providers and clients will respond to them. The most obvious incentives are those that reward outcomes. At present, these are mostly *dis*incentives for improvement. When payment is tied to a client's level of care (i.e., the more dependent, the more payment), the incentive is directed to deterring improvement. Even when payment is linked to items of service rather than to outcomes, there is a tendency to do more, rather than to encourage the client to do things for himself.

Measuring the quality of long-term care is quite different from measuring the quality of acute care (Kane and Kane 1988). Long-term care has been a highly regulated industry. Certification for participation in federal and state programs, licensing, and regular review efforts have shaped the industry. Indeed, one can argue that America's nursing homes are more reactive than proactive. Having been driven to adjust their behavior to meet the demands of the regulators, they are reluctant to initiate and to innovate.

A recent study by the Institute of Medicine (1986) pointed to the need for reforms in nursing home regulation. (Many of these reforms were incorporated into the nursing home reform provisions of the 1987 Omnibus Budget Reconciliation Act.) The study's authors made an important distinction between quality *assessment* and quality *assurance*. Too often most of the energy goes into measuring the deficiencies and little is devoted to doing something about them. Sometimes the fear of closing a facility in the face of heavy utilization leads to inaction, or even worse, to pouring additional money into an inadequate facility in the hopes of making it better. The rewards are thus perverted.

Some have argued that the test of medical care lies not in its adherence to orthodoxy but to the outcomes it achieves (Institute of Medicine Committee on Regulation of Nursing Homes 1986). However, outcomes are the result of several factors. Most important is the patient's initial condition; any outcome approach must adjust its findings on the basis of the clinically relevant parameters. Those who dislike using outcomes insist that too many factors are involved in determining the outcome; one can give good care and not always achieve a good result. In truth, using outcomes requires that one not look at individual cases, but at groups of cases to study the pattern of performance. Adjusting for case mix is not an easy task but is feasible. It is a critical part of many research designs to test the efficacy of an intervention. Extrapolating from the work on hospital mortality data points to the need for more precise data analysis, which considers factors other than primary diagnosis (Greenfield et al. 1988). In the world of long-term care, case-mix has been used as a basis for paying nursing homes (Schneider et al. 1988).

Especially in long-term care, it is possible to envision a system of reimbursement that would reward good outcomes, where the latter are defined as clients functioning better than might be expected statistically, given acceptable standard care. The key to such an approach is identifying reasonable expectations and using the ratio of observed/expected as the basis for determining the reward. The outcomes of LTC can be expressed along a continuum of domains, which include physiologic function, activities of daily living, comfort, cognition, affect, social activity, interpersonal activity, and satisfaction with care and environment. All of these can be reliably measured from data obtained directly from LTC clients (Kane et al. 1983). The weight assigned to any one of these is best derived from ascertaining the relative value placed on it by appropriate groups in society. These weighted results can be used in a calculation of the bonus or penalty applied to the basic costs of LTC; the organizations that achieve better than average outcomes would be paid more and those with consistently poorer outcomes less.

Under such a system the contribution of mental health services would best be appreciated if mental health outcomes were more heavily weighted. The incorporation of such services would presumably be influenced by the belief in their efficacy, especially in their ability to produce an overall improvement.

The issue of the values imputed to different types of persons requiring long-term care has special importance for dementia care. Not only is it more difficult to obtain information about such items as satisfaction from those with severe cognitive impairments, but the value placed on their quality of life is quite different. When diverse groups of respondents including family members, providers, regulators, and the general public were asked to rate the several outcome states for each of a series of patients with different levels of physical and mental impairment, virtually all groups studied rated the various outcome states consistently lower for demented clients than for clients who were physically impaired (Kane et al. 1986).

By relying on a ratio of observed to expected, the system is self-norming and avoids the dangers of market skimming by avoiding the difficult cases. Because a good outcome is defined not in absolute terms, but relative to what might be reasonably expected from good care, the clients with the worst prognosis offer the best chances of a successful finding.

While such a step as outcome-based reimbursement may be too difficult to take at once, an intermediate position would be to provide some rewards for better outcomes, or at least to remove the current disincentives. In the case of psychiatric care, the Medicare program presents strong disincentives for ambulatory care by severely restricting payment for these services. There is an understandable fear of uncontrolled utilization of such care, but this situation represents an exciting opportunity for innovative reimbursement strategies linked to evidence of effectiveness.

The time has come to test the effects of an outcome-based approach. Why not establish a randomized clinical trial in which one group of facilities was paid, in whole or in part, on this basis and the controls continued under traditional reimbursement? In both groups client outcomes would be assessed, but only the experimentals would get feedback in the form of more or less remuneration. The key question is whether such an incentive approach could produce the desired improvements in quality of care. Such a demonstration would need to be sustained for enough time to allow for the innovations hopefully stimulated to blossom. It would also need sufficient waivers of current regulations to permit new approaches to care.

Previous efforts to use outcome-based incentives failed for lack of a supportive environment and inadequate introduction of the concept (Meiners et al. 1985; Jones and Meiners 1986). An experiment conducted in San Diego was designed to see if nursing homes would respond to payment incentives for improving patient functioning and for discharging patients back to the community. However, the study utilized a complex formula for incentive reimbursement designed to meet expected additional costs but not so great as to be very attractive. Nursing home operators seemed to be very confused about how the bonus would apply and were generally unwilling to make a heavy investment in care for a demonstration project, which would not last long.

Although the enthusiasm for outcome measurement is still building, there is a growing sentiment that some information is better than none, and that consumers have a right to better information about the institutions that provide health care. One way to encourage better care may be to provide consumers with better information about the aggregate results of an institution (Ginsburg and Hammons 1988). Because most people are likely to have limited personal experience and even then may not be able to judge good quality care, information similar to that used to rate restaurants and other services should be of great value in choosing, or even agreeing to be sent to, a given facility. In the case of dementia victims, the deciding parties are more likely to be families, but the same principles hold.

At the same time, it is fair to note that there is no evidence that people have boycotted those hospitals cited as having high mortality rates in the published data on Medicare outcomes. Part of the lack of effect may be explained by the confusing way the data were released and the subsequent controversy around their validity.

A major disincentive to innovation is the fear of litigation. Much of medical practice today is driven by so-called defensive medicine. Such an atmosphere constrains innovation. Part of the conservative environment can be traced to the tradition of professional orthodoxy. In the absence of hard information on the effectiveness of therapy, there has been a strong sense of the importance of the therapist's credentials. A greater willingness to broaden the treatment tolerance in the context of better accountability for results achieved may encourage the needed innovations by changing the way standards of care are defined.

One important step in reforming the tort liability process might be to focus on paying for the consequences of the untoward event and not inflating the level of punitive damages. The latter might be expected to be managed better in a system of outcome accountability.

In the absence of reforms in the malpractice tort system, legal risk can be reduced by greater efforts by clinicians to explore in advance of treatment decisions with clients and their families the risks and benefits of alternative treatment approaches. Better documentation of understanding of the risks and evidence of deliberate choice will help allay accusations in retrospect.

Specifically identifying bad outcomes not directly linked to carelessness or incompetence and separating them in statistics on the overall performance of an individual or institution will help. Clinical outcomes can only be assessed rationally on averages, but legal reasoning is based on individual cases. The possibility of a bad outcome is always there and it can rarely be said for certain that a bad event could not have been prevented. The real test for society and for payers is whether there is a *pattern* of poor outcomes. For the individual there is a need to be compensated for damages suffered. In a rational system, compensation for bad outcomes of good care would come from pooled resources that reflected the pooling of risks.

Incentives also affect families. It is shortsighted to penalize those with families willing to bear some of the burden, and unfair to penalize those without families to take responsibility for care. Especially with regard to dementia, where families often play a central role, families providing care should be eligible for assistance as needed. Care planners should be given enough leeway to allow plans that offer indirect care to caregivers. Although some have advocated even paying family caregivers, as is done in some European countries, there is a very real danger in such a course. While for some families, the payment might indeed enable a working family member to stay at home to provide needed care, for many such payment would be simply a bonus for doing what they were doing anyway. Even with a system to monitor those who actually gave up productive work, there is a great propensity for exploitation. We rely heavily on families for long-term care services but seem unable to afford paying them for this work, nor is there any evidence that such payment is necessary.

Conversely, when assessing the effects of a program in dementia, it is important to distinguish benefits that accrue to families from those that may produce some secondary benefit for the dementia victim. It is not clear when family satisfaction or reduced caregiver burden is a reasonable outcome measure for dementia care; when it leads to better client outcomes, the decision is easy, but in the absence of such effects the picture is far from certain.

Constraints

In assessing the effectiveness of a treatment innovation it is important to be sure there is real treatment. In many instances the treatment as delivered is not as dramatically different as first intended because of conservative forces. Some of these have already been identified. Payment will limit the degree of innovation. Medicare and Medicaid waivers come with constraints that limit the total amount of resources actually or theoretically used, or impose some floors or ceilings on the amount of care to be given. For example, community care waivers require that care for an individual not exceed the cost of institutional care. In other cases, the kinds of providers eligible to be paid may be limited or limits are placed on the types of services that are reimbursable; for example, services to families may not be paid for even though a more stable family can serve as a more stable source of informal care. In other cases, the family may have to accept certain specific services in order to get other support they need. Payment changes in demonstration projects may not have the effect intended because the organization is reluctant to make major shifts in procedures and policy for the short periods of funded demonstrations.

We do not at present have sufficient legal protections to cover care given in innovative programs. Informed consent is designed to protect the innovator, but it is not certain how much protection such a procedure conveys, especially when the risks are not well known. The more the care process is codified in regulations, the more difficult it will be for innovative programs to deviate from those norms without incurring legal risks.

Eligibility criteria can influence who participates in an innovation. Functional information is often used as criteria for eligibility for services. The way the item is measured can be very important. Especially in the case of dementia, there is great concern that using the typical ADL dependencies may underestimate the need for services. Many dementia patients (as well as others, like some stroke victims) do not need physical assistance but do need supervising and cuing to perform a given task. One strategy is to use a different metric for the cognitively impaired, but this is cumbersome. It seems much simpler to expand the basic ADL measurement approach to include cuing as a level of assistance for everyone.

The failure to recognize the importance of cuing and supervision is especially troublesome in developing both eligibility criteria and payments schemes for care of demented clients. Ironically, supervision and encouragement generally require more time than simply doing the task for the patient. In fact, this kind of care forms the basis of what, under other circumstances, is recognized as rehabilitation.

When case-mix measures for long-term care are developed by linking staff time spent per client to levels of ADL and other markers, the dementia patients are often erroneously judged to require less care than the physically disabled precisely because the measures are skewed away from cuing and supervision. The dementia patients are rated as having few ADL deficiencies and hence needing little attention. It is little wonder then that systems like Resource Utilization Groups (RUGS) (Fries and Cooney 1985) used in New York State and similar approaches used in the half dozen or so other states that use case-mix as the basis for nursing home payment place dementia patients in the least costly category.

Assessing Effectiveness

Although the current watchword is efficiency (or cost-effectiveness), it is important to appreciate that one cannot be efficient until one is first effective. Ascertainment of effectiveness requires a shared perception of program goals and concordance that the measures used to translate goals into performance (or achievement) are true reflections of the constructs intended. Agreement must be established in advance of the findings. It is certain that those results that fail to meet the standards established will be challenged. Once the results are available, objectivity vanishes.

The issue of measuring effectiveness is clouded by two important, often confused issues. The first critical step is determining what is supposed to result. The second is finding an appropriate way to measure that result. The second step cannot occur without the first.

The problem of establishing reasonable goals is especially complicated in the case of dementia. Take, for example, the current effort to launch a major demonstration of respite care for the caregivers of persons with severe dementia. What is a reasonable outcome from such a venture? The very concept of respite suggests that the effort should affect the caregivers rather than the person with the disease. Any measures directed toward the dementia victim should be used only to establish that deteriorated function is not an untoward consequence of the intervention. However, it is easy to see how client functioning can quickly become a primary outcome and the emphasis shifted in that direction. Studies of day care often get trapped into looking for signs of improvement in patients when their purpose may be mainly respite for caregivers.

If the caregivers are the primary target, what kinds of changes are expected from them? At best, one might hope for a slowing of the rate of fatigue; but, here again, there is a propensity to look for more dramatic evidence of positive improvement. Any measure designed to show reduction in decline requires a strong control group because the measure is by definition relative.

One of the problems that arises in such demonstrations is the high level of expectations created. Any new program is usually introduced with great promises of making significant inroads. Because few persons can easily obtain resources for a program with admittedly modest goals, claims for expected benefit are often exaggerated and the test of the evaluation is posed against inflated expectations. Under such circumstances it is hard to show a substantial effect.

Outcome measures should be linked to the goals in terms of both content and metric. Great care should be taken to assure that the measures used are appropriate to both the fundamental question and to the population treated, and that they truly measure what their names imply. The literature is replete with misplaced measures, such as using life satisfaction to assess the impact of relocation (Kane and Kane 1981). In general, outcome measures are better when they can be easily understood. Scales do not tell the same tale as do discrete, familiar increments of behavior. It is easier, for example, to develop enthusiasm for a program that moves clients from immobile to mobile (or from disruptive to constructive behavior) than for one that produces fractional changes on a scale.

Fewer outcome measures are usually better than a lot. At best, multiple measures imply lack of clarity about the expected results and open the possibility of mixed pictures of effectiveness. At worst, there is a fear of selective reporting of only those measures that show desired results.

It is important to consider the metric used to reflect the level of performance on a given task. Functional data can be used for several purposes, each of which implies a different metric. Measuring client progress requires a scale that reflects levels of performance at once sensitive to change and indicative of greater independence. For example, walking a given distance in less time or feeding oneself with encouragement after being fed formerly are signs of improvement. Developing a care plan requires information expressed in terms of the human effort required to assist a client. For this purpose, it does not matter whether the time is spent supervising and encouraging the client or providing physical assistance. In fact, the latter may be cheaper because it usually can be done faster. Thus the same change can be an improvement in one system and no change, or even a worsening, in another. Moreover, a heavy person who requires the assistance of two helpers may function at the same level as a light person, but the care burden is doubled.

The basic factors that apply to clinical and health services research in general are especially germane with regard to neuropsychiatric efforts. Because the natural history of both depression and dementia is so varied, control groups are a must for any intervention. Because it is difficult to identify accurate prognostic factors, randomized clinical trials are strongly preferred over other approaches that rely on matching. In designing and analyzing the results of studies, it is important to assure comparability of the groups, especially with regard to the stage of the disease. Because duration and stage do not closely correlate, careful attention to standardized clinical assessment and grading is necessary.

One persistent problem with demonstration projects is the pressure of time. There is an urgency to begin measuring effects before the treatment has been in place long enough to make a difference, to say nothing of allowing for the developmental phase needed to refine the innovation. This propensity to measure early creates several important and often subtle problems. First, the treatment tested may be in the early stage when the caregivers are still feeling their way. In some cases this means studying an immature program, while in others it means studying the effects of enthusiasm for a new undertaking rather than the steady state level of performance of an established program. Cost-effectiveness measures may be misleading, because developmental costs may be much higher than eventual operating costs for the program in a steady state.

Time also plays an important role in determining the chance of seeing an effect. Much of the innovation in long-term care is built on an "investment" model, whereby additional resources are expended on the client early in the project with the anticipation that the benefits later will more than offset these initial costs. It is not always easy to predict when the lines will cross. The earlier in the client's course the outcomes are measured, the less the chance of finding an effect in this model. Downstream savings will be found only when there is enough time for them to emerge. Under the artificial pressure of a demonstration project, the push for showing outcomes may force premature assessment before the point of maximal effectiveness.

In some cases, demonstration projects cannot produce the impact of operational programs. When agency behavior needs to change to create the desired effect, it may be difficult to motivate providers to change their fundamental approach to a situation if the project is seen as only temporary. It may simply not be worth their while to make major changes in operational policy for a program expected to disappear in a few years. Thus, it may be hard to obtain a real measure of the programmatic impact. For this reason, it is always important in evaluating a demonstration to ascertain whether there really was a full treatment. Part of the evaluation effort must be directed toward obtaining measures of the existence and extent of the treatment or change that was sought. This evidence should not be confused with proof of effectiveness; it is simply evidence of the necessary condition under which to reasonably expect an impact.

In an era of fragmented funding, measures of cost savings must similarly distinguish who is saving money. Transferring fiscal responsibility is not equivalent to true savings. One program or group may benefit at the expense of another. For example, shifting funding responsibility from Medicare to Medicaid, or from professional agencies to families may not represent a net saving (see Chapters 5 and 7).

Finding a positive difference does not always mean that the treatment produced the better outcome. It is important to search diligently to determine what is the component of the independent variable (presumably the treatment) that really made the difference. For example, the several studies of the effectiveness of geriatric assessment using strong experimental designs generally show positive effects; but the variation in program content and staff suggest that the effect may be due to factors other than just assessment *per se* (Kane 1988). It may be that the key variable is the milieu created by bringing together people who are enthusiastic about the goals, or that simply believing that improvement is possible can often make it happen.

A final caution about the evaluation of demonstration projects is in order. Evaluation is essential to understanding whether the intervention worked. Often it costs more than the demonstration itself, because it involves collecting information on a control group as well as on those treated. Too often evaluation is an afterthought, developed after the program has begun, perhaps even after it has concluded. This situation is tragic and results in the loss of valuable information. For example, baseline data assuring that the control group is comparable to the experimental group cannot be easily reconstructed after the fact.

Good evaluations must be planned along with the projects. Often the evaluators can help the program developers by asking penetrating questions about the fundamental goals of the effort.

Some might urge that any demonstration be conducted at multiple sites to assure its generalizability, but prudence suggests that a new idea be tested first at one site, because demonstration funds are in scarce supply. After the initial concept has proven itself, replication is indicated. Then, the real test lies in the translation from a demonstration program staffed by dedicated innovators to a basic program operated by a more diverse group. A final evaluation should be conducted after a program has been broadly inaugurated. Since it must rely on designs that do not require random assignment to experimental and control groups, clients in programs should be sufficiently characterized diagnostically so that expected outcomes can be estimated.

Neuropsychiatric Application

This discussion has been restricted to dementia and depression, as the two major neuropsychiatric afflictions of the elderly. However, the approach described is relevant to other disorders, such as Parkinson's disease and stroke. For Parkinson's disease proper diagnosis and medical therapy can make an enormous difference in functional outcome. For stroke care, the picture is less clear. It is difficult to separate cleanly acute and chronic (or rehabilitative) care and to assess the true impact of each component, to say nothing of the importance of the therapist's credentials. However, this ignorance does not preclude strong enthusiasm. For example, although the information available to support the efficacy of stroke rehabilitation is not convincing, few are comfortable with the idea of foregoing such care, even as part of a randomized clinical trial.

In the area of rehabilitation there is persuasive clinical evidence that *individual elements* of care are helpful. For example, getting a patient to move his/her hand better may increase autonomy, or stretching limbs may prevent contractures. But evidence of overall effectiveness for a rehabilitative package, using outcome measures of everyday function, will rely on careful trials that randomize cases and use parallel observations for both experimental and control groups.

How does this theory apply to efforts in dementia and depression? Dementia presents a very challenging set of issues. There is no convincing evidence that neuropsychiatric care is particularly central to the course of dementia. Although there has arisen in the last several years a clamor of interest in the medical management of dementia among various specialties, beyond the point of diagnosis, the role of the physician is quite limited, although the potential for causing great harm through medical interventions, especially mismanaged drugs, is very real. The management of complications may involve some drug therapy, but most activities and environmental therapies can be provided by a variety of disciplines. At the same time, the physician has, by law and tradition, played a central role in authorizing many critical decisions about care. Thus the introduction of new approaches to managing dementia care must confront this history.

The absence of strong proof of the value of specific medical approaches should not be misinterpreted to imply any lack of interest in finding more effective and more humane ways to manage dementia victims, especially in their late stages. Much more in this area needs to be developed and tested. Nor should the medical community be discouraged from active involvement in that cause. Much seems to have happened simply by changing the way these patients were labelled, from dismissing their plight as an inevitable consequence of aging (as implied in the term "senility") to calling it a disease process, which can presumably be treated if not eventually cured.

At present, beyond scientific study there is often no reason to rush to identify dementia patients early in their disease course. For some, an early diagnosis offers an opportunity to plan better, to take legal steps to provide for a durable power of attorney or to establish a strategy for managing assets (Overman and Stoudemire 1988). This ability to get one's life in order while cognitive capacity is relatively intact must be weighed against the burden imposed by learning of the inevitable advance of a terrible and untreatable disease. At the heart of this moral dilemma is the difficulty of even asking a person if he wants to know, but sometimes the patient will simplify the task by asking the clinician directly. It does not seem the sort of problem suitable for empirical study.

The situation with depression seems different. The availability of effective therapy for many older patients suffering from this problem suggests a basis for active efforts to identify cases and bring them under treatment. There is some indication of physician apathy and ignorance about the general problems of caring for older patients (Radecki et al. 1988a, 1988b) (see also Chapter 4).

Because the major modality of treatment involves potent drugs, the physician has a central role to play. More work is needed to identify ways to encourage physicians to even consider depression as a diagnosis in the elderly. Complex screening tests may not be the answer. A question routinely asked as simple as, "Are you depressed?" may increase the detection rate.

For both dementia and depression, but probably more for the latter, more work needs to be done to ascertain what proportion of the care is better delivered in hospital and which can be given on an ambulatory basis. At present, economic incentives favor inpatient care. The exemption of psychiatric units from Medicare's prospective payment system combined with high copayments for outpatient treatment, creates an incentive to treat psychiatric conditions like depression on an inpatient basis.

We are left then with a series of challenges in both the near and far terms. While all look forward to prevention and cure, today's efforts must be directed toward better management. There are both large and small improvements to be made. Innovative approaches to management should be encouraged and disseminated, but larger policy changes are needed. Incentives for better care, primarily by creating a climate that rewards better care through recognizing its results, will help to shape a more humane and intensive care system. Plans for major innovations deserve careful scrutiny and intensive evaluation. The plans for the latter should go hand in glove with the former.

References

Becker PM, Feussner JR, Mulrow CD: The role of lumbar puncture in the evaluation of dementia: the Durham Veterans Administration/Duke University Study. Journal of the American Geriatrics Society 33:392-396, 1985

Eisenberg JM: Doctors' Decisions and the Cost of Medical Care. Ann Arbor, MI, Health Administration Press, 1986

Fries BE, Cooney LM: Resource utilization groups: a patient classification system for long-term care. Medical Care 23:110-122, 1985

Ginsburg PB, Hammons GT: Competition and the quality of care: the importance of information. Inquiry 25:108-118, 1988

Greenfield S, Aronow HU, Elashoff RM, et al: Flaws in mortality data: the hazards of ignoring comorbid disease. JAMA 260:2253-56, 1988

Hammerstrom DC, Zimmer B: The role of lumbar puncture in the evaluation of dementia: the University of Pittsburgh study. Journal of the American Geriatrics Society 33:397–400, 1985

Institute of Medicine Committee on Regulation of Nursing Homes: Improving the Quality of Care in Nursing Homes. Washington, DC, National Academy Press, 1986

Jones BJ, Meiners MR: Nursing Home Discharges: The Results of an Incentive Reimbursement Experiment. Long-term Care Studies Program Research Report. DHHS Publication No. (PHS) 86-3399. Washington, DC, National Center for Health Services Research and Health Care Technology Assessment, 1986

Kane RL: Beyond caring: the challenge to geriatrics. Journal of the American Geriatrics Society 36:467-472, 1988

Kane RA, Kane RL: Assessing the Elderly: A Practical Guide to Measurement. Lexington, MA, D. C. Heath, 1981

Kane RA, Kane RL: Long-term care: variations on a quality assurance theme. Inquiry 25:132-146, 1988

Kane RL, Bell RM, Riegler SZ, et al: Predicting the outcomes of nursing-home patients. Gerontologist 23:200-206, 1983

Kane RL, Bell RM, Riegler SZ: Value preferences for nursing-home outcomes. Gerontologist 26:303-308, 1986

Katzman R, Lasker B, Bernstein N: Advances in the diagnosis of dementia: accuracy of diagnosis and consequences of misdiagnosis of disorders causing dementia, in Aging and the Brain. Edited by Terry RD. New York, Raven Press, 1988

Larson EB, Reifler BV, Featherstone HJ, et al: Dementia in elderly outpatients: a prospective study. Annals of Internal Medicine 100:417-423, 1984

Larson EB, Reifler BV, Sumi SM, et al: Diagnostic tests in the evaluation of dementia: a prospective study of 200 elderly outpatients. Archives of Internal Medicine 146:1917-1922, 1986

Larson EB, Kukull WA, Buchner D, et al: Adverse drug reactions associated with global cognitive impairment in elderly persons. Annals of Internal Medicine 107:169-173, 1987

Lawton MP: Environmental approaches to research and treatment of Alzheimer's disease, in Alzheimer's Disease, Treatment and Family Stress: Directions for Research. Edited by Light E, Leibowitz B. Washington, National Institute of Mental Health, 1989

Lawton MP, Brody EM, Saperstein AR: A controlled study of respite service for caregivers of Alzheimer's patients. Gerontologist 29:8-16, 1989

Meiners MR, Thorburn P, Roddy PC, et al: Nursing Home Admissions: The Results of an Incentive Reimbursement Experiment. Long-term Care Studies Program Research Report. DHHS Publication No. (PHS) 86-3397. Washington, DC, National Center for Health Services Research and Health Care Technology Assessment, 1985

Montgomery RJV: Respite Care: Lessons from a controlled design study. Health Care Financing Review 1988 Annual Supplement, pp 133-138

Nelson A, Fogel B, Faust D: Bedside cognitive screening instruments: a critical assessment. The Journal of Nervous and Mental Disease 86:1359-1363, 1986

Overman W, Stoudemire A: Guidelines for legal and financial counseling of the Alzheimer's disease patient and their families. American Journal of Psychiatry 145:1495-1500, 1988

Radecki SE, Kane RL, Solomon DH, et al: Do physicians spend less time with older patients? Journal of the American Geriatrics Society 36: 713-718, 1988a

Radecki SE, Kane RL, Solomon DH, et al: Are physicians sensitive to the special problems of older patients? Journal of the American Geriatrics Society 36:719-725, 1988b

Schneider DP, Fries BE, Foley WJ, et al: Case mix for nursing home payment: resource utilization groups, version II. Health Care Financing Review 1988 Annual Supplement, pp 39-52

Siegler M: Pascal's wager and the hanging of crepe. N Engl J Med 293:853-857, 1975

12

The Relevance of
Case Management

Rosalie A. Kane, Ph.D.

Case management is widely hailed as the answer to multiple problems in health care and social services (Weil et al. 1985; Zawadski 1984; Steinberg and Carter 1983). Commonly, the general problems in delivering health care are separated into an interrelated and troublesome threesome: 1) maintaining adequate quality, 2) assuring appropriate and equitable access, and 3) controlling costs. In its various guises, case management—which can be construed as either a direct service or an administrative function—has been proposed to address all three nagging problems.

This chapter considers whether and how case management might be helpful for elderly neuropsychiatric patients. It addresses the following questions:

- What target group of elderly neuropsychiatric patients is likely to benefit from case management?
- What are reasonable goals of case management for elderly neuropsychiatric patients?
- What services should be available in a case-managed system for elderly neuropsychiatric patients ?
- Is case management different for chronically mentally ill people than for functionally impaired people (usually old) who need long-term care? Should it be different? If so, where do elderly neuropsychiatric patients fit?
- Is the care of elderly neuropsychiatric patients best managed in a separate program or in concert with other case management programs (e.g., for the frail elderly, or for the chronically mentally ill)?
- What are the advantages and disadvantages of different models of case management for elderly neuropsychiatric patients?

To approach these questions, this chapter offers a definition of case management, and it sketches the history of case management in health and human services (with an emphasis on the somewhat different ways case management has evolved in long-term care for functionally impaired old people compared to the chronically mentally ill), and discusses models of case management. With this frame-of-reference, this chapter concludes with specific issues about case management for elderly persons with neuropsychiatric disorders.

What Is Case Management?

Case management—sometimes called care management, case coordination, care coordination, resource coordination, or (with a different set of connotations) managed care—is a term that refers to coordination of services for a defined population group. Thus, case management embodies within its definition a focus on a population. To use the epidemiological construct, case management concerns itself with the denominator of the problem (i.e., the entire specified population) rather than just the numerator (i.e., those who present themselves for service at any given time).

The general purpose of this coordination of services is dual. On the one hand, a case management system ensures that people with identified needs receive all necessary diagnostic, curative, and supportive services. On the other hand, a case management system attempts to allocate services efficiently and fairly. These somewhat contradictory stances of the case manager are sometimes encapsulated by juxtaposing the terms "advocate" and "gatekeeper." Some case management veers towards advocacy and some emphasizes gatekeeping, but case management at its most difficult (and I would argue at its best) is an uneasy blend of the two (Kane 1988a).

Another way of approaching the definition of case management is by articulating its component functions. Here considerable consensus has emerged. Case management includes the following elements: casefinding (i.e., identification from the larger target population those who may be in need of assistance); comprehensive assessment (i.e., a multidimensional and systematic assessment of the client's physical, emotional, cognitive, and social well-being, and the adequacy of present formal and informal service to meet identified needs); care planning, implementation of the plan, monitoring both the adequacy of services under the plan and changes in the situation or need of the client; and reassessment at intervals (White 1988).

The case manager's power to implement the plan varies. In what is sometimes called a "broker model" of case management, the case manager's only tools may be expertise and persuasion. Implementation of plans requires the case manager to make referrals, to influence both clients and community organizations to accept the plan, and to help the client negotiate any complexities that ensue. The broker/case manager is more an advocate than a gatekeeper. In contrast, other case managers have authority to purchase services for the client, and the corollary power to decide whether the client is eligible for services and how much he or she needs. If implementation includes purchase of service, the case management program may well include a complex set of functions pertaining to the purchase of service—e.g., getting competitive bids, negotiating contracts, and establishing and enforcing quality standards among vendors (Christianson 1988).

When case managers have control over pursestrings, they can potentially exert a gradual influence on the system of care in a community as well as influence the care received by any single client (Austin 1989; Austin et al. 1985). When combined with modern information technology and a uniform approach to client assessment, the case managers can identify gaps and duplication in service. Some case management programs also make systematic efforts to develop resources where none exist—for example, by employing personnel for that purpose.

History and Development of Case Management

Case Management Elements in Social Work, Nursing, and Medicine

Case management is a relatively new term, but many of the functions embodied in modern case management are deeply embedded in established professions such as social work and nursing. This led one authority to question whether case management is merely "reinventing social work" (Austin 1987). Since their emergence as a professional group at the turn of the 20th century, social workers have typically focused on "the person-in-the environment." In addition to psychotherapy and counseling to help their clients make personal changes, social workers often try to render the physical and service environment more amenable to the client. They take a comprehensive view of the person and the family, referring clients to services beyond the scope of the agency where the social worker is employed. In that sense, for example, social workers in hospitals have long viewed themselves as case managers, with a particular emphasis on arranging aftercare. In an influential text on social work practice with the frail elderly, Silverstone and Burack-Weiss (1983) recommend what they call an "auxiliary function model" of social work practice. This requires the social worker to perform whatever case management is needed to address temporary or permanent inabilities of clients and their families to manage their own care.

Public health nurses and other visiting nurses have similarly had a long tradition of comprehensive, multidimensional assessment, referral, brokering of service, and advocacy on behalf of their clients. Even in hospital settings, there is a trend toward more comprehensive, holistic approaches among nurses. Several decades ago, at least some hospitals explored the role of the "primary care nurse." This notion was premised on the idea that one nurse should be responsible for coordinating a patient's entire nursing care: getting to know that patient, and advocating for him or her in the increasingly impersonal and complex hospital system. Now that case management has become a staple of programs for the elderly, nursing educators have developed materials to illustrate the natural compatibilities between older concepts of "nursing diagnosis" and the newer notions of case management (Harkness et al. 1987).

Finally, there is even a view that some physicians can or should serve as case managers. With the increase in medical subspecialization that characterized the 1960s and beyond, it became at least plausible to consider the family practitioner or internist as a first-stop manager of care who assesses the patient's ongoing needs and makes referrals to medical and nonmedical specialists as needed. Until the advent of much more recent practice arrangements, however, the rhetoric of the primary care physician as case manager was not matched by clear incentives that would encourage patients or the medical community to foster a managed pattern of care.

This familiarity of social workers and nurses with the techniques of case management (such as comprehensive assessment, monitoring, service arranging, advocacy) is both an advantage and a disadvantage in the development of case-managed care systems. On the one hand, it means that social workers and nurses are vocationally and temperamentally fit to act as case managers. On the other hand, it promotes confusion about the emerging role of case manager in both long-term care and mental health, a belittling of the distinctive knowledge and skills needed to do the job well, and inattention to the built-in procedures for communication, tracking, and safeguarding of client interests needed in case-managed care. If all social workers and nurses think that they do case management as part of their regular work, this attitude impedes the effectiveness of those case management systems designed to truly coordinate a wide array of services across organizations, disciplines, and even service systems (the latter including health care, social services, aging services, and mental health).

Population-Based Models

Although social workers, nurses, and, to a lesser extent, physicians have long performed some of the functions of case managers, the patterns discussed so far do not involve the continuity and responsibility over time that is almost always associated with case management today. They also fail to reflect the responsibility and authority that falls to case managers who have control over service dollars.

Early models of population-based case management can be identified. The vocational rehabilitation counselor, for example, has typically been responsible for a group of people. The group could be defined by geography, disability, or service site (e.g., all dischargees from a particular general, rehabilitation, or psychiatric hospital). Rehabilitation counselors have budgets and broad discretionary authority to spend money to promote vocational rehabilitation. For example, they may purchase shelter, health care, training and education, or special equipment. Rehabilitation counselors have had to decide how to allocate these resources based on both the problems and needs of the client and the likelihood of an effective outcome. Ideally, both need for rehabilitation and potential to benefit from it have been necessary criteria for a rehabilitation counselor to purchase services.

Another model for case management is found in the nation's child welfare system. Until they reach adulthood, departments of child welfare are responsible for the safety and development of minor children who are wards of the state—a responsibility that can persist for many years. To that end, the child welfare worker can arrange and purchase a wide range of services and is responsible for monitoring their quality. The list of services includes day schools and residential schools, foster care, medical and psychiatric treatment, summer camps and other recreational services, and basic necessities such as clothing.

It is somewhat ironic that case management for the frail elderly and the chronically mentally ill is being discovered at the same time as the child welfare system (which is case management except in name) is breaking down. Child welfare authorities are ruefully recognizing how the system contributes to discontinuities in the lives of the children under their care—the frequent changes in responsible social worker; the lack of monitoring and tracking so that children get "lost in the system"; the shortages of adequate foster care, day care, and other services that are the building blocks of the system; the ambiguities about the proper relationship between the child welfare system and the child's own family members, if they exist; the inadequacies of budgets to meet needs; and the sheer pressures of numbers exerted by huge caseloads. As the chapter now turns to case management for functionally impaired older adults, for chronically mentally ill people, and for the subset of both groups who are elderly neuropsychiatric patients, the experience of case management in the child welfare system stands as a cautionary tale of what can go wrong in a case-managed service system.

Case management has been mandated in the field of developmental disability for more than a decade. The 1975 Developmental Disability Act (PL94-103) established case management in federal law as a necessary service to help developmentally disabled people live in the least restrictive atmosphere, and, through "habilitation" efforts, flourish as much as possible despite many inherent limitations. Developmental disability was first defined categorically to include mental retardation, cerebral palsy, epilepsy, or other substantial neurological handicapping conditions. In 1978, a new federal definition defined it more broadly to include a wide range of people suffering from functionally impairing conditions with onset before age twenty-two (Caires and Weil 1985).

In many states, a specialized network of regional centers for the developmentally disabled has been created as a focal point for integrating educational, vocational, housing, and treatment efforts on behalf of the population. Case managers, typically in partnership with parents or other family, coordinate and oversee the habilitation plan and purchase services as much as their funding limitations permit. Arguably, the developmentally disabled compose a group with needs so unique that they are best met through a specialized system of case management. One must ask whether all or any subset of elderly neuropsychiatric patients also need a separate system of case management.

Case Management in Long-Term Care

In the long-term care field, case management is indeed a growth industry. Very quickly after the passage of Medicare and Medicaid in 1965, the high and rapidly rising costs of care became apparent. Both Medicare and Medicaid waiver authority became available to test whether expansion of community-based services could stem the use of more expensive hospital and/or nursing home care. Typically, the new benefits were mediated by case managers, whose services can be covered as an item under the waiver. For a brief period in the late 1960s and early 1970s, a humanitarian desire to promote home care and a cost-conscious desire to seek less costly approaches converged. Early projects seemed to confirm that functionally impaired older persons whose disabilities made them technically eligible for nursing homes could be maintained at home at lower costs. Certainly the home-based services usually cost less than the going nursing home rates. Thus it seemed possible to provide care in a more desirable form and simultaneously save money.

By the mid-1970s, a second generation of controlled studies of case-managed, community-based, long-term care was well under way. These studies tended to show no difference in functional status, use of nursing homes, or other outcomes for those receiving the additional services (Austin et al. 1985; Austin 1987; Haskins et al. 1984). Moreover, because of the additional services and the case management, the experimental group members tended to generate higher costs without receiving any obvious offsetting benefits.

The culmination of social experiments on case management in long-term care was the National Long-Term Care Channeling Demonstration, a randomized study that took place in 10 states. Channeling was tested in two forms—a basic model wherein the case managers brokered services, and a "financial control model," wherein the case managers were able to spend a proportion of the costs of nursing home care in purchase of services for their clients. Neither model showed marked beneficial effects on use of institutions or other client outcomes, and, as expected, the financial control model was more expensive than the basic model (Carcagno and Kemper 1988).

Analysts now realize that the case management and community services had been imperfectly targeted. Some clients were unlikely ever to enter nursing homes, or unlikely to generate high costs through long stays in nursing homes. Not all people disabled enough to be eligible for nursing home care actually use it—for every person in a nursing home several equally disabled persons reside in the community. Furthermore, for some older people, nursing home care is cheaper than home care (Kane and Kane 1987). The break-even point at which public costs of maintaining a person at home equals that of maintaining a person in a nursing home depends on 1) the amount of service that the older person needs; 2) the amount of volunteered family care and privately purchased care available to meet that need; 3) the extent to which the housing costs and living expenses of the community dweller are publicly subsidized; and 4) the price established for both community care and nursing home care (Weissert et al. 1988).

Thus, the direct substitution of home care for nursing home care proved an oversimplistic and largely illusory goal, especially in the artificial context of a time-limited demonstration project (Kane 1988b). Nonetheless, community-based long-term care is a worthwhile goal in its own right, and case management seems to be a necessary element to use community-care benefits parsimoniously and equitably. The Omnibus Budget Reconciliation Act of 1981 (OBRA) for the first time created Medicaid waivers (2176 waivers) that permitted states to develop operational (i.e., nondemonstration) programs of community-based long-term care. Case management is a part of almost all the waivers granted thus far. The move from "project" to "program" presents an opportunity to use case management to reshape the incentives of all community care providers and to upgrade the quality of services. Some states are well under way in the process of using 2176 waivers to develop statewide approaches to community-based long-term care. At about the same time, the Robert Wood Johnson Foundation financed a demonstration effort to encourage hospitals to undertake case management and community-based long-term care (Capitman et al. 1987).

Meanwhile, the several decades of experience with demonstration projects under Medicare and Medicaid waivers (including some multi-site projects like Channeling) vastly increased collective experience with case management programs under a variety of auspices and programmatic conditions. These include hospitals, area agencies on aging, health departments, and social service agencies (Capitman 1986; Capitman et al. 1986; Pelham and Clark 1986; Miller 1988; Phillips et al. 1988). A considerable body of conventional wisdom has emerged about the best ways of organizing case management for particular purposes—for example, approaches to care planning (Schneider 1987) or to assisting clients when they are in the hospital (Peters 1986). Various groups have attempted to promulgate standards for training and performance of case managers (National Council on Aging 1988). The question of standards and "best approaches" is confounded. Over the years, various professional groups, health care providers, and community agencies have developed a vested interest in case management. The multiplicity of organizations doing case management in many communities led a consortium of foundations headed by the Commonwealth Fund and the Pew Memorial Trust to fund a series of 22 nationwide demonstration projects designed to improve the overall system of managed care within large United States cities (Hughes and Weissert 1987). Essentially, these projects strive to coordinate the coordinators (that is, the case managers) with the goal of eliminating duplication, filling gaps, or reaching hard-to-reach clientele.

Case management projects described thus far have attempted to rationalize and coordinate services across agencies. At the same time, parallel efforts have developed to create consolidated service organizations that, on a capitated payment basis, provide both acute and long-term care for enrollees. The Social Health Maintenance Organizations (S/HMOs) are the best known of these efforts: The service agency receives an annual sum from the Medicare program for each enrollee plus an enrollment fee. In exchange, the agency provides all benefits available under Medicare and other needed services from a list of expanded long-term care benefits. Case managers employed by the S/HMOs are responsible for screening to identify people from the pool of members who need the additional services. They undertake comprehensive assessments, develop care plans, implement the plans (including purchase of service), and monitor the services (Leutz et al., 1985). Like other case managers, those in the S/HMOs combine an advocacy and a gatekeeping function, the latter actively focused on keeping a provider organization which is at financial risk in the black rather than on making the most of a fixed Medicaid or other allocation. Finally, most proposals for long-term care insurance also have a case management component to determine whether the beneficiary's condition warrants the long-term care benefit and to make and implement plans. Typically, the insurance company contracts with one or more local agencies to provide these functions.

Case Management in Mental Health

Case management seems to be as much a buzz-word in mental health as it is in long-term care (Caragonne 1980; Intagliata 1982; Honnard 1985). The development of case management in mental health has followed a parallel track with similar justifications: both the frail elderly and the chronically mentally ill are considered vulnerable populations. Additionally, many of these people have intrinsic difficulties in organizing services for themselves. Both groups are served by fragmented programs characterized by gaps and duplications and confusing eligibilities. In contrast to case management for the frail elderly which was seen as a route to preventing unnecessary or premature institutionalization in nursing homes, case management for the chronically mentally ill was largely conceived as a corrective for a public policy that, in the 1960s, had released many chronically mentally ill patients from state mental hospitals into unprotecting and disregarding communities. Community mental health centers (CMHCs) failed to follow-up adequately with this group of hospital dischargees, who were often left with no tangible support (in the form of housing, income, or job assistance) or emotional support for community life. To some extent, psychodynamically oriented mental health professionals disparaged work with the chronically mentally ill, seeking clientele more amenable to insight and change.

Case management has been targeted largely to chronic schizophrenics or other severely and persistently mentally ill persons. For example, case management was integral to the National Institute of Mental Health's Community Support Programs (CSPs). CSPs attempted to provide support, stability, and timely service to chronically mentally ill people, thus helping them to function in the community and staving off unnecessary hospitalization (Turner and TenHoor 1982). More recently, the Robert Wood Johnson Foundation (1986) competitively awarded nine projects to serve the chronically mentally ill in American cities with populations greater than 250,000. These programs combine case management at the individual level and systems development at the community level (including promoting housing opportunities and interagency cooperation). Currently under development and evaluation, some of these projects incorporate experimental designs and even prepayment. Prepayment schemes resemble the consolidated HMO-like models emerging in long-term care, but offer less clarity about which services should be included in the capitated benefits.

Although chronic schizophrenics are the most frequent group targeted for case management in mental health, another younger population can be identified as in need of more continuity of service. Patients in this group often are chemically dependent or dually diagnosed as both mentally ill and chemically dependent. They seem to receive little help from community mental health authorities. Some separate case management programs have been developed for this particular subgroup, but are beyond the scope of this review.

In mental health, case management most often refers to a service provided by supportive, paraprofessional personnel who, by definition, do no psychotherapy. They assess, make care plans, arrange services, negotiate with payers, and sometimes purchase services. Their focus is to assist the patients in coping with reality rather than symptomatology. They may be prepared at the master's level, but more often have only bachelor's level preparation—and in a variety of fields. They are referred to as "generalists" (Intagliata 1982). With relatively small caseloads (for example, thirty), they are expected to provide continuity and a comprehensive approach to patient and family. Sometimes, they literally provide concrete services such as transportation in a rural state (Fisher et al. 1988).

A small study of case managers showed that they could indeed become extremely involved in labor-intensive work in the client's support system, and sometimes became primary support figures themselves (Baker and Weiss 1984). Shueman (1987) differentiates between a rehabilitative model of case management (wherein a more professionally trained case manager arranges therapy on a time-limited basis) and supportive case management (that is expected to continue indefinitely and where the goals are maintenance rather than rehabilitation). In either model, Shueman argues for targeting to appropriate clientele, developing mechanisms for evaluating providers, and developing an information system to track client outcomes and other data. All of this is reminiscent of case management in long-term care.

Case management in mental health differs from case management in long-term care in several ways: There is not such a strong tradition of uniform assessments with standardized assessment instruments, paraprofessionals as case managers seem to be the norm, and health services research on case management in mental health is less often done and is less sophisticated.

Some authors are skeptical about the efficacy and utility of mental health case management compared to other potential expenditures (Franklin 1988; Ashley 1988). They point to the high costs of case management, and the untested assumptions that it is helpful. Ashley questions whether a paraprofessional is capable of determining when hospitalizations or therapeutic help are needed. Citing the multiple conflicting goals of case management (advocacy, safety, and lowered costs), she argues that a paraprofessional case manager lacks the background to judge which services are needed and may act inappropriately to curb expenditures. Along the same lines, Lamb (1980) also argues for case managers who are therapists as well as brokers of services.

Two controlled studies of case management in different environments report similar unimpressive results. Franklin et al. (1987) randomized chronically mentally ill persons into an experimental group receiving case management and a control group receiving regular services. Virtually no differences were found at a one-year follow-up. However, with about half the experimental group unlocated or uninterviewed at follow-up, one cannot help but conclude that the case management implemented proved a weak intervention. Fisher et al. (1988) compared services and outcomes for those receiving and not receiving case management in rural Mississippi. They also attempted to link the outcomes to the specific activities of the case managers, the latter falling into five categories 1) assessment/treatment planning; 2) linkage/referral; 3) follow-up/monitoring; 4) advocacy; and 5) direct transportation. All case management services together accounted for less than 3% of the overall variance in patient outcomes. The hypothesis that linkage/referral and advocacy would be associated most with patient change was rejected; in fact, case managers did very little of either activity. The authors point to lack of vocational, housing, and other services to manage as a possible explanation.

Variation in Case Management Models

All of the experience with case management derived from long-term care, mental health, and other service sectors has resulted in extraordinarily varied practices. It remains for some classifier to develop a full typology of all the species and subspecies of case management. Without attempting such an exhaustive listing, case management varies in at least the following ways:

- The scope of services managed—for example, whether they cross agency and service sector lines, whether case management continues when a client is in a nursing home, and whether case managers have anything at all to do with acute-care services;
- The duration of case management—for example, some case management is construed as time-limited and cases are closed when no services are needed, whereas in other programs, case management is construed as a continuous process for persons with functional disabilities whether or not they need services.
- The amount of authority that case managers have to establish eligibility for entitlements and/or to purchase services for clients.
- The extent to which the case management is separated from or integrated with service delivery. (Some commentators feel strongly that conflicts of interest arise when agencies likely to benefit from case manager's decisions also do the case management.)
- The way case management is reimbursed. (Case management is sometimes perceived as a service for which public reimbursement and private payment should be made. In contrast, it is sometimes perceived as an administrative cost.)
- Whether case management is a single-entry or multiple-entry system—that is, whether one particular organization (geographically decentralized but administratively unified) acts as the entry point for case-managed services in a state or community, com-

pared to a system in which a variety of agencies can be delegated to perform case management functions.

- Whether the functions of case management—that is, casefinding, assessment, care planning, implementation, and monitoring are done by a single case manager or organization, or parcelled out (e.g., a hospital does the initial assessment for hospitalized patients and a home health agency for community patients, followed by assignment to different organizations for ongoing monitoring of the plans).
- The frequency and established triggers for reassessment.
- The assumptions of the program about how much family contributions will be encouraged or required before formal services are purchased.
- The extent to which the program will purchase services from private persons or untraditional vendors. (Some case management programs insist on dealing with agencies with which they hold formal contracts, whereas at the other end of the spectrum some case management programs will authorize payments to neighbors for care or transportation.)
- The intensity of personal involvement between case manager and client, which can range from a clinically significant relationship to an impersonal relationship of reviewing plans and authorizing expenditures.
- The extent to which clients' own preferences are incorporated into the plans.

Given this variation, the confusion about what case management is or should be is unsurprising. Part of the difficulty arises because the consolidating, rationalizing force inherent in a system of case management will inevitably cause dislocations for community agencies and in some cases threaten their autonomy or established modus operandi. As Havens (1986) discusses, boundary-crossing is a necessary, occupational hazard of case management. Political compromise and skirmishing for position frequently occur in the evolution of case management programs, and produce the sometimes odd configurations that exist. Other dilemmas arise over how the case managers should balance the responsibility for ensuring high quality of service with the challenge of giving clients the flexible kind of care they want—and at reasonable prices. Relying on agencies defers the responsibility for quality to another organization, but can lead to less flexible, more expensive patterns of care. The appropriate stance of case management to a client's family is another delicate issue. Seltzer and Mayer (1987) describe an approach in which they train family members to act as case managers.

This could potentially lead to cost-effective and high quality service, but care must be taken to respect client autonomy and confidentiality in the process. When clients are intellectually competent, it is questionable whether their family members should be put in the role of their case managers.

Elderly Neuropsychiatric Patients

Who Are They?

This long preamble leads to considering old people with mental health problems, and their need for case management. Distinct populations can be identified:

- Chronically mentally ill old people, most of whom experienced onset of psychiatric symptoms when younger;
- Old people with irreversible senile dementia, attributable to Alzheimer's disease and other disorders;
- Old people with treatable psychiatric disorders such as severe reactive depression or a range of less severe diagnoses;
- Old people without cognitive impairment living in settings where they are deprived of privacy, stimulation, and even identity, a description that characterizes life in too many United States nursing homes. (These old people are likely to become withdrawn, lethargic, and depressed as a normal rather than pathological reaction to severe stress.)

With groups as divergent as these, no single approach to case management is likely to be useful, nor is it likely that all persons falling under the broad heading of old people with neuropsychiatric problems would benefit by case management at all. On the other hand, some groups—particularly the chronically mentally ill and those with advanced or mid-stage senile dementia—are precisely the kind of vulnerable groups for whom case management makes sense.

How Are Elderly Neuropsychiatric Patients Served?

There is widespread agreement that the elderly have not been well served by mental health programs (Light et al. 1986). Despite the high prevalence of depression and anxiety among people over 65 (and often with first onset after age 65), organized mental health services (both CMHCs and private practitioners) see fewer older people than would be expected given their representation in the population. Despite the large number of interpersonal problems experienced by older people or couples and their adult children, they are less likely to be seen in family therapy than younger clients and families. Ageism and therapeutic nihilism about the likelihood for change in the old have contributed to this imbalance.

The separation of service jurisdictions also has been a problem. Typically, CMHCs have had little interaction with aging programs run under the Older Americans Act—although this is changing. Typically, too, mental health services for nursing home residents have been limited to very perfunctory consultation, without recognition of the heterogeneity of neuropsychiatric problems found in nursing homes—some of which are amenable to individual therapies and approaches and some to environmental change (Kane 1986). Model programs of outreach to nursing homes (e.g., Gurian 1982) have been few and far between. Describing services for persons with senile dementia, Kane (1986) pointed out that the client could have a very different service trajectory depending on whether he or she first came to the attention of a medical program, a mental health program, an aging program, or a social service program (such as adult protective services). Ideally, one would like to see that client routed to whatever diagnostic, treatment, and supportive programs are most suited to his/her needs.

In 1986, NIMH established Community Support Program Grants for the elderly (Community Services Systems Branch 1986). The 16 projects funded under this initiative are designed to develop and test model programs to better serve elderly neuropsychiatric patients. Case management is a feature of all the projects, but a review of program descriptions suggests that little else is constant. Target groups vary, from inner city, single-room occupancy dwellers and "skid-row" populations to isolated rural elders to ethnic minority group members who have typically underutilized mental health services. Lead agencies involved at the local level include hospitals, CMHCs, home care agencies, day care centers, nursing homes, housing units, and a variety of others. In some instances, the emphasis is on training indigenous paraprofessional personnel. Diagnostic targeting seems to lean toward schizophrenics and other persons with early onset chronic mental illness, but some projects are earmarked to address senile dementia. Although a very useful set of programs for model development, this demonstration seems to illustrate the lack of consensus about the priorities in mental health programming for the elderly and the appropriate target groups. Even the age definition of elderly mentally ill is unclear. Some projects include people in their 50s as part of their "aging" clientele.

With the increased attention to Alzheimer's disease and other dementias (largely a result of the effective educational work of the

Alzheimer's Disease and Related Disorders Association [ADRDA], some authorities propose a specialized system of case management, linkage, and referral designed especially for Alzheimer's disease. Advocates of this approach point out that traditional service systems have failed the people with senile dementia (U.S. Congress 1987). At present, the Office of Technology Assessment is preparing recommendations for the United States Congress about an improved service system for senile dementia. It is too early to judge the position of the report. My own view is that persons with Alzheimer's disease are a subset of those needing health services and long-term care. They are likely to be disadvantaged if they are isolated in a separate system. On the other hand, this population provides the most severe test of the effectiveness of a service system. Case-managed long-term care programs should be judged by how well they can meet the needs of those with senile dementia. Referrals for specialized diagnostic workups and services should be readily available (Kane 1985).

Conclusion

Having mapped the moving terrain of case management in health and human services and described the multiple models that have emerged in long-term care, mental health, and elsewhere, let's return to the original questions about case management for elderly neuropsychiatric patients. Without venturing definitive answers to questions about which elderly neuropsychiatric patients need case management and in what form, some guidelines for making that determination can be offered. For the sake of discussion, I propose the following:

- Not all older persons with mental health problems need case management. Elderly persons should be able to receive effective psychotherapies, drug treatment, and other mental health services in CMHCs and the private sector just as people of all ages. To ensure that this happens, systematic barriers to access and payment should be addressed, as well as any lingering attitudinal barriers on the part of mental health providers.
- Chronically mentally ill persons can probably benefit from case management, although this has not been proven yet in the research literature. Refinement of case-managed programs requires fuller consideration of target groups, the type of services that should be included in the case-managed program, and the relationship of the case manager to the primary therapist. When such problems are resolved, it seems that elderly people with

chronic mental impairments, such as schizophrenia, but without physical disability could be well-served by the same programs as their younger counterparts. Indeed they may come into old age with a case manager already in place.

- Persons with Alzheimer's disease and other dementias are probably better served through a long-term care program because inevitably patients need skilled medical services and long-term care services during the long course of their disability. Case-managed long-term care programs will need better links to legal and financial planning services and will need to eliminate arbitrary ages of eligibility to properly serve a dementia population. It will also be important for case managers to be aware of mental health needs of family caregivers for persons with dementia and to make appropriate referrals. Program rules may need to be changed to permit purchase of mental health services for these family caregivers, but surely the regular mental health system—without benefit of case management—can rise to the occasion of helping a spouse or adult child cope with the emotional toll of dementia in a loved one.
- It is important to render unto case management what belongs to case management. If service systems are unduly fragmented or hard to locate, some corrections could surely be introduced into the services themselves. And if public policy creates situations for older people where depression is the only "normal" response, those situations should be corrected before we create case management bureaucracies to handle the results.
- Any case management program for elderly neuropsychiatric patients should pay particular attention to persons in board and care homes—many of them unlicensed and most of them relatively unstaffed. This is an important target group of older people with chronic mental impairments.
- Any case management program for long-term care should attempt to integrate seniors in nursing homes into care planning. If we truly abandon the quest for "alternatives" to the nursing home, we may come to regard nursing homes as addresses where some seniors live for long periods of time and many seniors live for short periods of time. Their lives and their need for service go on. It would be useful to break down the barriers between nursing homes and the so-called community. Within this set of propositions, many researchable questions are nested. However health and human services are organized, there will always be need for collaboration. However services and benefits are constructed, no person, discipline, or organization is likely to be able to do everything to address complex human needs of persons

with longstanding dependencies, be they physical or mental. The job of case management is to ease these transitions and barriers, and to help clients negotiate the system when their own physical or mental abilities stand in their way. But case management is not a panacea for everything wrong with a service delivery system. It should never be used as a quick fix to justify the status quo and avoid improving basic service delivery patterns.

References

Ashley A: Case management: the need to define goals. Hospital and Community Psychiatry 39:499-500, 1988

Austin CD: Case management: reinventing social work? Presentation at the Professional Symposium of the National Association of Social Workers, New Orleans 1987

Austin CD: Case management components, models, and delivery system contexts, in Health Care of the Elderly. Edited by Peterson M, White D. Newbury Park, Calif, Sage Publications, 1989

Austin CD, Low J, Roberts EA, et al: Case Management: A Critical Review. Seattle, Pacific Northwest Long-Term Care Gerontology Center, University of Washington, 1985

Baker F, Weiss RS: The nature of case manager support. Hospital and Community Psychiatry 35:925-928, 1984

Caires KB, Weil M: Developmentally disabled persons and their families, in Case Management In Human Services Practice. San Francisco, Jossey-Bass, 1985

Capitman JA: Community-based long-term care models, target groups, and impacts on service use. The Gerontologist 26:389-397, 1986

Capitman JA, Haskins B, Bernstein J: Case management approaches in community-oriented long-term care demonstrations. The Gerontologist 26:398-404, 1986

Capitman J, MacAdam M, Yee D: Case management in the Robert Wood Johnson Foundation Program for Hospital Initiatives in Long-Term Care. Generations 12:62-65, 1987

Caragonne P: A Comparative Analysis of Twenty-Two Settings Using Case Management Components. Report of the Case Management Research Project, Austin, TX, 1980

Carcagno GJ, Kemper P: The evaluation of the National Long-Term Care Demonstration, 1: an overview of the channeling demonstration and its evaluation. Health Services Research 23:1-22, 1988

Christianson J: Purchase of service by case management agencies. Generations 12:19-22, 1988

Community Services Systems Branch: Summaries of Elderly Community Support Program Grants (unpublished report). Bethesda, MD, National Institute of Mental Health, December 1986

Fisher G, Landis D, Clark K: Case management service provision and client change. Community Mental Health Journal 24:143-142, 1988

Franklin JL: Case management: a dissenting view. Hospital and Community Psychiatry 39:921, 1988

Franklin JL, Solovitz B, Mason M, et al: An evaluation of case management. American Journal of Public Health 77:674-678, 1987

Gurian B: Mental health outreach and consultation services for the elderly. Hospital and Community Psychiatry 33:142-147, 1982

Harkness EG, Redford LJ, Connors JR, et al: Nursing Assessment And Management Of The Frail Elderly: A Curriculum of Eight Modules on Case Management. Third Revision. Kansas City, KS, University of Kansas School of Nursing, 1987

Haskins B, Capitman J, Bernstein J, et al: Final Report: Evaluation of Community Oriented Long-Term Care Demonstration Projects. Berkeley, CA, Berkeley Planning Associates, 1984

Havens B: Boundary Crossing: An Organizational Challenge for Community-Based Long-Term Care Service Agencies. Managing Home Care For The Elderly: Lessons from Community-Based Agencies. New York, Springer Publishing Company, 1986

Honnard R: The chronically mentally ill in the community, in Case Management in Human Services Practice. San Francisco, Jossey-Bass, 1985

Hughes S, Weissert W: Living at home: variations on a case management theme. Generations 12:66-67, 1987

Intagliata J: Improving the quality of community care for the chronically mentally disabled: the role of case management. Schizophrenia Bulletin 8:655-674, 1982

Kane RA: Toward a public policy for senile dementia, in The Dementias: Policy and Management. Edited by Gilhooley M, Birren J, Zarit S. Englewood Cliffs, NJ, Prentice-Hall, 1985

Kane RA: Mental health in nursing homes: behavioral and social research, in Mental Health in Nursing Homes: Agenda for Research. Edited by Harper MS, Lebowitz B. Washington, DC, U.S. Government Printing Office, 1986

Kane RA: Case management: ethical pitfalls on the road to high quality managed care. Quality Review Bulletin 14:161-166, 1988a

Kane RA: The noblest experiment of them all: learning from the National Channeling Demonstration. Health Services Research 23:189-198, 1988b

Kane RA, Kane RL: Long-Term Care: Principles, Programs and Policies. New York, Springer Publishing Company, 1987

Lamb HR: Therapist case managers: more than brokers of services. Hospital and Community Psychiatry 31:762-764, 1980

Leutz WN, Greenberg JN, Abrahams R, et al: Changing Health Care for an Aging Society. Lexington, MA, D. C. Heath, 1985

Light E, Lebowitz BD, Bailey F: CMHCs and elderly services: an analysis of direct and indirect services and service delivery sites. Community Mental Health Journal 22:294-302, 1986

Miller LS: Increasing efficiency in community-based, long-term care for the frail elderly. Social Work Research and Abstracts 24:7-14, 1988

National Council on the Aging: Case Management Standards: Guidelines for Practice. Washington, National Council on the Aging, 1988

Pelham AO, Clark WF: Managing Home Care for the Elderly: Lessons from Community-Based Agencies. New York, Springer Publishing Company, 1986

Peters B: The Ten Commandments of Case Management During Hospitalization: A Practice Perspective, in Managing Home Care for the Elderly: Lessons From Community-Based Agencies. New York, Springer Publishing Company, 1986

Phillips B, Kemper P, Applebaum R: The evaluation of the national long-term care demonstration, 4: case management under channeling. Health Services Research 23:67-82, 1988

Robert Wood Johnson Foundation, Program for the Chronically Mentally Ill: Program Abstracts. Princeton, NJ, Robert Wood Johnson Foundation, 1987

Schneider B: Care planning. Generations 12:16-18, 1987

Seltzer MM, Mayer JB: Families as case managers: a team approach for serving the elderly. Generations 12:26-30, 1987

Shueman SA: A Model of Case Management for Mental Health Services. Quality Review Bulletin 13:314-317, 1987

Silverstone B, Burack-Weiss A: Social Work Practice with the Frail Elderly: An Auxiliary Model. Springfield, IL, Charles C Thomas, 1983

Steinberg RM, Carter GW: Case management and the elderly. Lexington, Mass, D. C. Health, 1983

Turner J, TenHoor W: The NIMH community support program: pilot approaches to a needed social reform. Schizophrenia Bulletin 4: 655-674, 1982

Weil M, Karls JM, and Associates: Case Management in Human Service Practice. San Francisco, Jossey-Bass, 1985

Weissert WG, Cready CM, Pawelak JE: The past and future of home and community based long-term care. The Milbank Memorial Fund Quarterly 66:309-388, 1988

White M: Case management, in Encyclopedia of Aging. New York, Springer Publishing Company, 1988

U.S. Congress, Office of Technology Assessment: Losing A Million Minds. Washington, DC, U.S. Congress, 1987

Zawadski RT (ed): Community-Based Systems of Long-Term Care. New York, Haworth Press, 1984

13

Managed Care

Terrie Wetle, Ph.D.
Hal Mark, Ph.D.

The crisis of care for elderly psychiatric patients has impelled policy makers to explore new avenues for providing care. One such approach is "managed care." In this chapter we briefly review the clinical characteristics of elderly psychiatric patients, the financial and utilization data which are available based upon early managed care studies, and the applicability of various managed care tools as they apply to this population. We argue that current managed care arrangements have failed to develop any distinctive programmatic accommodations for the unique and substantial needs of the elderly mentally ill, but that future managed care arrangements may succeed in doing so. We conclude with a discussion of the issues which bear upon the likelihood that managed care may adequately serve this population. Specifically, we address the possibility of attaining operational efficiencies, improved coordination of care, the provision of a more complete array of services, and the ability to monitor quality of care.

Prevalence of Psychiatric Illness Among the Elderly

Identification of elderly persons with mental health problems is not an easy task. Few population-based studies are reported, and even fewer use methodologies which give confidence in the validity or generalizability of results (Bliwise et al. 1987; Blessed et al. 1982). Nonetheless, reviews of studies with appropriate methodologies indicate high prevalence rates for various types of mental illness and cognitive impairment among the elderly population. Details on the prevalence of mental illnesses and neuropsychiatric disorders are provided in Chapters 1 and 4.

While the prevalence rates of many individual disorders (e.g., depression) have been estimated, it is currently difficult to predict the number of elderly individuals who would benefit from mental health services (Bliwise 1987). Nineteen percent of elderly responding to a national survey indicated that they could use professional mental health assistance (Douvan et al. 1978), and it is estimated that more than 60% of the elderly with mental health care needs were not receiving treatment (Shapiro et al. 1985). Burns and Taube (in Chapter 4) offer the more conservative estimate of 37% for unmet need in the community. Overall, major issues in the treatment of mental health problems in geriatric patients are identification of patients, adequate screening and diagnosis, and access to appropriate services. Recent data indicate that elderly individuals respond well to appropriate treatments, but they may require more intensive management because of concomitant physical illnesses and increased likelihood of negative reactions to medications (Bliwise 1987; see also Chapter 3). Moreover, because of the prevalence of multiple health and social problems, elderly patients are likely to require the services from several disciplines and a number of different agencies or programs (Besdine 1988a, 1988b; Wetle 1988b).

Financing Psychiatric Care for the Elderly

As described in Chapter 5, the current system of finance for services to psychiatric patients is fragmented, complex, and very confusing (Marmor 1988; Foley and Sharfstein 1983). There is no comprehensive policy covering the geriatric mental health patient, and payment for services is provided via a noncoordinated array of federal, state, and private sources (Rice 1987; Scheffler 1985; Wetle 1988b). While many of the problems faced by geriatric patients are common to other psychiatric patients, the aged have additional concerns because of the patchwork of financing for geriatric services in general. Details of the financing system are provided by Goldman and Frank in Chapter 5, and by Sharfstein in Chapter 6. However, because of their special relevance to managed care, we will review here the distinctive features of health maintenance organizations.

Health maintenance organizations (HMOs) integrate traditional insurance and the health care delivery functions into one organization. HMOs share four basic features; 1) contractual responsibility for assuring delivery of a stated range of services, 2) a voluntarily enrolled population, 3) enrollees pay a fixed monthly payment, independent of use of services, 4) the HMO assumes financial risk or gain (Luft 1981). Based upon early plans for Los Angeles city workers in 1929 and Kaiser construction workers in the late 1930s, the Federal HMO Act (P.L. 93-222) was passed in 1973. There are three models of HMOs. In the Staff/Group model the

HMO employs physicians to provide services exclusively to plan enrollees. In the Closed Panel model, physicians contract to provide services to enrollees on a capitated basis but may serve other patients as well. In the Independent Practice Association (IPA) model, physicians work in their own settings but bill the IPA on a discounted fee-for-service or capitated basis (Luft 1981).

It has been argued that HMOs achieve cost savings as compared to the fee-for-service system, and that these cost savings are based on several factors (Luft 1978). First, because physicians are not paid for each unit of service performed, there is no financial incentive to overprovide service. Second, there is a financial incentive to maintain the health of enrollees, and thereby decrease utilization (Arnould 1984). Also, because there is an opportunity to "manage care," it is possible that cost savings would accrue by the substitution of less expensive for more expensive services (e.g., outpatient for inpatient, or lower-paid health professionals for physicians) (Bonanno and Wetle 1984). Indeed, experience indicates that major cost savings are achieved primarily through reductions in hospital utilization, which is 15 to 40% less than in a fee-for-service system (Luft 1981). Although it has been argued that these savings were attributable to the enrollment of healthier populations into HMOs, a randomized study comparing the cost and utilization experience of HMOs and various fee-for-service plans suggests that annual expenditures, hospital admission rates, and total hospital days were significantly lower in HMOs compared to the fee-for-service plans, even when controlling for the health status of patients (Manning et al. 1984).

Although some Medicare beneficiaries were enrolled in prepaid health plans in the 1960s, the plans were reimbursed only for Part B services on a noncapitated basis (Iglehart 1985). Since 1972, Medicare has permitted direct, capitated prepayment to Health Maintenance Organizations (HMOs) for both Part A and Part B. In 1982 Congress, in the Tax Equity and Fiscal Responsibility Act (TEFRA), authorized that prepaid care be available to all elders by amending the Social Security Act to allow prospective capitation payments at 95% of the average Medicare costs for Medicare beneficiaries of the same age and sex living in that community (Schlesinger and Wetle 1988). By June of 1986, 132 HMOs had enrolled 630,000 Medicare beneficiaries on a prepaid basis (Ellwood 1986).

There are several potential advantages to enrolling Medicare beneficiaries into HMOs. Cost containment could lead to overall savings to the Medicare program, as well as to improve services to the elderly, if indeed savings are converted into added benefits. In the past, when such cost savings have occurred, HMOs have chosen either to reduce copayment requirements for enrollees or to cover ancillary medical expenses such as for eyeglasses, dental care, or prescription drugs (Iglehart 1985; Rossiter et al. 1985; Ellwood 1986). Moreover, the centralized record-keeping and administrative systems of HMOs provide enhanced opportunities for improved case management, particularly for elderly patients with chronic diseases and multiple health problems (Bonanno and Wetle 1984). Unfortunately, although some HMOs have developed case-management systems for Medicare enrollees, most Medicare HMOs programs have fallen short of developing systems particularly suited to the needs of the elderly (Iversen and Polich 1985; Schlesinger 1986). Special demonstrations of "enhanced" HMOs such as the Social/Health Maintenance Organization (S/HMO) projects supported by HCFA over the past several years indicate that it is possible to develop models of care with a broad array of needed services, but that such models are likely to have substantial start-up costs (Greenberg et al. 1988) (see Chapter 10 for details of the S/HMO and related plans).

Mental Health Benefits and Utilization in Prepaid Plans

Few data exist regarding the use of psychiatric services, in particular by HMO Medicare enrollees (Rossiter et al. 1988), but studies of general HMO enrollee utilization are informative. Federally certified HMOs are required to provide short-term (not to exceed 20 visits) outpatient evaluative and crisis intervention mental health services; and medical treatment and referral services for alcohol and drug problems. In comparing the annual mean HMO physical and mental health service utilization costs for years 1978 and 1982, Levin and colleagues (1988) showed that across the 304 responding HMOs, coverage for HMO mental health services has remained relatively constant (median mental health benefits remained at 30 hospital days per member/year and 20 ambulatory visits per member/year). Turning to utilization, while mean general hospital days and number of admissions decreased (446 days versus 375 days/1,000 members and 87 admissions versus 74 admissions/1,000 members), hospital admissions and days for mental health services increased during the 4-year period (32 days versus 37 days/1,000 members and 3.00 versus 3.27 admissions/1,000 members). Use of both general ambulatory encounters (about 4.4 per member) and mental health ambulatory services (about 0.3 encounters per member) remained constant over the study period (Levin 1988).

Developing a clear understanding of HMO utilization is complicated by the observation that patients with higher levels of general health service utilization are more likely to report psychiatric or mental health symptoms (McFarland et al. 1985), but are not likely to be treated for mental illness. If offered, treatment is by nonspecialists (Freeborn et al., in press). Focusing simply on psychiatric services within the HMO will provide a biased underestimate of overall service use by patients with mental health service needs. Moreover, these data suggest that a more comprehensive approach to management of these patients might result in more appropriate trade-offs among services (see Chapter 8 on cost-offsets).

Managed Care Problems with the Elderly Mentally Ill

We will use the term *managed care* broadly to refer to several varieties of alternative delivery systems. This definition includes organizational arrangements such as PPOs or IPAs, as well as managed care "tools" such as precertification or case management. The "managed care revolution" as it has recently been called (Health Affairs 1988), is likely to have a significant impact upon the elderly mentally ill much as it will other populations requiring health care services. All of the various forms of managed care, however, will not be equally applicable to elderly psychiatric patients.

Some managed care tools and techniques encounter specific difficulties when applied to psychiatric patients. One such tool is diagnostic-related groups (DRGs) which have proven to be such a poor predictor of length of psychiatric stay that they have been waivered from the system (Schumacher et al. 1986). The fact that the DRGs don't "work" when applied to psychiatric care has attracted the attention of many health service researchers and brought forth a variety of proposed substitutions for the DRG system (Frank et al. 1986). In the absence of an applicable DRG system, psychiatric inpatient costs have gone up by as much as 30% a year and at least one major payer (CHAMPUS) is proposing a nationwide flat per diem rate as a substitute for psychiatric DRGs (Medicine and Health, July 18 1988). Provider representatives fear that the CHAMPUS system may be adopted by other payers and use words such as "disastrous" to describe its potential effect. It is impossible to anticipate what form of prospective payment system will be adopted for psychiatric services. Those who provide inpatient psychiatric care, however, should not assume that the current DRG exemption they enjoy will last forever. Annual increases of 30% generate a "something has to be done" mentality which could lead to the adoption of an imperfect or inequitable system.

Precertification is another managed care arrangement which is growing in importance for general medical admissions. However, it has been of little value in limiting unnecessary psychiatric admissions, because of frequent difficulties in obtaining objective diagnostic data regarding both the specific diagnosis and the severity of illness for psychiatric admissions. As a consequence, there is seldom sufficient justification for denying an admission. For this reason, it is doubtful that precertification will ever become a major factor in psychiatric care.

Related to precertification procedures are concurrent review programs. This cost containment technique is applied after the patient is admitted and is intended to save money by reducing the length of stay. A recent large scale study of the effects of utilization review programs on general medical services concluded that these efforts reduce inpatient days by 8% and hospital costs by almost 12% (Feldstein et al. 1988). Such efforts, however, are contentious and adversarial and are increasingly controversial. In a recent statement before the Institute of Medicine, the American Hospital Association noted that the Mayo Clinic must now respond to more than 1,000 private review agencies (American Hospital Association 1988). They went on to comment that "Using the utilization review function to camouflage arbitrary coverage restrictions can lead to clinical standards set by insurance agents rather than by qualified clinicians, raising serious questions about the effect of external utilization review on access to and delivery of needed care" (American Hospital Association 1988). Concurrent review procedures applied to psychiatric patients suffer from the same data deficiencies which hinder precertification efforts. Similarly, retrospective reviews and claims audits are of little value because psychiatrists leave few tracks, (i.e., unlike a "medical" admission wherein the record will contain lab reports, x-rays, etc., there is often little in the record of a psychiatric patient which is useful for the purpose of assessing the adequacy of the care provided or the necessity of the number of days of hospitalization). Nonetheless, Medicare through its fiscal intermediaries continues to review patient charts looking for "key phrases" which indicate the necessity for continued hospitalization.

Case management is also an important managed care tool with particular relevance for the elderly psychiatric patient. Unfortunately, the term "case management" has been used to describe several different functions. In the private sector, case management may refer to a concurrent review function which is intended to save money through "gatekeeping" (American Hospital Association 1988). Alternatively, it may refer to the direct, hands-on coordination of services for a seriously ill, high cost patient. In the public sector, case management takes on a quite different meaning. Here, it usually refers to the management of a patient who is living in the community but needs help. This public sector form has been referred to as "aggressive case management" or even "outpatient commitment" (Wines 1988). Even greater confusion occurs when these public sector case management functions are referred to as "advocacy" which may come into direct conflict with other responsibilities such as gatekeeping (Wetle 1988a). Notwithstanding the multiple definitions, several functions of case management are important tools of managed care and are particularly relevant to any chronically ill population including the elderly mentally ill. The full therapeutic potential of case management is achieved when it is bundled together with the provision of services, with a focus on management for the patient rather than for the provider (see Chapter 12 for a detailed and scholarly analysis of these issues).

In addition to these managed care tools, a variety of organizational arrangements are also part of the "managed care revolution." Some of these hybrids such as IPAs, open-end HMOs, and what are coming to be called "modified indemnity" plans are not likely to be as relevant for the elderly mentally ill, given their focus on acute care and general medical-surgical services. Serving the elderly mentally ill requires a greater specialization of staffing and/or subcontracts, neither of which is attractive unless a large enough number of enrollees are involved to permit achieving economies of scale. Typically, these organizations operate in a highly competitive environment focused on enrollment of persons who are under the age of 65 and employed. A second reason for excluding the more loosely constituted alternative delivery systems is that as organizations, they represent more of a marketing alliance than a focal point for an effective management control function. In the absence of a credible management control capability, it is not likely that such organizations would deal effectively with either the chronicity of the elderly population or their multiple needs. The managed care entities which are most likely to be successful in serving the elderly mentally ill are those which are prepared to bundle together the services which are required along with the management of those services. This distinction is an important one in that the elderly mentally ill are not likely to be informed buyers on their own.

Two examples of such arrangements are staff model HMO or a PPO sponsored by a large hospital. Either would have the size and diversity of staff to make the type of broad-based commitment that would be required to adequately serve this population. Smaller, less specialized, managed care entities are more likely to concentrate on managing costs rather than meeting specific patient care needs and, as a result, would probably have quality and underservice problems.

A rapidly growing managed care trend relative to specialty services is known as a "carve out" arrangement. The services involved (e.g., pharmacy, rehabilitation, mental health services) need to be of the kind that are easily separated from the balance of the health care benefit. A carve out usually involves a discount in exchange for priority or sole access to an enrolled population. To the provider it is a way to maintain market share, census, and revenue. To the employer and the beneficiaries, it represents an acceptable compromise with the needs of cost containment in that some free choice of provider is exchanged for cost savings.

For the elderly mentally ill "carve outs" may offer an important advantage, a greater likelihood to receive more specialized care. To the provider entity which holds the carve out contract, serving the needs of the enrolled population efficiently is the difference between making and losing money. Elderly beneficiaries with chronic psychiatric problems are at risk for recurrent hospitalizations. A well designed program to maintain the stability and health status of this population could easily pay for itself in the context of a carve out arrangement (Lurie 1987).

There have, however, been concerns raised regarding psychiatric "carve outs." One such problem is the potential loss of coordination between the more traditional medical services and the psychiatric services offered via carve out arrangements. This may be a particular problem for elderly patients, who are more likely to have comorbidities, and who are more likely to suffer adverse drug reactions. These reactions may involve negative responses to psychotropic medications or cognitive or behavioral changes as a result of physical illness or the treatments for such illnesses.

The managed care movement, in general, has other problems specific to the elderly. A high variation in the estimates of the cost of care for individual elderly patients results in capitation pricing problems. Estimates of cost which vary too widely increase the risk which is assumed by providers and decrease their willingness to enter into such arrangements. Secondly, the elderly mentally ill require substantial social support services. In the past, it has been uncommon for "health care dollars" to be used to pay for social services. However, in the long run, if the needs they represent are not met, greater "medical" cost may be incurred (Wetle and Pearson 1986). Multiple year capitation arrangements may create incentives to bundle together social services and medical care. A third problem derives from the fact that the elderly suffer comorbidities more frequently than a younger population and this adds to the problem of cost estimation. A possible solution may be to "split off" the top 5% of catastrophically ill patients and negotiate a separate, more flexible, financial arrangement specifically for these patients. This would have the effect of keeping the per member per month rate lower and more stable for the other 95% of the population.

Structural Problems with Benefit Coordination

With multiple payer sources competing for the prerogative of "last dollar coverage," the elderly and mentally ill population faces major problems with benefit coordination and cost shifting. The locus of financial responsibility for the elderly, particularly the elderly mentally ill, has never been clear, and as policies come and go, (e.g., deinstitutionalization) this responsibility is constantly shifting. A century ago the mentally ill elderly lived out their years on county poor farms. Then, until the mid 1950s, they resided in state hospitals. As the state hospitals responded to "Community Mental Health" (and the growing availability of neuroleptic drugs), the elderly mentally ill migrated to skilled nursing facilities (Koran and Sharfstein 1986). Now because of a new interpretation of an old Medicaid regulation (relating to "institutions for mental diseases") the number of elderly with primary psychiatric diagnoses is decreasing (Ready 1989). Where they will go next is unclear and, sadly, many of them are on the streets. Private sector support for the services required by this population is equally muddled. Many have no coverage at all once they reach the age of 65; others have some coverage "coordinated" with Medicare; and only the most fortunate have substantial major medical coverage which goes well beyond Medicare.

Two significant limitations characterize all private sector coverage for mental illness. These are annual or lifetime benefit limitations and significant copayment restrictions, typically limited to half of the cost of the service. Retirees who are fortunate enough to have some continuing coverage may soon feel the hot breath of managed care due to a change in the standardized rules of accounting relating to the liability of self-insured companies (Karamon 1988). The Financial Accounting Standards Board (FASB) now requires that a company's liability for the cost of retiree health care benefits be reflected on the annual balance sheet as a deduction from assets. Previously, such obligations were recognized only in the year in which expenditures occurred. The FASB however has reasoned that, inasmuch as these expenses represent a claim against company assets, they should be documented on the books as such. This seemingly minor accounting change has increased attention to the growing private sector responsibility for post-retirement health care costs in particular, and to the cost of health care services for the elderly more generally. Despite the level of private coverage, elderly chronic mentally ill inevitably "graduate" into the public sector. The entire question of funding responsibility for this population is hopelessly confused, yet any effective long-term improvement will require coordination and focusing of financial resources.

The EPO Model and Risk-Based Management Incentives

We have argued that the special needs and characteristics of the elderly mentally ill limit the applicability of most managed care arrangements. In this section, we will suggest that if managed care concepts are to be successfully used in serving this population three criteria must be met: 1) Services and their management must be bundled together; 2) There is a utilization management capacity sufficient for the provider to assume a full service at-risk responsibility; and 3) Provision must be made for social support services.

The incentive for preventive and wellness programs resides in the fact that the exclusive provider organization (EPO) is at risk over time. In the context of this type of financial arrangement, any acute care expenses which might have been avoided by "preventive services" represent an instance of bad management.

The staffing pattern for the EPO, the affiliations, subcontracts, programs, etc. are all to be determined by the EPO. The objective of risk-based case management is to create an environment in which caregivers will be innovative and creative, but will also be aware of the cost implications of their decisions. What structural and organizational arrangements work best will depend upon the needs of the population contracted for and the resources which the EPO has available to it.

EPOs can be any kind of organization with sufficient clinical and fiscal capability to be a creditable contractor. Most potential EPOs will be either hospitals or have existing contractual arrangements with hospitals. However, regardless of what general arrangements exist, when a patient who is covered by the provisions of a risk-based EPO contract needs to be hospitalized, the EPO makes every effort to retain full control. In this context, the hospital is a subcontractor providing only a portion of the care for which the EPO is responsible. If the hospital in question is not a part of the EPO structure, then the patients will be referred there only so long as the EPO is satisfied with the hospital's performance.

The elderly mentally ill have needs that are complex, multifaceted, on-going, and likely to change over time. There is a much greater likelihood of continuity in the provision of needed services if a single organization has responsibility for provision. By creating linkage between the provision of services and the responsibility for the management of those services, the current fragmentation of an unmanaged fee-for-service system can be addressed. In addition to having a focal point of organizational responsibility, it is also necessary to have a management function, sufficient to accept risk-based contractual arrangements. As previously noted, many so-called managed care plans are only loosely conceived marketing and claims processing arrangements with, perhaps, a token utilization review program tacked on. There is not a sufficient degree of management control in these sorts of arrangements, as many insolvent IPAs have discovered. For this reason loosely constituted managed care arrangements, while quite common, are not likely to meet the needs of a difficult-to-serve population. Finally, for the elderly with psychiatric problems, medical and hospital care alone is not sufficient. The provider with a contract responsibility to serve this population must be prepared to offer a range of social support and health-related services. Traditional limitations on benefits are penny-wise and pound-foolish. Elderly mentally ill beneficiaries who receive adequate medical care but then deteriorate due to isolation or poor nutrition will inevitably require additional, and avoidable, medical and/or hospital services. Given the high expense of these intrusive interventions, it is likely that the net cost is greater than if an adequate range of services had been provided in the first place.

The type of managed care "plan" most likely to meet these criteria is an EPO (Finney 1985). The EPO "arrangement" involves a marketing/management trade-off wherein the provider organization gains exclusive access to a defined population in exchange for assuming the financial risk of a discounted fixed price per enrollee. The beneficiary is "locked in" and any unauthorized out-of-plan service must be paid for out-of-pocket. The EPO, however, is locked-in, as well, in that they assume full financial responsibility to provide for the needs of the (enrolled) population. The unique applicability of the EPO arrangement as it applies to the elderly mentally ill lies in the incentive to serve all of the needs of covered beneficiaries since to do otherwise is likely to be more costly in the long run.

As with other capitation agreements, EPO contracts would have to be carefully monitored since certain "perverse" incentives could lead to underservice. Such reviews of quality and appropriateness of care could be made the centerpiece of annual contract renegotiations. EPOs with an investment in staff and facilities (as well as a desired continuity in service) will wish to "look good" in order to maintain volume and cash flow and therefore focus attention on quality of care. This incentive for contract renewals may counterbalance the tendency to save money by underserving the enrollees. This "assumption," however, will remain only a hopeful expectation until its validity is established in carefully designed demonstration projects.

Although all elderly might benefit from these proposals, the seriously mentally ill are the target group for the demonstration project described below. Such a demonstration project would require the following: a financially credible provider organization willing to accept at-risk arrangements, the identification of a cohort of elderly mentally ill who could be expected to benefit from the proposed arrangement, and an agreement on the part of insurance companies and other payers to pool their resources and contract exclusively with the EPO. In addition, it would be necessary to constitute an independent evaluation component. The evaluation would address the following questions: Is it possible to better serve the elderly mentally ill without increased costs by bundling services over time on an at-risk basis? Is 12 months an appropriate time period to create the intended clinical and administrative incentives while keeping the financial risk at an acceptable level? What factors are associated with the greatest variation in year-to-year cost estimations? And, what strategies (e.g., alternative levels of care) are adopted by the EPO to fulfill its service delivery responsibility within the limits of the contracted level of funding? A significant by-product of the demonstration would be the development of cost estimating methodologies specific to the types of services required by the elderly mentally ill.

Some Reasons for Optimism

Overall we are hopeful that the elderly psychiatric population can benefit from "the managed care revolution" (Health Affairs 1988). This optimistic outlook is based upon several factors. First, although Medicare is a major player relative to health care services for the elderly, it does not now adequately serve the needs of the mentally ill elderly. However, policy options are being discussed which could benefit this population albeit indirectly (e.g., expanded funding for home health care) (Greenberg et al. 1988). For the elderly mentally ill to benefit directly from Medicare reforms, resolution of the confusion regarding which level of government should be financially responsible for this population is necessary. Shifting of patients (and costs) from one public payer to another will continue until there is clear public policy coordinating state and federal service payment. One approach to addressing this dilemma is suggested by the On Lok demonstrations which "pool" public monies from Medicare, Medicaid, and state funds. A similar demonstration which pooled mental health funds and general financing to contract for services with a managed care entity could be designed. Quality of care, coordination of services, cost, and quality of life indicators would all require monitoring, but if favorable, such a demonstration would suggest that it is possible to better serve this population by re-bundling services and funding.

Secondly, there is a possibility that the elderly mentally ill could benefit from the developing political interest in the "catastrophically ill." HR 2470 liberalized payment for outpatient prescription drugs, but continued the exclusion of psychiatric hospitals and nursing homes relative to the new hospital benefit which, after a $564 deductible, provided unlimited free care (Anonymous 1988). However, more than 30 other "catastrophic health care" bills have been introduced in Congress, and such financing was an issue in the 1988 election campaign. Again, the issue of state versus federal responsibility for the mentally ill has to be addressed, but if managed care options can prove to be an effective way to serve special populations with expensive and continuing needs, then EPO contracts may be incorporated into some of these proposals.

A third factor which may generate managed care options relative to the elderly is contained in a little-known change in the standardized rules for accounting proposed by the Financial Accounting Standards Board (FASB). The new FASB rules would require employers to include in their day-to-day budgeting (and annual reports) the cost of future retiree health care benefits as opposed to the current rules which only report the responsibility for the current year (Coile 1988). The proposed changes are serving to focus a new attention on retiree health care benefits (Karamon 1988). Certainly, not all of the elderly mentally ill have this coverage but renewed efforts to manage the costs incurred by retirees may indirectly benefit the mentally ill, particularly if managed care options of the kind we have discussed are brought to bear on this new "problem."

Finally, and most importantly, the needs of the elderly mentally ill are ongoing and continuous. Many of the mental illnesses of the elderly are chronic or reoccurring. We have suggested that those cost containment technologies which "work best" with a chronically ill population are those which require attention to continuity of care and a liberally defined spectrum of services. Managed care arrangements are far more likely to develop this broader focus of care than traditionally organized systems which concentrate upon acute care and episodes of illness. The state hospitals or nursing homes, which managed care plans could conceivably replace, have dealt with the needs of chronically ill patients, but they have been paid by days and visits similar to an acute care population. Managed care, together with the growing pressures to find new solutions, has the potential to change this, by offering new incentives to avoid or shorten institutional stays.

Problems and Concerns

By introducing a centralized organizational focus and a management control function, it is assumed that inefficiencies will be reduced and the money saved can be redirected to other services such as social supports. This assumption needs to be tested. It may well be that even if the management function is superior, we may discover that the inefficiencies counted upon to provide the "margin" are not there. The argument can be made that there is a basic underutilization of long-term psychiatric services (Frisman et al. 1989). If this is so, then there is little "fat" in the system and it is unlikely that any amount of management oversight will be able to attain the expected efficiencies. To some extent, this issue is being tested in the social HMO demonstration projects. It may well turn out that for the elderly and chronically ill (because they are underserved to begin with) access to more and better services will cost more money regardless of how they are organized, managed, or delivered.

Secondly, there are valid concerns about what has been termed the "woodwork" effect (i.e., that as more social support services are made available, more recipients "appear" to take advantage of them). There are limited data on the cost and cost potential of social support services. If an EPO, motivated by an at-risk arrangement, seeks to cut total costs by spending more on social supports, can cost-efficient trade-offs occur between social services and other more expensive care or is the social support budget an ever-thirsty "sponge"? This is a serious concern, which like the cost/efficiency issue discussed above, needs to be addressed by well-designed demonstration projects. The available secondary source data regarding social support costs are flawed in many ways. The pertinent data are not integrated, and there are too many separate "providers" to allow efficient coordination. Many social service "transactions" are never recorded, and, of those that are, the cost data tend to be inadequate because such services are typically highly subsidized. If funds were available to pay the "true" cost of social services it may well be that the total would be much greater than the estimated costs we have available to us now. Again, appropriately designed demonstration projects are required to explore this issue.

Finally, risk assumption arrangements of the kind discussed here inevitably generate some incentives that can result in under-service (Schlesigner 1986). Revenue is fixed by contractual agreement; therefore, any services which can be withheld represent costs which are avoided particularly in the short run. For this reason it is essential to build in clinically effective quality assurance mechanisms. The incentive to renew contracts may serve to assure quality of care, however, an independent assessment would be useful to insure that this is not a simply "targeted minimum." Here as well, much could be learned from a demonstration project. Having a closed management loop and longitudinal data would provide a unique opportunity to develop quality measures which would go beyond the episode-of-care based measures which are common today. Quality of life, patient satisfaction, and medical cost offset data could also be developed in the context of an EPO demonstration project.

Summary and Conclusion

Elderly Americans suffer from mental illnesses which are quite likely to go untreated or to be treated by less than appropriate care. Because of factors associated with retirement, lifetime benefit limitations, and biases within the system, elderly patients migrate from an acute care, medically based health services system to one which is badly fragmented, underfunded, lacking in coordination, and more oriented to custody than to treatment. There is agreement that something must be done, and that the current system of care has failed the elderly psychiatric patient. It is possible that the options discussed herein offer opportunities to improve quality of care while responsibly managing costs of those services.

References

American Hospital Association: Statement on Private Utilization Review Before the Institute of Medicine. Washington, DC, June 6, 1988

Anonymous: Mentally ill should benefit from newly passed Medicare Catastrophic Bill. Psychiatric News, July 1, 1988

Arnould R: Do HMOs produce services more efficiently? Inquiry 21:3, 1984

Besdine RW: Clinical approach to the elderly patient, in Geriatric Medicine. Edited by Rowe JW, Besdine RW. Boston, Little, Brown, 1988a

Besdine RW: Dementia and delirium, in Geriatric Medicine. Edited by Rowe JW, Besdine RW. Boston, Little, Brown, 1988b

Blessed G, Wilson ID: The contemporary history of mental disorder in old age. British Journal of Psychiatry 141:59-67, 1982

Bliwise NG: The psychotherapeutic effectiveness of treatments for psychiatric illness in late life, in Serving the Mentally Ill Elderly. Edited by Lurie EE, Swan JH. Lexington, MA, D. C. Heath and Company, 1987

Bliwise NG, McCall ME, Swan S: The epidemiology of mental illness in late life, in Serving the Mentally Ill Elderly. Edited by Lurie EE, Swan JH. Lexington, MA, D. C. Heath and Company, 1987

Bonanno JB, Wetle TW: HMO enrollment of Medicare recipients: an analysis of incentives and barriers. Journal of Health Politics, Policy and Law 9:41-62, 1984

Coile RC: Managed care may be only solution to crisis in retiree benefits. Managed Care Outlook 1:1-3, 1988

Douvan E, Kulka R, Veroff J: Study of modern living, 1976: Report to respondents. Ann Arbor, MI, Institute for Social Research, University of Michigan, 1978

Ellwood DA: Medicare risk contracting: promise and problems. Health Affairs 5:183-189, 1986

Feldstein PJ, Wickizew TM, Wheeler JC: The effects of utilization review programs on health care use and expenditures. The New England Journal of Medicine 318:1310-1314, 1988

Finney RD: Today's medicine buyer: a change from the last to know and the first to pay, in The New Healthcare Market: A Guide to PPOs for Purchasers, Payors and Providers. Edited by Boaland P. Homewood, IL, Dow Jones-Irwin, 1985

Foley HA, Sharfstein SS: Madness in Government: Who Cares for the Mentally Ill. Washington, DC, American Psychiatric Press, 1983

Freeborn DK, Pope CR, Mullooly J, et al: Consistently high users of medical care among the elderly. Portland, Ore, Center for Health Research, Kaiser Permanente (in press)

Frerichs RR, Aneshensel CS, Clark VA: Prevalence of depression in Los Angeles County. American Journal of Epidemiology 113:267-271, 1981

Frisman LK, McGuire TC: The economics of long-term care for the mentally ill. Journal of Social Issues 45:119-130, 1989

Greenberg J, Leutz W, Greenlick M, et al: The social HMO demonstration: early experience. Health Affairs 7:66-79, 1988

Health Affairs (entire volume devoted to managed care), Volume 7, 1988

Iglehart JK: Medicare turns to HMOs. N Engl J Med 312:132-137, 1985

Iversen LH, Polich CL: The Future of Medicare and HMOs. Excelsior, MN, Interstudy, 1985

Karamon G: Limits seen on retiree health care: companies study a cap for retiree health care. The New York Times, August 22, 1988, p D1, D4

Koran LM, Sharfstein SS: Mental health services, in Health Care Delivery in the United States. Edited by Jonas S. New York, Springer, 1986

Levin BL, Glasser JH, Jaffee CL: National trends in coverage and utilization of mental health, alcohol, and substance abuse services within managed health care systems. American Journal of Public Health 78:1222-1223, 1988

How do health maintenance organizations achieve their savings? New England Journal of Medicine 298:1136, 1978

Luft H: Health Maintenance Organizations: Dimensions of Performance. New York, John Wiley, 1981

Lurie EE: The interrelationship of physical and mental illness in the elderly, in Serving the Mentally Ill Elderly. Edited by Lurie EE, Swan JH. Lexington, MA, D. C. Heath and Company, 1987

Manning WG, Leibowitz A, Goldberg GA, et al: A controlled trial of the effect of a prepaid group practice on the use of services. New England Journal of Medicine 310:1505–1510, 1984

Marmor TR: The political and economic context of mental health care in the United States (unpublished manuscript). New Haven, CT, Yale School of Organization and Management, 1988

McFarland BH, Freeborn DK, Mullooly JP, et al: Utilization patterns among long term enrollees in a prepaid group practice HMO. Medical Care 23:1221-1233, 1985

Medicine and health: CHAMPUS psychiatric reforms draw fire. Perspectives, July 18, 1988

Ready T: Nursing homes sue U.S. to halt limits on admitting mentally ill. Health Week 3(8):4, 1989

Rice T: An economic assessment of health care coverage for the elderly. Milbank Quarterly 65:487-520, 1987

Rossiter L, Friedlob A, Langwell K: Exploring benefits of risk-based contracting under Medicare. Health Care Financing Review 39:42-57, 1985

Rossiter LF, Nelson LM, Adamache KW: Service use and costs for Medicare beneficiaries in risk based HMOs and CMPs: some interim results from the National Medicare Competition Evaluation. American Journal of Public Health 78:937-943, 1988

Scheffler RM: Mental health services: new policies and estimates. Generations 9:33-35, 1985

Schlesinger M: On the limits of expanding health care reform: chronic care in prepaid settings. Milbank Quarterly 64:189-215, 1986

Schlesinger M, Drumheller PB: Medicare and innovative insurance plans, in Renewing the Promise: Medicare and Its Reform. Edited by Blumenthal D, Schlesinger M, Drumheller PB. New York, Oxford University Press, 1988

Schlesinger M, Wetle T: Medicare's coverage of health services, in Renewing the Promise: Medicare and Its Reform. Edited by Blumenthal D, Schlesinger M, Drumheller PB. New York, Oxford University Press, 1988

Schumacher DN, Namerow MJ, Parker B, et al: Prospective payment for psychiatry—feasibility and impact. New England Journal of Medicine 315:1331-1336, 1986

Shapiro S, Skinner EA, Kramer M, et al: Measuring need for mental health services in a general population. Medical Care 23:1033-1043, 1985

Wetle T, Pearson DA: Long term care, in Health Care Delivery in the United States, 3rd ed. Edited by Jonas S. New York, Springer, 1986

Wetle T: Ethical Issues in Geriatric Medicine. Edited by Rowe JW, Besdine RW. Boston, Little Brown, 1988a

Wetle T: The social and service context of geriatric care, in Geriatric Medicine. Edited by Rowe JW, Besdine RW. Boston, Little, Brown, 1988b

Wines M: After 30 years mental institutions may be as empty as they'll ever be. The New York Times, September 4, 1988

14

Chronic Mental Illness

Linda H. Aiken, Ph.D.

The general well-being of elderly Americans has improved substantially over the past two decades both in real terms and in comparison to other age groups (Preston 1984). The proportion of the elderly with incomes below poverty has fallen from more than one-third in 1960 to less than 15% today. Americans 65 years and older are less likely to be poor today than persons of younger ages. This improved picture for the over-65 age group as a whole, of course, does obscure some of the large variations in income among the elderly. For example, almost one-third of the over-85 age group and one-half of blacks over 65 are characterized as living below the near-poverty level. Near poverty is defined as 125% of the poverty income level. Thus, while some subgroups within the larger elderly population still have insufficient incomes, particularly when large medical expenditures are required, the majority are faring better than in years past.

Access to health care has improved dramatically for the elderly over the past two decades (Aiken and Bays 1984). In 1960, half the elderly had no health insurance; today almost all are eligible to receive health care benefits under the Medicare program. This is in sharp contrast to the 37 million Americans under 65 with no health insurance coverage. The long-standing differences in use of hospital and physician care between the poor and nonpoor elderly have been largely eliminated since the introduction of Medicare. Moreover, the poor elderly appear to receive comparable amounts of care throughout the United States regardless of place of residence due to the almost universal coverage of Medicare. In contrast, the nonelderly poor have substantially different medical care utilization patterns by state, reflecting the lack of uniformity in eligibility and benefits in the Medicaid program (Blendon et al. 1986).

Improvements in health have accompanied greater access to health services and the improved economic position of the elderly.

Since 1968, age-adjusted death rates for people 65 years of age and over have declined for all of the leading causes of death except cancer.

It is within a context of substantial overall improvement in access to health care and economic well-being of the elderly that we examine how well the elderly with serious and chronic mental illness have fared.

Mental Illness in the Elderly

Specific criteria for defining chronic mental illness are lacking. The patients affected are heterogeneous, suffer from a variety of distinct disorders, and have illnesses that follow different and unpredictable courses (Mechanic 1989). Three dimensions of illness have been used to differentiate the chronically mentally ill from those with other kinds of problems: diagnosis, disability, and duration (NIMH 1987). Diagnostically, the chronically mentally ill category includes schizophrenia, major affective disorders, paranoid disorders and other psychoses. The term chronic mental illness usually conveys a history of serious, episodic, acute episodes plus continuing residual disability of long duration.

Technically, nonpsychotic organic mental disorders among the elderly such as senile dementia of the Alzheimer's type could be included in the definition. However, because the problems of caring for these patients are significantly different, they are not usually included in discussions of the chronically mentally ill, and will not be the focus of this chapter.

The President's Commission on Mental Health estimated that from 600,000 to 1,250,000 elderly persons suffered from serious chronic mental illness, primarily organic mental disorders including dementias (PCMH 1978). The NIMH Epidemiologic Catchment Area (ECA) project confirmed severe cognitive impairment to be the most prevalent form of mental disorder in persons 65 years of age and over (NIMH 1985, p. 5).

It is estimated from the NIMH Epidemiological Catchment Area project that the prevalence of disorders meeting DSM-III criteria in the general population range from 15 to 23% (Myers et al. 1984). Rates of disorder were lower in the group over age 45, with the exception of cognitive impairment, which is substantially higher among the elderly.

Prior to the NIMH Epidemiological Catchment Area project, there were no studies or surveys that could be used as a reliable and valid basis for estimating the prevalence of mental disorders among the population 65 years of age and over (Redick and Taube 1980).

If the one-year period prevalence rate of 15% estimated for the total population is applied to the 65 and over population as a minimum estimate of prevalence for the age group, then some 4 million elderly would be estimated to be in need of mental health services in a one-year period.

Various authors have found age-specific prevalence rates of schizophrenia and related psychoses among the elderly to be in the range of 3 to 5 per 1,000 population at risk. Applying these estimates to population data indicate that approximately 85,000 to 145,000 persons over the age of 65 in the United States probably suffer from these disorders (Kay and Bergmann 1980). It is widely held that the period of risk for schizophrenia ceases at about the age of 45. However, case register data show that new referrals still occur after the age of 70 (Kay and Bergmann 1980). The incidence and prevalence of paranoid psychoses of late onset are probably underestimated because they are often diagnosed as organic brain syndromes (Gurland et al. 1976).

The amount of serious mental illness in the population depends on the rate of incidence, the size of the population at risk, and the duration of illness. Large relative increases are occurring in numbers of persons in age groups at high risk for developing mental disorders—young adulthood when the risk of schizophrenia is greatest and old age when the risk of dementia is greatest (Kramer 1983). Hence, can we expect an increase in the number of people with mental disorders in the future. Additionally, there will be changes in the racial composition of the seriously mentally ill as well. Between 1980 and 2005, a 5% increase in schizophrenia is expected for whites but a 39% increase can be expected for blacks due to an increase of blacks in the age groups at greatest risk (Kramer 1983).

As the current large cohort of adults between the ages of 20 and 45 reaches old age, the number of elderly with chronic mental illness can be expected to increase substantially. However, evidence from longitudinal studies of the clinical trajectory of schizophrenia has begun to refute the commonly held view of schizophrenia as an intractable condition with an inevitable deteriorating course (Mechanic 1989, p. 119).

A long-term follow-up averaging 32 years has been conducted of members of a cohort of once profoundly ill, back ward, chronic patients from the Vermont State Hospital who were determined to have met DSM-III criteria for schizophrenia (Harding et al. 1987a). These patients were provided with a comprehensive rehabilitation program and released to the community 20 to 25 years ago. The 5- to 10-year follow-up study found that two-thirds were out of the hospital but required heavy support by the mental health system in order to remain in the community. Most follow-up studies have ended at this point, leaving the impression of continuing disability and heavy service need. However, follow-up of this cohort twenty or more years following discharge found widely heterogeneous patterns of social, occupational, and psychological functioning; one-half to two-thirds had achieved considerable improvement or recovered. The Vermont study corroborates similar results from four other long-term studies of schizophrenia: three in Europe and another U.S. study in Iowa (Harding et al. 1987b).

We do not know to what extent improved functioning over time is due to the natural course of the disease or the impact of successful treatment. On balance, the evidence suggests that appropriately managed programs of care can improve both short- and long-term outcomes (Kiesler and Sibulkin 1987). Hence, our success in providing appropriate care for the chronically mentally ill of all ages will likely affect the magnitude of disability and need in future cohorts of elderly.

Patterns of Mental Health Services Utilization

When data on utilization of psychiatric services by the elderly are compared with estimates of prevalence of mental illness, it would appear that only a small proportion of those needing services are actually receiving them, at least in the specialty mental health sector. In 1975, only 5% of admissions to all psychiatric services including public mental hospitals, private psychiatric hospitals, general hospital psychiatric inpatient units, community mental health centers, and outpatient psychiatric services were for persons 65 years of age or older (Redick and Taube 1980). In 1980, persons age 65 and older accounted for only 7% of admissions to all hospital psychiatric inpatient settings (NIMH 1987, p. 64) compared to 33% of all hospital admissions.

While there seems to be a general consensus that there is substantial unmet need for mental health services among the elderly (Redick and Taube 1980), the magnitude is difficult to determine for several reasons. The elderly more commonly use the general medical care system than mental health specialty care, and are thus less likely to obtain a psychiatric diagnosis. Clinicians (and researchers) have difficulty making a psychiatric diagnosis in the elderly because many of the criteria used in younger age groups such as employment and role function are not as applicable, and others relating to physiological changes such as weight, sleep, and activity are difficult to interpret. The ECA findings suggest that the elderly report fewer symptoms of psychological distress. It is not clear yet whether the elderly actually have less symptomatology or whether the findings are methodological artifacts. In any event, there is little or no evidence that the elderly with serious chronic mental illness have substantially better access to services appropriate to their unique needs as a result of Medicare than do the chronically mentally ill of younger age groups.

Care of the Chronically Mentally Ill

Despite considerable improvements in access to health care for most Americans over the past two decades, the chronically mentally ill remain a neglected and often incapacitated group. Most depend exclusively on underfinanced, fragmented, and often inaccessible public services. The social welfare and health programs initiated in the 1960s that were so important in improving the well-being of most of the elderly and many of the nation's poor—Medicare, Medicaid, Supplemental Security Income (SSI), Social Security Disability Insurance (SSDI), food stamps, public housing assistance—have not been nearly as effective in improving the well-being of the chronically mentally ill. The most visible evidence of this failure is the large and growing numbers of homeless mentally ill in the nation's large cities, most of whom do not receive benefits from any of these programs (Rossi and Wright 1987).

Prior to 1955 when deinstitutionalization began, serious chronic mental illness was treated almost solely in public psychiatric hospitals. These "total institutions" controlled most aspects of patients' daily activities as well as providing medical care. A variety of social, technological, legal, and financial factors led to reductions in patient populations in public mental hospitals from 560,000 patients in 1955 to 116,000 today (Mechanic and Aiken 1987). The availability of neuroleptic drugs offered the potential of outpatient treatment. Civil commitment laws came under greater scrutiny by legal advocates for the mentally ill. And institutions became increasingly expensive for state governments to operate.

The enactment of the new social programs of the sixties offered the potential of shifting more of the costs of the care of the mentally ill from state budgets to the federal government. The importance of these new programs as a stimulus to deinstitutionalization is reflected in the rate at which patient populations in state hospitals declined. Between 1955 and 1965 when neuroleptics were already available, the reduction in patient census proceeded at a rate of about 1.5% per year. After the launching of the Great Society Programs of the mid-sixties, the resident population in state hospitals began to fall by 6% a year (Gronfein 1985). But the promise of these new social programs for improved community-based care for the seriously mentally ill was greater than the reality.

The care of the chronically mentally ill is primarily a task of maintenance of function that requires some control of the life circumstances of patients, and the ability to maintain continuity of care. Effective community care involves the ability to respond to needs ranging from appropriate housing to the medical management of acute psychiatric illnesses. In essence, the challenge for community mental health is one of recreating the functions and responsibilities of a mental hospital but in a community context.

It was originally envisioned that community mental health centers could provide appropriate care for patients following hospitalization. But in reality community mental health centers do not control the services necessary to even approximate the care received by the seriously mentally ill in public hospitals. Community mental health centers have no control over housing, income maintenance, or medical insurance. Moreover, these programs are under the control of different agencies, often at different levels of government making coordination extremely difficult. Even within the mental health sector, inpatient and outpatient services often are controlled by totally separate organizations making longitudinal care of patients a haphazard process.

Case management often is the proposed solution to the fragmented services and benefit structure that currently exists. However, in most instances, case management is not embedded in an infrastructure that controls the resources required. Therefore, it has a limited impact on substantially improving the quality of care and patient outcomes (Mechanic and Aiken 1987; Franklin et al. 1987).

In the absence of a functioning community system of services, institutions remain a major source of care for many of the chronically mentally ill. As length of stay in mental hospitals was reduced, admissions increased. Now the majority of all admissions to public mental hospitals are readmissions (Bassuk and Gerson 1978). Three decades after the beginning of deinstitutionalization, public mental hospitals continue to account for almost two-thirds of state mental health expenditures (NIMH 1987, p. 162).

The treatment of psychiatric disorders among the chronically mentally ill shifted increasingly to acute general hospitals and nursing homes as use of public mental hospitals declined. Since 1969, expenditures (in constant dollars) have more than doubled for general hospital psychiatric services, offsetting totally the somewhat lower expenditures for public mental hospitals. In 1984, there were 1.7 million discharges from short-stay hospitals with primary diagnoses of mental illness (NIMH 1985).

The introduction of Medicaid in 1966 created the opportunity to shift long-term chronic patients from state hospitals to lower cost nursing homes where the federal government shared the expense (Swan 1987). Between 1965 and 1979, the number of elderly patients in state mental hospitals dropped from 773 per 100,000 to 164 per 100,000, a decrease of 79% reflecting increased placement of aged residents in nursing homes and the release of others to the community (NIMH 1986, p. 12) Nursing homes are now the largest single institutional setting for the care of the mentally ill in this country, exceeding the number of mentally ill in state mental institutions by some 600,000 (NIMH 1986, p. 1). It is estimated that another 175,000 to 300,000 mentally ill reside in board and care facilities (National Conference of State Legislatures 1988).

Analysis of data from the 1977 National Nursing Home Survey yielded estimates of 668,000 chronic mentally ill patients residing in nursing homes (Goldman et al. 1986). Of this total number of mentally ill, 72,000 were chronically mentally ill only, 35,000 had both physical and mental diagnoses, and 561,000 suffered from dementia of which three-quarters also had physical disorders. Persons with a diagnosis of mental retardation but no other mental disorders were excluded from the above estimate. This analysis revealed a bimodal group of patients in nursing homes with substantial differences between patients with only chronic mental illness (CMI) and those with physical impairments and dementia. The CMI group were younger, more mobile, and had less need for assistance with basic activities of daily living. While the majority received psychiatric medication, fewer than 10% received psychotherapy and other psychiatric therapies. Other studies also document little involvement of psychiatrists and other mental health specialists in nursing home care despite the high prevalence of mental disorder (Borson et al. 1987; Tourigny-Rivard and Drury 1987).

These studies and others raise questions regarding the appropriateness of care of the CMI provided in institutions primarily organized to provide care for the functionally dependent elderly and which have few psychiatric services. Since its introduction in 1984, the Medicare Prospective Payment System in the past several years has increased the incentives for general hospitals to discharge elderly medical and surgical patients to nursing homes at an earlier stage of recovery from acute illness. As a result, the case mix in nursing homes is changing in the direction of a more medically and functionally impaired population (Aiken et al. 1985). Even less attention to psychiatric impairment may be one consequence of the heavy demands placed on the staff in nursing homes because of the changing case mix.

Impact of Health Policy on Patterns of Care

Insurance coverage for psychiatric illness has always been incomplete; coverage has been markedly inferior to that for physical illness and has favored inpatient care (Bassuk and Gerson 1978). This tradition was followed in the design of Medicare in which severe limits were placed on outpatient psychiatric care ($250 reimbursement for $500 of outpatient care) and a lifetime maximum number of 190 psychiatric hospital inpatient days were allowed. These limits have been widely criticized for encouraging expensive hospital care when outpatient services would have been as effective, and for severely limiting the elderly's access to specialty mental health services. After increasing the cap on outpatient mental health services to $450 in 1988 and $1100 in 1989, the Congress finally removed the dollar limit on outpatient mental health treatment altogether, beginning in 1990. However, Medicare beneficiaries are still required to pay 50% of their outpatient mental health treatment costs, substantially more than the 20% copayment required for other medical treatment, and the lifetime limit on inpatient care was retained.

Medicare is a program designed to finance short-term acute care for the elderly. However, most expenditures reimburse care for chronic conditions like heart disease, cancer, stroke, diabetes, and end stage renal disease. Acute psychotic episodes of chronic mental illness are the psychiatric analogues of hospitalization for diabetic acidosis but are not recognized as such by Medicare. Because of restrictive psychiatric benefits under Medicare, the elderly chronically mentally ill have much the same problems obtaining access to appropriate psychiatric care as younger patients without Medicare. The primary difference is that Medicare patients have good coverage of general medical and hospital care which may substitute, in some respects, for specialty psychiatric care.

Federal health and social welfare policies have been formulated on the premise that care of the chronically mentally ill is a state and local government responsibility. When the dominant setting for care was the state mental hospital, this distinction between state and federal responsibility was less troublesome than it is now that the vast majority of chronically mentally ill persons live in community settings. The continued adherence to this policy in the context of a very different pattern of care results in inefficient resource utilization and poor clinical outcomes.

Medicaid, although not designed for the mentally ill, has become a major funder of mental health services. In total outlays, Medicaid is second only to direct state appropriations for mental health services (Searight and Handal 1986, p. 159). Restrictions originally imposed to limit the shifting of state obligations for the care of the chronically mentally ill to the federal government have had major adverse consequences for the development of a rational system of high quality and cost-effective mental health services.

Mentally ill people between the ages of 21 and 65 are not eligible for Medicaid if they are hospitalized in facilities that care for mental disorders exclusively. This restriction includes residential treatment centers such as halfway houses and other settings that provide specialty psychiatric services. However, Medicaid benefits are available for inpatient care in general hospitals and in nursing homes that are not predominantly psychiatric facilities. These provisions have adversely affected the cost and quality of care of the mentally ill by promoting the use of expensive general hospital care when less costly alternatives would have been as or more effective. They also encouraged the institutionalization of thousands of mentally ill in nursing homes with almost no mental health services. Moreover, Medicaid predominantly covers care that is delivered in traditional office or clinic settings despite evidence that outreach services to the community have been demonstrated to be more effective for many of the chronically mentally ill.

Supplemental Security Income (SSI), established in 1972, is a critical resource in developing community-based care for the chronically mentally ill. SSI provides subsistence income and eligibility for Medicaid, subsidized housing, and other benefits. Chronic psychiatric patients account for an estimated 10%–12% of all SSI beneficiaries and are thought to account for up to 20% in some states (Searight and Handal 1986). However, the eligibility and benefits structure of SSI are not optimal for the chronically mentally ill.

Eligibility for SSI is based largely on disability. Additionally, people 65 years of age or over can also qualify on the basis of financial need. The requirement that mentally ill persons must be designated disabled in order to access these resources is counterintuitive for those for whom vocational rehabilitation is an objective. Moreover, the clinical course of chronic mental illness with periods of reasonable functioning alternating with disability complicates disability determination (Okpaku 1985). The disability determination process requires a level of patient participation that is often unrealistic given the nature of mental illness. Therefore, many individuals who could qualify are unable to complete the process. SSI eligibility is lost by patients who require state institutional care for any period of time. Then, the arduous disability determination process must begin all over again after discharge. Inasmuch as state hospitals are not well integrated with community-based services, patients are often discharged without SSI benefits and without adequate follow-up to ensure that the disability determination process is completed.

The large numbers of homeless mentally ill are evidence of the failure of SSI to help many of those most in need. In one of the most rigorous studies of the homeless undertaken to date, Rossi and Wright (1987) found that 23% of the homeless had been patients in a mental hospital at some time. Of those, more than half had been hospitalized more than once. In total, four out of five homeless persons had some form of disability; however, only one in four received welfare, general assistance, or disability payments.

Policy Directions for the Future

Public tolerance for the failures of the mental health system to provide decent services for the mentally ill is diminishing. There are frequent debates about reinstitutionalizing the chronically mentally ill. However, the number of mentally ill people has grown tremendously since deinstitutionalization began in 1950 due to demographic and population shifts. The establishment of a comparable institutional system would require an investment considerably greater than current expenditures. Thus, it appears that community-based psychiatric care is here to stay. That being the case, our agenda should focus on how to reshape current programs and on how to redirect existing resources to build a more effective community-based system.

A key element in any effort to improve community care is to capture hospital funds for programs of managed care at the local level. These programs must be responsible for both inpatient and outpatient services for defined populations (Mechanic and Aiken 1987). This effort will require the development of a strong local organizational structure that can give coherence to the system of services that will necessarily depend upon many different providers and different revenue sources. Ideally, such an organization would be rooted in local government, either as an operating component of city or county government, as a public authority, or a nonprofit corporation linked to local government (Walsh and Leigland 1986). Local government sponsorship is essential for several reasons. Local government sponsorship would be most effective because it controls many of the key services and resources that are critical to effective community-based mental health: emergency response systems, the criminal justice system, public general hospitals, subsidized housing, and tax revenues.

With the possible exception of several small states, state government is not optimally organized to provide direct services at the community level. Operating state-run hospitals is a very different business than the provision of local services which often involve many different local service provider organizations. State governments must be convinced to delegate the authority and responsibility for public mental health services to local communities while maintaining their longstanding financial obligations to the mentally ill.

The federally sponsored community mental health centers were based on the catchment area concept. It is now clear that this method is ineffective as the major organizing framework for public mental health services. The most successful programs have been in smaller communities where a single community mental health center covers the entire population, such as the successful model program developed in Dane County, Wisconsin (Stein and Test 1980). In large cities with as many as 10 or more community mental health centers, central planning is often absent. Some services are provided in every center while specialty services for relatively small population groups such as the elderly, children, and the homeless may be missing altogether. Moreover, single CMHCs in big cities usually lack sufficient influence on other local services to develop an integrated services structure necessary for maintaining the chronically mentally ill in community settings. The development of an effective central authority or infrastructure would do much to increase the effectiveness of CMHCs.

The development of community-based mental health services has been severely hampered by underfinancing. The only practical way to solve this problem is to target the "slack" in the system and redirect those resources to building a community system. The slack is primarily in resources devoted to institutional care. Two strategies are necessary. First, local mental health authorities must have control over both outpatient and inpatient mental health funds derived from state appropriations. A consolidated state mental health budget allocated on a formula basis to the counties was a critical element in the development of the highly successful Dane County program (Stein 1989). In recognition of the need to give local mental health boards more flexibility in developing a continuum of services that best meets local needs, Ohio has recently passed similar legislation. In these arrangements, savings achieved by preventing unnecessary hospitalization are available to finance innovative community care models for persons with severe mental illnesses.

The second strategy involves more effective use of Medicaid. Medicaid expenditures for general hospital care for the severely mentally ill are substantial and they are growing. In 1980, Medicaid was the principal source of payment for 23% of all psychiatric admissions to general hospitals and for 7% of all admissions to private psychiatric hospitals (NIMH 1985). A rough estimate suggests that in 1980 Medicaid was the principal source of payment for 1.3 million bed-days in general hospitals and private psychiatric institutions for patients with chronic mental illnesses (Mechanic and Aiken 1987).

The chronically mentally ill are often brought by police to emergency rooms where they are seen by medical staff who know little about their medical history, and who tend to follow a conservative approach of hospitalization, often financed by Medicaid. Other patients use emergency rooms as a point of entry into the mental health system. In Philadelphia, for example, persons who frequently use psychiatric emergency services account for only 20% of the unduplicated caseload but they use 60% of all service hours and they constitute 55% of all admissions (Surles and McGurrin 1987). Many of these admissions could be prevented in a well-organized system of managed care. The savings achieved could be invested in the development of a continuum of services in the community.

Medicaid reform, in combination with consolidated and decentralized state funding, could substantially improve the effective utilization of resources already being spent on the severely mentally ill. Capitation, although fraught with complexities, offers great potential as a strategy for consolidation of funding and control over expenditures (Mechanic and Aiken 1989). Existing efforts to use some form of capitation in mental health can be divided into those that mainstream the mentally ill into existing HMOs where they receive the range of medical and psychiatric benefits typically provided, and others that establish in one form or another a "mental health HMO" for designated beneficiaries (Christianson 1988).

Efforts to mainstream the mentally ill into HMOs have not proven to be successful (Mechanic and Aiken 1989). Considering that HMOs are not typically organized to deal with the range of problems that the seriously mentally ill present, this outcome is not surprising. Also, the pressures on typical HMO practitioners are such that it is unlikely that the special needs of the severely mentally ill will receive the necessary attention (Schlesinger 1986). The use of capitated approaches for public mental health services show considerably more promise (Mechanic and Aiken 1989). Rhode Island and Rochester, NY, have implemented mental health capitation, and other states and locales have proposals at various stages of development. These include Philadelphia, South Carolina, and Arizona. Most efforts have concentrated on discharging long-stay mental hospital patients to the community and capturing the funds formerly spent on their hospital care for the development of community services. At this time, none of these efforts capitates Medicaid. However, Medicaid capitation forms the basis of the Philadelphia plan to build a managed care system for the most severely mentally ill. Medicaid capitation offers the best potential of capturing new funds for community care for the mentally ill who already reside in the community. This is especially the case in states that have high utilization of Medicaid-financed general hospital care for the mentally ill.

Medicaid capitation provides greater control over resources which enables savings on inpatient care to be reinvested in the development of community services. It also allows the development of provider incentives to encourage more cost-effective decision-making, and it provides much greater flexibility in the services provided. Capitation is a strategy for bypassing many of the restrictive regulations that make it difficult to provide care for patients in nontraditional settings. Medicaid capitation requires federal waivers which traditionally have been difficult to obtain. The 1986 Omnibus Budget Reconciliation Act (OBRA) included provisions to allow the 9 cities participating in the Robert Wood Johnson Foundation/HUD demonstration (Aiken et al. 1986) to apply for such waivers. This may set a precedent for applications from other states.

Some states have used other strategies to achieve greater flexibility in Medicaid funding for community-based services (National Conference of State Legislatures 1988). Recent changes in Medicaid show some signs of allowing for greater flexibility in Medicaid-covered services under various state options. For example, reimbursement for case management for the seriously mentally ill was added in 1985. Clinic options have been used creatively by some states, most notably Colorado, to fund a range of ambulatory services for the mentally ill. Four states have used Home and Community-Based Waivers ("2176 waivers") designed originally to reduce nursing home utilization by the elderly, to fund community mental health care for the mentally ill who otherwise would have required institutional care. Because the emphasis was on substituting community services for nursing home care rather than general hospital care, the 2176 waivers have been of limited utility in mental health (Laudicina and Burwell 1988). OBRA changes in 1986 make it easier to meet the cost-effectiveness test and thus obtain approval for 2176 waivers for the CMI. Patients who are at risk for periodic hospitalization because current community-based services are not sufficient are now included along with those at risk for nursing home care.

A discussion of policy directions to improve mental health services for the chronically mentally ill would not be complete without discussion of Social Security disability policies and housing. The shift from hospital-based to community-based systems cannot be accomplished without resources to provide income maintenance, housing, and medical benefits to the severely mentally ill. These services are tied to SSI, which makes disability policies and their implementation critical to building community mental health services. The new disability criteria for mental illness developed by the Social Security Administration should improve the reliability and validity of disability determination. However, the process of disability determination for the mentally ill needs major revisions. The determination process is long and requires multiple steps and perseverance by the applicant. Social Security workers who administer SSI are typically located in offices organized to serve elderly social security beneficiaries, a group that is very different from the mentally ill. There are few, if any, outreach services designed specifically to bring the disability determination process to the places where the disabled mentally ill are likely to be. A pilot program in New York City which provided outreach by SSA workers to shelters and clinics for the homeless proved to be very successful in obtaining SSI and related resources to truly disabled persons who had not been successful in completing the process themselves. An innovative expedited review process conducted primarily by phone in Ohio showed similar results (for discussion of these pilot efforts see National Conference of State Legislatures 1988). Recent budget cuts in Social Security make it unlikely that these successful outreach and expedited review programs will be widely available without the designation of specific personnel to undertake them.

Housing is a critical element in developing alternatives to hospital care. Despite evidence that homelessness is a major problem among the mentally ill and that housing is an integral part of any therapeutic care plan, mental health agencies have limited available housing placements. A survey conducted in the nation's 60 largest cities revealed that as little as 5% to 10% of the estimated housing needed was available (Aiken 1987).

Many chronically mentally ill are eligible for subsidized housing. However, housing authorities have little understanding of their needs, and thus the mentally ill receive little attention in the development of public housing priorities. This problem could be overcome by greater targeting of existing funds within HUD to ensure that local housing authorities would establish joint programs with mental health agencies. Moreover, mental health agencies have not developed the expertise necessary to garner available housing resources for their clients. The development of a strong central mental health authority should make it possible for more housing expertise to be included within mental health. This will allow for the collective influence of the mental health system to be used more effectively to influence the distribution of existing public subsidies and to interest private developers in joint ventures to increase housing stock.

The challenge is not simply developing more housing placements, but integrating mental health services and housing. This includes incorporating the mentally ill that are already housed outside the mental health services system. The large numbers of chronically mentally ill in board and care facilities, many of whom are elderly, represent a group that may be receiving little, if any, psychiatric care.

Innovative programs designed specifically for the mentally ill elderly who do not have significant physical disabilities or degenerative illnesses such as Alzheimer's disease have been limited. The chronically mentally ill are not perceived to be good candidates for innovative programs designed to integrate acute and long-term medical care, such as social health maintenance organizations or life care communities. These initiatives, for the most part, are insurance programs that limit the entry of persons with preexisting conditions or who are Medicaid beneficiaries at the time of admission. On Lok in San Francisco is a social health maintenance organization designed specifically for elderly Medicaid patients. A demonstration is currently underway to try to replicate the On Lok model in other communities. If the demonstration is successful, the On Lok model would offer potential for improved care for elderly persons disabled by serious mental illness if psychiatric services were among those offered.

The recent nursing home reform legislation illustrates the dilemmas created by the absence of appropriate service models for the mentally ill elderly. The Omnibus Budget Reconciliation Act of 1987 included provisions that for the first time require that the mentally ill in long-term care settings receive active psychiatric treatment. The new legislation was developed in response to the concerns that many mentally ill individuals had been institutionalized in nursing homes that provided little or no treatment for their primary problem. Nursing homes that admit patients needing active psychiatric care risk losing federal Medicaid payments unless such care is available. The likely result is that nursing homes will discharge patients with primary diagnoses of mental illness. In most states, the primary alternatives to nursing home care for the seriously mentally ill are state psychiatric hospitals or board and care facilities. Neither setting is optimal. Thus, because there are so few appropriate models of care for the mentally ill elderly, efforts to improve their care like the nursing home reform legislation may actually result in a less appropriate placement, at least in the short term.

The mentally ill elderly are a neglected and vulnerable group whose needs are obfuscated by those of younger chronically mentally ill persons on the one hand, and by the elderly with predominantly physical disabilities on the other. Current reimbursement policies mitigate against the development of innovative programs for the mentally ill elderly. Sustained efforts are needed to revise reimbursement policies to support the development of more appropriate services for this group. In the interim, there is sufficient flexibility within existing financing arrangements for the development and testing of more creative approaches. Perhaps one of the positive outcomes of the nursing home reform legislation will be to serve as a catalyst for improved models of care for the seriously mentally ill elderly.

References

Aiken LH: Unmet needs of the chronically mentally ill. Image: Journal of Nursing Scholarship 19:121-125, 1987

Aiken LH, Bays KD: The Medicare debate: round one. New England Journal of Medicine 311:1196-1200, 1984

Aiken LH, Mezey MD, Lynaugh JE, et al: Teaching nursing homes: prospects for improving long-term care. Geriatrics 33:196-201, 1985

Aiken LH, Somers SA, Shore MF: Private foundations in health affairs: a case study of the development of a national initiative for the chronically mentally ill. American Psychologist 41:1290-1295, 1986

Bassuk EL, Gerson S: Deinstitutionalization and mental health services. Scientific American 238:46-53, 1978

Blendon RJ, Aiken LH, Freeman HE, et al: Uncompensated care by hospitals or public insurance for the poor: does it make a difference? New England Journal of Medicine 14:1160-1163, 1986

Borson S, Liptzin B, Nininger J, et al: Psychiatry and the nursing home. American Journal of Psychiatry 144:1412-1418, 1987

Christianson J: Capitation of mental health care in public programs, in Advances in Health Economics and Health. Services Research Vol. 8. Edited by Scheffler R, Rossiter L. Greenwich, CT, JAI Press, 1988

Franklin JL, Solovitz B, Mason M, et al: An evaluation of case management. American Journal of Public Health 77:674-678, 1987

Goldman HH, Feder J, Scanlon W: Chronic mental patients in nursing homes: reexamining data from the National Nursing Home Survey. Hospital and Community Psychiatry 37:269-272, 1986

Gronfein W: Incentives and intentions in mental health policy: a comparison of the Medicaid and Community Mental Health programs. Journal of Health and Social Behavior 26:192-206, 1985

Gurland B, Fleiss J, Goldberg K, et al: A semi-structured clinical interview for the assessment of diagnosis and mental state in the elderly: the Geriatric Mental State Schedule, II: a factor analysis. Psychological Medicine 6:451-459, 1976

Harding CM, Brooks GW, Ashikaga T, et al: The Vermont longitudinal study of persons with severe mental illness, II: long-term outcome of subjects who retrospectively met DSM-III criteria for schizophrenia. American Journal of Psychiatry 144:727-735, 1987a

Harding CM, Zubin J, Strauss JS: Chronicity in schizophrenia: fact, partial fact, or artifact? Hospital and Community Psychiatry 38:477-486, 1987b

Kay WK, Bergmann K: Epidemiology of mental disorders among the aged in the community, in Handbook of Mental Health and Aging. Edited by Birren JE, Sloane RB. Englewood Cliffs, NJ, Prentice-Hall, 1980

Kiesler CA, Sibulkin AE: Mental Hospitalization: Myths and Facts About a National Crisis. Newbury Park, CA, Sage Publications, 1987

Kramer M: The continuing challenge: the rising prevalence of mental disorders, associated chronic diseases and disabling conditions. American Journal of Social Psychiatry 3:13-24, 1983

Laudicina SC, Burwell B: A profile of Medicaid home and community-based care waivers 1985: findings of a national survey. Journal of Health Politics, Policy and Law 13:525-546, 1988

Mechanic D: Mental Health and Social Policy, 3rd ed. Englewood Cliffs, NJ, Prentice-Hall, 1989

Mechanic D, Aiken LH: Improving care for the chronically mentally ill. New England Journal of Medicine 317:1634-1642, 1987

Mechanic D, Aiken LH: Integrating Mental Health Services Through Capitation. San Francisco, Jossey-Bass, 1989

Myers JK, Weissman MM, Tischler GL, et al: Six-month prevalence of psychiatric disorders in three communities. Archives of General Psychiatry 41:959-967, 1984

National Conference of State Legislatures: Mental Health Financing and Programming: A Legislator's Guide. Washington, DC, National Conference of State Legislatures, 1988

National Institute of Mental Health: Mental Health, United States 1985. DHHS Publication (ADM) 85-1378. Washington, DC, U.S. Government Printing Office, 1985

National Institute of Mental Health: Mental Illness in Nursing Homes: Agenda for Research. DHHS Publication (ADM) 86-1459. Washington, DC, U.S. Government Printing Office, 1986

National Institute of Mental Health: Mental Health, United States 1987. DHHS Publication (ADM) 87-1518. Washington, DC, U.S. Government Printing Office, 1987

Okpaku SA: A profile of clients referred for psychiatric evaluation for Social Security Disability Income and Supplemental Security Income: implications for psychiatry. American Journal of Psychiatry 142:1037-1043, 1985

President's Commission on Mental Health: Final Report, Vol 1. Washington, DC, U.S. Government Printing Office, 1978

Preston SH: Children and the elderly: divergent paths for America's dependents. Demography 21:435-457, 1984

Redick RW, Taube C: Demography and mental health care of the aged, in Handbook of Mental Health and Aging. Edited by Birren JE, Sloane RB. Englewood Cliffs, NJ, Prentice-Hall, 1980

Rossi PH, Wright JD: The determinants of homelessness. Health Affairs 6:19-32, 1987

Schlesinger M: On the limits of expanding health care reform: chronic care in prepaid settings. Milbank Memorial Fund Quarterly 64:189-215, 1986

Searight HR, Handal PJ: Psychiatric deinstitutionalization: the possibilities and the reality. Psychiatric Quarterly 58:153-166, 1986

Stein LI: Wisconsin's system of mental health financing, in Integrating Mental Health Services Through Capitation. Edited by Mechanic D, Aiken LH. San Francisco, Jossey-Bass, 1989

Stein LI, Test MA: Alternatives to mental hospital treatment. Archives of General Psychiatry 37:393-397, 1980

Surles RC, McGurrin MC: Increased use of psychiatric emergency services by young chronic mentally ill patients. Hospital and Community Psychiatry 38:401-405, 1987

Swan JH: The substitution of nursing home for inpatient psychiatric care. Community Mental Health Journal 23:3-18, 1987

Tourigny-Rivard M, Drury M: The effects of monthly psychiatric consultation in a nursing home. Gerontology 27:363-366, 1987

Walsh AH, Leigland J: Public Authorities for Mental Health Programs. New York, Institute of Public Administration, 1986

15

Present and Future Solutions

Barry S. Fogel, M.D.
Gary L. Gottlieb, M.D., M.B.A.
Antonio Furino, Ph.D.

The contributions to this volume, in exploring access and financing for neuropsychiatric care for the elderly, have depicted a heterogeneous problem for which solutions will require initiatives at all levels of government, as well as within the private sector. We will begin this chapter by recapitulating some of the major conclusions and recommendations of the contributors. Then, we will discuss several recent or pending Congressional initiatives. We will conclude by offering three ideas for future policy development: 1) improving identification and recognition of neuropsychiatric problems; 2) generalizing the idea of case management; and 3) developing new programs on a regional basis through public/private/academic collaboration.

Readers desiring more detailed policy recommendations will find them in the noted chapters. Those desiring a more qualitative feel for how decision-makers and advocates think about the issues may find it in Appendix I ("A Window on the Debate").

Conclusions and Recommendations

1. The neuropsychiatric disorders of late life are widely prevalent. They are underdiagnosed and undertreated. Their identification and treatment definitely will improve older Americans' quality of life. In certain subpopulations, neuropsychiatric care may improve physical function, avert institutionalization, and save on total health care expenditures. Among the healthiest elderly, neuropsychiatric care may augment economic productivity (Chapters 1, 2, 3, 4, and 8).

2. Much of the treatment of acute neuropsychiatric disorders, such as depression and prescription drug psychotoxicity, will take place in the general health sector. Therefore, primary care physicians must be better trained in the recognition, differential diagnosis, and treatment of mental health problems. Institutions serving the health needs of the elderly must make use of psychiatric consultation. Physician payments, especially by Medicare, must offer nonpsychiatric physicians incentives to properly evaluate their patients' mental health problems. Payments to psychiatrists must be sufficient to promote psychiatrists' involvement with the elderly. The claims of other mental health provider groups for Medicare reimbursement deserve serious attention, ideally including empirical studies of the unique contributions of each discipline and appropriate structures for multidisciplinary treatment of specific problems. Patients' copayments must be kept low, to avoid discouraging patients from seeking treatment. Consultations to nursing homes, in particular, must be adequately reimbursed, as nursing home residents are dramatically underserved (Chapters 4, 7, 8, and 9).

3. Even when payment for services is adequate, there is a shortage of human resources in geriatric psychiatry and related mental health disciplines. Both public funds and private foundations should underwrite more intensive training of mental health professionals in the care of the elderly mentally ill (Chapters 4 and 10).

4. State governments have traditionally taken responsibility for the chronically mentally ill. They should retain responsibility for patients with long-standing mental illnesses when they grow old, rather than attempt to shift costs and responsibilities to the federal government and to nursing homes. On the other hand, the care of elderly people with dementia or with late-onset mental disorders, who are accustomed to obtaining care from the general health care system, should not be shifted to an already overburdened state mental health system (Chapters 5 and 14).

5. Innovation in the development of new models for service delivery to the elderly must be encouraged. Promoting access while controlling costs and quality will require skillful management and organizational design, rather than a fragmented and chaotic service system. Funding for innovative care models includes adequate funds for proper program evaluation, and data collection for evaluation should be built into the program design. Because of the wide prevalence of mental disorders in the elderly, mental health measures should be incorporated in demonstration projects and evaluations. Economic outcome measures also

are essential. State and federal regulatory agencies should cooperate in minimizing the legal and regulatory barriers to innovation and service design, when projects are designed with proper safeguards for patient protection (Chapters 8, 9, and 11).

6. Managed care systems such as exclusive provider organizations, and comprehensive long-term care systems such as continuing care retirement communities, offer an exciting option for building in better access to mental health services at a containable cost. However, the potential of such systems for improving the integration of physical and mental health care is threatened by their tendency to "carve out" mental health benefits, or to exclude institutional long-term care from the services for which the health plan is at risk. Among the elderly, physical health, mental health, and the needs for social and supportive services interact, and the effect of one factor on another may occur over months or years. Putting providers at risk for the largest range of services over the longest range of time offers the best incentives for discovering and exploiting potential cost-offsetting effects of timely mental health interventions (Chapters 10, 11, 12, and 13).

The Present Policy Environment

At the present time, federal and state governments share with private industry common preoccupations: the containment of cost and the management of risk. When those preoccupations cannot be addressed by better management, they are addressed by efforts to shift costs to other payers or to shift risks to providers, subcontractors, or insurance companies. When health care policy is primarily driven by budgetary considerations, new ideas for providing service to underserved populations are evaluated with greater weight to fiscal than to clinical criteria. Also, potentially money-saving proposals often are seen with skepticism and left untested to avoid the risk of an unsuccessful outcome, and possible blame for overspending. Nonetheless, within an environment that may appear hostile to innovation, there are dedicated and caring individuals who recognize the problems of underserved populations and poorly organized care. These hard-working public servants offer opportunities for implementing innovative programs, provided that the incremental costs are modest and the risks are manageable.

The current federal legislative environment seems inhospitable to any sweeping expansion of benefits for older people. Such benefits cannot come out of general funds in a time of massive budget deficits, and citizens' response to the Catastrophic Coverage Act suggests that special levies on the elderly are politically unacceptable. In the short term, therefore, federal initiatives are likely to be limited to small incremental changes—modifications of existing programs, research within demonstration projects, and perhaps the incorporation of neuropsychiatric elements within existing programs. The next five sections discuss examples of current federal legislative efforts.

The Nursing Home Reform
Provisions of OBRA 1987

In the 1987 Omnibus Budget Reconciliation Act (OBRA), a large section was devoted to nursing home reform. The most controversial section concerns a requirement that patients not be admitted to nursing facilities (NFs) if they suffer from a mental illness (MI) requiring active treatment, unless they have a medical illness or disability otherwise requiring nursing care, and the facility provides the active treatment needed for the MI at other than federal expense. Furthermore, NFs receiving Medicaid funds are required to review their residents annually and to make alternative dispositions for those residents who have mental illnesses, when the illnesses require active treatment that cannot be provided in the NF, or if they do not have concurrent physical problems or advanced age that would otherwise require NF care. (While there are further details and exceptions, they are not addressed here. The interested reader may consult OBRA 1987 and OBRA 1989 for details, or may review one of the excellent summaries of the provision, such as that prepared by the National Mental Health Association [NMHA 1988].)

This provision of OBRA, known by the acronym PASARR (Pre-Admission Screening—Annual Resident Review), has the obvious purpose of reversing the trend for chronically mentally ill patients to be shifted from state hospitals and related institutions into nursing homes funded primarily by Medicaid. In this respect, its result is cost shifting, although the goal is more nobly expressed as assurance that residents receive needed psychiatric care. The cost-shifting emphasis is clear from the statement in the legislation that the existence of alternate dispositions may not be taken into account when conducting the screening process. Therefore, a mentally ill patient in a nursing home might have to be discharged, even if a more suitable disposition did not exist. The intention is to force states to develop suitable alternative dispositions for the chronically mentally ill, other than Medicaid-funded nursing homes. In the short term, many mentally ill patients, estimated to number at least 20,000 and perhaps as many as 200,000, will suffer some dislocation

(NMHA 1988), while the cost of their care will be shifted back to states, localities, and families.

Simultaneously, other provisions of OBRA 1987 require nursing facilities to provide medically related social services to attain or maintain "the highest practicable level of physical, mental, or psychosocial well-being of each resident," and to comprehensively assess residents' psychosocial status, cognitive status, and psychotropic drug therapy (Federal Register 1989). Residents who display psychosocial adjustment difficulties are to receive appropriate treatment for remotivation and re-orientation, and the development of new difficulties by residents with withdrawn, angry, or depressed behavior is to be regarded as a negative outcome measure under the new regulations. Therefore, routine care in NFs is supposed to pay significant attention to cognitive and behavioral, i.e., neuropsychiatric, dimensions of care. Evidently, the recipients of this care are not to be seen as "mentally ill" and the services they receive are not to be seen as "active treatment."

The impact of PASARR will depend greatly on how the notion of active treatment is defined. If active treatment is defined as the kind of services that would be provided in a psychiatric hospital, the impact of PASARR would simply be to eject from nursing homes people who should not be there in the first place. On the other hand, if active treatment also includes that combination of medication management and social support that is the treatment of choice for many late-life depressions, PASARR would be a strong disincentive for NFs to ever diagnose or treat the secondary depressions that are known to occur in at least one-third of nursing home residents.

Fortunately, it is likely that the Health Care Financing Administration (HCFA) will develop a narrow definition of active treatment. Their May 1989 draft definition defines active treatment as involving "24-hour supervision by mental health professionals," and specifically excludes intermittent psychiatric services for medication adjustment, etc. (HCFA 1989). Strong political and legal pressure has been placed on HCFA by state mental health authorities and by the nursing home industry to define active treatment as narrowly as possible, to prevent the dislocation of large numbers of patients with its attendant human and economic costs.

The PASARR debate dramatically illustrates the fragmentation of the neuropsychiatric care problem between the problem of the chronically mentally ill grown old, and the problem of secondary mental illnesses such as depression, delirium, or stress reactions occurring in elderly people with physical illness. PASARR was designed to keep funding for the care of the former group a state responsibility, as it has been traditionally. Doing this without discouraging the diagnosis and treatment of mental comorbidities in "medical" nursing home patients proved to be a subtle challenge for the regulation-writers at HCFA.

Whatever the precise language of the final regulations, it is likely that there will be a number of patients who will require both NF care for a medical problem or physical disability, and active treatment for mental illness, even under a narrow definition of active treatment. Service to this population will offer a meaningful opportunity for innovative collaboration between state mental health authorities and nursing facilities, which are primarily in the private sector. At a lesser cost than developing new specialized facilities for the elderly mentally ill, state mental health authorities could design "add-on" programs for service provision and staff training to enable NFs to meet the treatment needs of their mentally ill residents without discharging them. It remains to be seen whether states will have the flexibility to do this. A strong incentive is that some components of add-on treatment services might be independently reimbursable by Medicare or Medicaid, as long as they were not billed by the NF itself.

Finally, OBRA 1987 mandates the development of a national uniform data set for nursing facilities, to aid in quality assurance. To the extent that measures of cognitive function, mood, and behavior are incorporated into the data set, it may become a valuable tool for raising consciousness of neuropsychiatric issues in NF operators and medical directors. The question remains open, however, whether feedback on outcome itself will improve care, unless there are outcome-based incentives for care providers.

Direct Medicare Reimbursement for Psychologists and Clinical Social Workers: Provisions of OBRA 1989

In OBRA 1989, several changes were made in Medicare reimbursement for mental health services. Psychologists became entitled to direct Medicare reimbursement for diagnostic and therapeutic services, and social workers became entitled to reimbursement for clinical services rendered outside of hospital and nursing home settings, where social work services are regarded as included in the daily bed rate. OBRA 1989 also eliminated the annual cap on reimbursement for outpatient mental health services, but did not eliminate the 50% copayment applicable to those services.

In the debate prior to the passage of these provisions, controversy focused on how much medical involvement should be required when nonphysician providers treat mental disorders in elderly or disabled people. OBRA 1989 requires that the Secretary of HHS develop criteria under which a psychologist must agree to consult with a patient's attending physician (OBRA 1989; Section 6113). The suggestions for the content of such requirements for consultation ranged from simple notification of the attending physician to a full medical reevaluation of potential organic causes of the patient's mental symptoms. Psychiatrists advocated more stringent requirements, while psychologists emphasized their diagnostic skills as independent doctoral-level practitioners, and the adequacy of their judgment regarding the need for medical, neurological, and psychiatric input (Buie 1989). The sense of the conferees was that the required consultation should be limited to notification of the primary physician, unless the patient objected to such notification.

The passage of these provisions raises several nontrivial issues of health policy. First, the clinical and economic implications of enfranchising a new class of providers are unknown. Certainly, access to care will be increased, but it is not clear for whom care will be improved. If the change in Medicare reimbursement has the result that psychologists in large numbers begin providing consultation to nursing homes, and, as a consequence, behavioral disturbances are better managed with fewer neuroleptic drugs, the change will be highly successful. If, however, the impact is a great increase in utilization of outpatient psychological services by elderly people for problems they previously handled satisfactorily without professional help, the legislation will have the adverse outcome of withdrawing resources from other areas of greater need. The uncertainty suggests that a follow-up analysis of claims made by psychologists and social workers for the treatment of Medicare beneficiaries might be valuable. Second, the legislation raises the issue of what actually are the barriers to access to care for elderly persons with neuropsychiatric disorders. For years, the psychologists and the clinical social workers have agreed that availability and choice of providers is an important factor. If other factors, such as stigma, nonidentification of problems, or high copayments are the major barriers to access, granting Medicare vendorship to psychologists and social workers will have a relatively small effect. Third, the psychiatrists' concern about care quality is also linked to an empirically testable issue on which we have no data. However, it may be possible to determine through systematic study whether psychologists with well-defined back-up by physicians produce more or less cost-worthy care than psychologists practicing independently for problems such as organic mental syndromes and psychotoxicity of prescription drugs.

One potential approach to the quality of care issue in expanding vendorship would be to operationally define an adequate medical evaluation for an elderly person with a behavioral disorder, and would require that any vendor of Medicare mental health services address the medical dimension of the problem and document its status. A possible set of criteria is offered in Table 15-1. The argument for such criteria would be that they would prompt all care providers, including nonpsychiatric physicians and psychiatrists themselves, to give systematic attention to organic factors and drug toxicity, and to consider pharmacologic as well as nonpharmacologic interventions to treat late-life mental disorders. The disadvantage would be that the criteria could inject an additional costly layer of evaluation that may not be required in all cases. Since it is likely that HHS will *not* develop particularly stringent requirements for medical evaluation of Medicare patients receiving nonphysician mental health services, prospective evaluation of the quality of care received by such patients might help to settle the question of whether the additional costs of requiring comprehensive medical reevaluation on all patients would be justified.

Physician Payment Reform

As discussed in Chapters 6 and 7, Congress is committed to revise Medicare payment schedules that put a relatively greater value on primary care services and on "cognitive services" provided by medical specialists, a relatively lesser value on diagnostic and surgical procedures. The revaluation of services will be based in part on the Harvard Relative Value Study, commissioned by Congress and recently completed. The preliminary report on the study suggests that psychiatrists' reimbursement is unlikely to change significantly under Resource-Based Relative Value Scales (RBRVS) (Hsaio et al. 1988). This may reflect a choice of case examples for psychiatry in the Relative Value Study that were not representative of psychiatric practice, and certainly not representative of practice with multi-problem medically ill elderly psychiatric patients (Chapters 6 and 7).

Before its ultimate adoption and implementation, the RBRVS will undoubtedly be subject to political influences. Discussion of the relative value scale and related issues of procedure coding afford advocates an opportunity to raise legislators' and regulators' consciousness about unique features of neuropsychiatric care for the elderly: 1) The usual elderly psychiatric patient has one or more medical problems and is on one or more nonpsychiatric medications. Therefore, the choice of psychotropic drug can be subtle,

Table 15–1.   Criteria for evaluation of medical aspects of mental health problems of the elderly

The provision of quality mental health services to the elderly requires adequate consideration of medical aspects of diagnosis and treatment, because of the high prevalence of combined medical and psychiatric illness in old age, and because of the widespread use of prescription drugs by the elderly, many of which have significant effects on mental state. The criteria are listed below:

1. The patient's medical problem list, complete medication list, and recent laboratory data will be reviewed to identify factors possibly causal of or contributory to the patient's mental or behavioral complaint. The drug list will include over-the-counter drugs, as well as alcohol and caffeine. If the patient has not had a recent physical examination or laboratory screening, an examination and screening will be performed relevant to the patient's complaints, general physical health, and epidemiologic risk factors. If causal or contributory problems are identified, a plan of remediation will be developed.
2. The patient will be screened for common neurologic disorders frequently associated with mental and behavioral symptoms. This screening will include at the minimum an evaluation of the patient's gait, memory, cognitive abilities, speech and language, hearing, and vision. Abnormalities will be evaluated further as clinically indicated, and an assessment will be made as to whether they are causal of or contributory to the patient's mental or behavioral problems. For problems identified as causal or contributory, a plan of remediation will be developed.
3. The appropriateness of psychotropic medication for the treatment of the patient's mental or behavioral problem will be considered. Consideration will be given to both pharmacological and nonpharmacological treatments of the patient's problem.
4. The evaluation described in items 1, 2, and 3 will be repeated if there is a significant deterioration in the patient's condition, or if the patient does not respond as expected to treatment.
5. When treatment is provided by a mental health professional separate from the physician who provides the diagnostic services described in items 1 through 4, the treating mental health professional will maintain patient records that include the report of the medical evaluation described in items 1 through 4.

involving considerable knowledge and experience, as well as the assumption of a significant risk of adverse outcome. 2) In working with elderly neuropsychiatric patients, a great deal of education and explanation is necessary for the patient and family to overcome issues of stigma and misinformation. Educational activities, while not formally regarded as psychotherapy, are both time-consuming and inseparable from good psychiatric practice. 3) Differential diagnoses of elderly psychiatric patients often involve numerous organic considerations, and may require the integration of substantial physical examination and laboratory data, as well as detailed mental status information and developmental history. The cognitive task of integrating information from several domains is complex and difficult. 4) Even the apparently simple issue of adjusting medication can be more time-intensive for a frail elderly patient than for a younger patient, as it may involve overcoming sensory and cognitive impairments to assure that the patient has understood the prescription. Also, the evaluation for side effects must be more meticulous, given the risk of serious adverse outcomes such as falls and disturbances of heart rhythm.

Both coding and reimbursement should be based on recognition that geriatric psychiatry involves time-consuming services that are not psychotherapy, and that the assumption of risk in aggressively treating psychopathology in the elderly is comparable with the risk assumed by cardiologists or other medical specialists in treating many of the disorders in their domain. Reimbursement must take into account time, complexity, and risk or there will continue to be financial disincentives for psychiatrists to grapple with the neuropsychiatric problems of the elderly. The use of the same code and reimbursement for adjusting antihypertensive medication in an otherwise healthy 65-year-old and for monitoring an antidepressant drug in an 80-year-old with a mild dementia and a cardiac arrhythmia is questionable. Discrepancies of this kind should be addressed in the final form of the RBRVS.

National Regulation of Private Long-Term Care Insurance

Over the past few years, private insurers have begun to develop products insuring individuals against the financial risks of prolonged institutional long-term care. Although the cost of these policies is high and the market is as yet small, it is obvious that these products have good prospects for growth in the future. With this growth in mind, the National Association of Insurance Commissioners (NAIC) developed model state regulations for long-term care insurance plans to promote fair competition and to protect consumers from unscrupulous practices by insurance companies. State regulations modeled on the NAIC regulation had been passed by over 15 states as of January 1989, and were pending in six others (NAIC 1989).

A curious feature of the NAIC model regulation is that it permits exclusion of benefits for disability caused by mental disorders. Table 15-2 lists the exclusions for mental disorders permitted in the NAIC model regulation. It should be noted that Alzheimer's

Table 15–2. An excerpt from the Long-Term Care Insurance Model Act

B. Limitations and Exclusions. No policy may be delivered or issued for delivery in this state as long-term care insurance if such policy limits or excludes coverage by type of illness, treatment, medical condition or accident, except as follows:

(2) Mental or nervous disorders; however, this shall not permit exclusion or limitation of benefits on the basis of Alzheimer's Disease;

(3) Alcoholism and drug addiction;

(4) Illness, treatment or medical condition arising out of:

(d) suicide (sane or insane), attempted suicide or intentionally self-inflicted injury;

disease and related disorders are not regarded as mental illness by the NAIC, but that common secondary mental problems of chronically ill patients, such as major depression and organic mood disorders, *would* be regarded as mental illnesses.

The NAIC exclusions presumably could be interpreted to deny long-term care benefits to a subscriber who had a secondary depression following a stroke. Or, the self-inflicted injury clause could be used to deny benefits to an elderly person recovering from a burn that occurred when, because of dementia, he neglected to shut off a stove.

The evident intent of the exclusions in the NAIC model regulation was to prevent long-term care insurance from being used to subsidize nursing facilities as dumping grounds for individuals with intractable mental illnesses. However, given the high prevalence of comorbid physical and mental illness in old age, opportunities for misinterpretation and exploitation abound. Congressman Fortney Stark had this in mind, among other considerations, in a recently introduced bill—HR 1325—to establish a national standard for private long-term care insurance. Mr. Stark's bill modifies the NAIC regulations to prevent insurance companies from excluding coverage when mental disorders are secondary complications of physical illnesses or disabilities. Modifications, displayed in Table 15-3, implement a neuropsychiatric perspective, and represent an advance over the traditional "carving out" of benefits related to mental disorders that is characteristic of the insurance industry (see Appendix I).

At the time of this writing, the fate of Stark's bill is uncertain. The bill, if passed, would advance the interests of elderly neuropsychiatric patients by clearly articulating that cognitive and emotional problems may be an integral part of physical illness in late life, rather than a separate and stigmatized problem.

Table 15–3.   Excerpts from H.R. 1325

(iii)   Subsection B of Section 6 (relating to limitations and exclusions), except that—
   (I)   the limitation or exclusion permitted under paragraph (2) of such Subsection shall not apply to a dementing disorder, an organic mental disorder, a mental disorder which is not the primary reason for long-term or extended care, or a mental disorder which results from or complicates a primary physical illness;
   (III)   paragraph (4)(d) of such Subsection shall not apply to attempted suicide or intentionally self-inflicted injury due in whole or in part to organically-based disturbances in mood or impulse control and shall, specifically, not apply to self-injurious behavior occurring in the setting of delirium, dementia, prescription drug toxicity, severe pain, or organically-based mood disturbance;

Long-Term Care Legislation

In the 101st Congress, bills to provide federal financing of institutional long-term care for functionally impaired elderly have been introduced by Senators Kennedy and Mitchell, and Congressmen Stark and Waxman. While these bills differ in details of scope and financing, they all share a common focus on impaired function as the basis of entitlement to federally funded care, and they all provide support for noninstitutional care alternatives, based at home or in the community. In the current environment of fiscal austerity, it is unlikely that any of these bills will pass in the 101st Congress, but they represent the current evolution of thinking on the issue.

   The adoption of functional impairment as a standard for entitlement to care offers an opportunity to introduce neuropsychiatric concerns while avoiding the stigma associated with mental illness. Specifically, advocates for improved neuropsychiatric care can observe that conditions such as depression, delirium, psychotoxicity of medications, and inadequately treated psychosis impair patients' physical and instrumental function—their ability to cope independently without supervision or direct care. These disorders create excess disability no matter what physical illness an individual suffers from, and with the exception of dementia, they may be more reversible than the patient's physical impairments.

   A reasonable position for advocates in discussions of federally supported long-term care is that evaluation for eligibility for federally supported long-term care should include appropriate neuropsychiatric assessment. If a treatable neuropsychiatric problem is discovered that might contribute substantially to the patient's functional impairments, that treatment should be fully funded, as it might obviate a much greater long-term care liability for the federal government. If the evaluation were required as a precondition for utilization of the federal benefit, the evaluation itself probably would not be stigmatized. If treatment of the neuropsychiatric comorbidity were an integral part of a general treatment plan, its implementation could be made a requirement for continued federal support for long-term care services. In this way, the mechanism of financing could be used to promote access to care. Services would automatically be focused on a high-risk group where cost-offsetting effects would be expected to be greatest (see Chapter 8).

Ideas for the Future

Given the present legislative environment and the universe of needs described by the contributors of this volume, we offer three guiding ideas for approaching the future. The first is the importance of problem recognition.

Improving Identification and Recognition of Neuropsychiatric Problems

A common theme among the authors of the preceding chapters is that there is a difference in how providers and patients perceive clinical needs and the nature of care appropriate to address them. The patient with depression-causing somatic complaints, or the family struggling with a relative who became paranoid on account of prescription drug toxicity, are examples. When problems are not recognized, effective interventions cannot be provided. On a population basis, lack of problem recognition reduces the size of effective demand for appropriate services, particularly for the earlier stages of neuropsychiatric disorders where appropriate diagnosis and treatment might produce the largest economic benefits.

The process that leads to medical care often begins well before the first encounter with a health care provider. It begins with someone, a person or his caretaker, perceiving a problem for which health services might be helpful. A decision must be made to seek health services. This may involve obtaining information about what services are available, and acquiring the means to pay for them. Eventually, access to services is obtained and a first encounter with a health care provider takes place.

This encounter triggers a shift in the decision process, after which primary control over resource utilization passes from consumers to providers. Patients' right to choose their treatment is effectively constrained by the information and advice given by the care provider. The symptomatic person, upon becoming a patient, may receive acute or long-term treatment, of either simple or complex nature, the latter involving multiple diagnoses, treatments, providers, or institutions. The chain of decisions initiated after the symptomatic person becomes a patient may or may not be relevant to the original problem identified by the individual or the caretaker, and the prescribed treatment will not necessarily address the original need. (The example of aggressive laboratory workup of somatic symptoms of an untreated depression offers a poignant example.)

Four phases, beginning with the perception of need and ending with the delivery of treatment, are depicted in Table 15-4. On an aggregate basis, the process shown explains how a population's needs are transformed into effective demand for services. Inaccuracies in the recognition of problems either by patients or by providers, or impairments in access to care may lead to demand for services that do not optimally address needs.

The four phases can be identified as: 1) initial perception of a need by the individual or family; 2) access to available services; 3) problem recognition by the provider, eventually leading to a diagnosis; and 4) treatment. Emphasis in research and policy is usually placed on the fourth stage and on the diagnostic stage of the third stage. Yet, an efficient system of health care delivery that translate needs into effective demand for appropriate and cost-effective services cannot be designed or implemented without attention to all four stages of the process beginning with need and ending with treatment.

Specifically regarding the size of effective demand for neuropsychiatric services, there is, apart from discriminatory limits on third-party payment, the fact that patients and families often deny mental disorders, or misattribute their symptoms and signs to physical illness, environmental circumstances, or old age itself (see Chapters 1 and 2). Furthermore, unjustified pessimism may exist about the prognosis, particularly for late-life depression, complicated bereavement, and confusional states. Regrettably, there is still stigma attached to mental illness, and patients may feel put down by a psychiatric diagnosis, even when repeated explanations are made that mental symptoms may be of organic or "medical" origin.

Once a search for service begins, barriers are encountered that include not only an overall shortage and geographical maldistribution of geriatric mental health specialists, but also difficulty in obtaining accurate information on how to select an appropriate care provider. Alternatively, the patient or family seeks care from a primary care physician who, as Burns and Taube pointed out in Chapter 4, may misidentify the problem or address it superficially,

Table 15–4.　The path from need to treatment

Stages	Influences
1. Need perception	• Severity and visibility of problem • Cultural and familial attitudes • Personality • Denial and misattribution • Knowledge of disorders
2. Access to services	• Proximity and transportation • Cost to client • Habits and traditions of service use • Gatekeepers • Information about services
3. Problem recognition and diagnosis	• Setting of service • Presenting complaint • Duration and structure of encounter • Provider-client relationship • Caretakers' involvement • Providers' knowledge, skills, and attitudes
4. Treatment	• Scientific evidence of efficacy • Traditions of the provider's specialty • Financial incentives • Availability of treatment components • Acceptability to client and caretaker

for example, by prescribing a tranquilizer. Even if an appropriate care provider is engaged and correctly perceives the nature of the patient's problem, treatment may require a series of encounters in which medical and social interventions are continued and perhaps modified until the desired result is obtained. Along the way, barriers of stigma, geographical access, and financing may again interfere. Even if they do not, there must be a commitment of patient and provider to pursue treatment until a mutually satisfactory outcome is obtained. This commitment is based on a shared recognition of the nature of the problem and of the appropriateness of the treatment. If a primary physician, for example, only tentatively accepts that depression is real, treatable, and of great importance to function and well-being, he or she may abandon treatment if an initial drug trial is unsuccessful. Likewise, if a patient and family do not have a full understanding of a neuropsychiatric problem, they too may become disillusioned, either giving up their pursuit of treatment, or shopping around for a new physician or diagnosis.

Therefore, at each of the four phases mentioned in this discussion, there are opportunities for intervention, and associated opportunities for research. For example, much can be done to educate the public about the neuropsychiatric disorders of late life. In addition to salutary efforts by advocacy groups such as the Alzheimer's Disease and Related Disorders Association (ADRDA), more can be done through other channels of adult education, including the mass media. If the content of these educational efforts emphasized the role of brain function in mediating the mental problems of late life, the problems would be destigmatized and seen as potentially remediable, rather than merely as signs of personal weakness or failure. Furthermore, education in the responsible use of prescription drugs and over-the-counter drugs, and greater awareness of their potential for mental side effects, can enable consumers to protect themselves from drug toxicities. These efforts would further destigmatize mental problems by disseminating knowledge about the most *conspicuously organic* kind of mental disorder in old age.

Regarding initial access to care providers, state and local departments of elderly affairs, once adequately informed about needs and cost-worthy interventions for them, can develop information and outreach resources for various kinds of medical and psychosocial services available to individuals with neuropsychiatric problems. These can be accompanied by information to enable patients and their families to evaluate the quality of the services they receive, and to make rational choices among different service providers, with nondogmatic discussion of their potential strengths and weaknesses.

Primary care physicians need to be a major focus of educational interventions. Their training must go well beyond simple continuing medical education on how to prescribe the latest antidepressant drug. A central issue in primary care physicians' treatment of the elderly is *lack of awareness* of the great importance of neuropsychiatric issues to elderly patients and their families. Changes in behavior and personality frighten families, and alterations in mood, energy, appetite, and sleeping habits are disturbing to patients. A drug that produces its desired medical effect at the price of causing confusion or memory loss will probably be unacceptable to most elderly people, but they may not volunteer that their memory and mood are affected unless the physicians ask the right questions.

The issue is not just one of rote knowledge of specific facts—it is one of an attitude toward recognition of the problem. If a problem such as depression is recognized in the fullest sense by a primary care physician, that physician will seek for his or her patient whatever medical or psychological treatment is necessary to resolve that depression. When the diagnostic or therapeutic needs go beyond the physician's personal skills, an appropriate referral will be made. (Even when the physician is unsure of exactly where or how to refer, full recognition of the problem will motivate the physician to obtain the information on behalf of the patient.) All of this will happen quite naturally, *provided that the problem is fully recognized*. Therefore, educational intervention, hopefully beginning at the earliest level in medical school, should focus on making recognition of neuropsychiatric problems a basic skill possessed by all physicians who will work with the elderly.

Opportunities for research and demonstration projects exist for all of these areas of intervention. For example, to better understand whether finances, proximity, or stigma have the most to do with elderly people not using neuropsychiatric services, one could survey a large elderly population, establish the presence of need, and inquire directly as to why people have or have not sought services. Then, a cost-benefit analysis of needed services not obtained could invest the findings with policy relevance.

Another study might determine how frequently elderly people who have begun treatment for depression discontinue it prematurely, and develop hypotheses to explain why it happens. All of these approaches are relatively inexpensive but strategically valuable in converting neuropsychiatric *need* into effective *demand*, an economic reality expressed by millions of consumers willing to mobilize their financial resources, their energy, and their political power.

Generalizing the Idea of Case Management

Several chapters of this book have suggested that case management, with or without financial control, can facilitate patients getting the services they need in a timely and coordinated fashion. Case management is generally seen as something to be employed when patients need a complex mix of services that would be difficult to arrange efficiently without a "broker," or when there would be a tendency to substitute more expensive services (e.g., inpatient care) for less expensive services unless an experienced hand were guiding the process of selection. Case management for coordination has tended to focus on refractory, complex or multi-problem patients, while case management for cost control has been used in prepaid health plans, even for patients with less-difficult problems.

The notion of case management, however, can be generalized to a concept of the *management function* of medical care. This function comprises a variety of information management, referral, and decision-making functions that are necessary when care involves multiple options and multiple providers. In this sense, a physician exercises a management function when he chooses to prescribe a generic rather than a brand name prescription drug. Risks and benefits of generic prescription are weighed by the physician, a decision is made, and a referral made to a provider of the drug in question. Other less trivial examples may include a physician's role in helping a patient choose a nursing home or a subspecialist consultant. A still more complex function would be the physician's role of reviewing the entire list of medications the patient is taking and screening them for potential adverse interactions.

In general, Americans accustomed to fee-for-service medicine expect that management functions will be carried out by the physician, or perhaps be shared by the physician and the patient. Special problems arise in the care of the elderly with neuropsychiatric problems, particularly if these problems are combined with multiple physical illnesses and disabilities: The physician may lack the knowledge, skills, attitudes, or time to perform the management function adequately if it reaches an excessive level of complexity. The patient may lack the cognitive or emotional capacity to participate fully in his or her part of the management function. In this situation, care is left to be managed badly, or informal managers are brought in, such as concerned family members, geriatric specialists, geriatric social workers, etc. The central point is that whether or not a patient receives formal case management or participates in a managed care system, medical care has a management function that is performed more or less well.

Requirements for the patient's effective participation in care management include the intellectual capacity to appreciate the problems, the judgment to make good decisions, and sufficient knowledge to understand problems and treatment options. If the patient lacks these prerequisites, family caretakers, if they possess them, can function as care managers. However, this requires satisfactory interpersonal relations between patient and family. Finally, the attending physician must be sufficiently informed about the issues of geriatric care, neuropsychiatric disorders, and the services available to offer the patient and family appropriate counsel on a full range of choices.

Because the neuropsychiatric disorders of late life often impair intellect and judgment, and because of limitations on physicians' specialized knowledge, time, and perhaps communication skills, it often happens that elderly patients and their physicians require assistance from specialists in the management function when dealing with neuropsychiatric problems. Physicians, nonmedical health service providers, social service providers, and lay people all can learn many of the components of managing care for the elderly. The dissemination of management knowledge and skills offers significant hope of rationalizing services by improving the management of care, and thus bringing effective economic demand more in accord with patients' actual needs. Opportunity exists both for outcome research and for educational research on the development of care management functions.

Developing New Programs on a Regional Basis

For reasons both fiscal and political, it is unlikely that the federal government will be the source of major new innovation in neuropsychiatric care. Perhaps this is appropriate, because different regions of the United States face quite different challenges. There are significant regional differences in the supply of health care workers, in the age distribution of the population, and in wealth—the latter being related to the implementation of Medicaid benefits and the funding of state mental health systems. Expectations, needs, and effective demand vary among regions and depend on such factors as the educational level of the population, its ethnic composition, and its level of poverty or wealth. The role of the private sector differs also among regions. In some New England states, there are few proprietary hospitals, while in some Sunbelt states, these institutions predominate. Psychiatrists are in shorter supply in the South and Midwest and in rural areas than on the two coasts and in urban areas. Some regions are better endowed than others with established homes for the aged and other institutions directed toward elderly people. The predominant third-party carriers and Medicare intermediaries may have differing levels of openness to innovation. Finally, the legal climate, including the prevalence of malpractice suits and the fear of litigation, differs from state to state, as evidenced by the wide variation in liability insurance rates.

Because of this variation and ongoing efforts to contain federal support of health care, regional planning may be more rational and efficient than a single federal plan. In regional planning, the private sector can develop service packages for those most able to buy—whether they be state agencies or affluent consumers with discretionary income to spend on customized health care services. Academic institutions, besides performing their traditional functions of research and formal training, can be involved in educational and outreach efforts. Private industry, as distinct from the health care industry, can participate in regional planning. Private industry is at risk, because of its responsibility for retiree health benefits, an increasing number of elderly workers in some regions, and the indirect impact of neuropsychiatric problems on family caretakers who may currently be middle-aged members of the workforce. Industry must be regarded as an interested party in regional planning efforts. Even when the initial contribution is small, the involvement of major local industries is crucial to developing the kind of shift in perspective necessary to create a more effective system of care.

States, perhaps in collaboration across regions, should also re-examine legal and regulatory barriers to innovation in the provision of services to impaired elderly people. Tort reform initiatives might consider limiting the liability of nursing homes for accidents that occur when patients are granted more autonomy, with due consideration and acceptance of the risk of injury. Regulations in some states that require all general hospital psychiatric units to accept dangerous and involuntary patients might be modified to permit specialized geropsychiatric units to treat frail elderly in a safer and less threatening setting where they are not exposed to young and acutely psychotic patients. Licensing and certification rules might be changed to allow the development of hybrid facilities for functionally impaired elderly with concurrent behavioral problems, that permit active treatment of the behavioral problems without the necessity of transfer to another facility. Finally, states could work collaboratively to fully exploit Medicare and Medicaid waiver programs, and assist local agencies and private providers in making the most of existing federally funded programs. All of these efforts might be accomplished efficiently by states providing resources across regions with common concerns and constraints.

References

Buie J: Medicare win looms closer after hearing. APA Monitor 20:1, 17, 1989

Federal Register: Rules and regulations. Federal Register. 54:5316-5373, 1989

Health Care Financing Administration (HCFA): State Medicaid Manual, Part 4. HCFA Publication 45-4. Washington, DC, Health Care Financing Administration, 1989

Hsaio WC, Braun P, Becker E, et al: A National Study of Resource-Based Relative Value Scales for Physician Services: Final Report. Boston, Harvard School of Public Health, 1988

National Association of Insurance Commissioners: Long-Term Care Insurance Model Act, 1989

National Mental Health Association: Nursing Home Reform Legislation of 1987: What MHAs Can Do (pamphlet). Alexandria, Va, National Mental Health Association, December 1988

Appendix I

A Window on the Debate: Dialogues from the National Conference

Edited by Barry S. Fogel, M.D.

Improved services for elderly people with neuropsychiatric problems will require effort from four different sectors of the health care system: state and local government agencies, private providers ranging from HMOs to hospitals to individual practitioners, federal Medicare and Medicaid programs, and the health insurance industry. In addition, both the medical research community and the health services research community will have a role to play. At the National Conference on Access and Financing for Neuropsychiatric Care for the Elderly, groups comprised of policymakers, advocates, providers, and researchers engaged in dialogue focusing on each of the four main sectors. With a large problem, a multiplicity of strongly held viewpoints, and about two hours to meet, no consensus was expected. It was hoped, however, that major issues and viewpoints would be better defined, and that some priorities for services research would be identified.

In the following reports of working groups, a brief summary of shared perceptions of reality, prevalent opinions, and services research priorities is offered. These are followed by edited vignettes of actual dialogue. To offer the greatest freedom to conference participants, it was agreed at the conference that dialogue would not be attributed to specific individuals. For this reason, speakers are identified generically, by their professional roles.

State and Local Agencies

Shared Perceptions of Reality

1. There is extreme diversity among states and localities regarding the resources they commit to the mentally ill. This implies that new federal policies are likely to help some public mental health systems and have an adverse impact on others.
2. The traditional responsibility of the public sector mental health systems has been the care of the severely and chronically mentally ill; psychiatric complications of medical illness have not been in their ambit.
3. Development of new services within public sector mental health systems usually is at the expense of established services, given overall constraints on resources.
4. It is possible to have any two, but not three, of the following simultaneously: deregulation, cost containment, and equity of access.
5. Unless informed clearly by the state and local agencies that will be affected, members of Congress are often unclear about the likely winners and losers from particular pieces of health policy legislation.
6. Local agencies prefer state funding and local control; state agencies prefer federal funding and state control.
7. Cost-shifting is universal: States shift patients to Medicare-funded acute hospitals whenever they can, while federal policy aims to move patients from Medicaid-funded nursing facilities to state-funded mental health facilities.

Prevalent Opinions

1. Any expansion of the role of state mental health systems in the care of the elderly should be accompanied by new resources, lest new services be at the expense of the chronically mentally ill who have traditionally relied upon state systems.
2. Patients with psychiatric complications of medical illness and no prior mental illness should be treated within the general health sector.
3. Patients with chronic mental illness who develop medical illness in old age should not be treated in public sector mental health systems, because their care is expensive and will take funds away from other clients.
4. Too much local autonomy in the provision of public mental health services leads to gross inequality among localities; states

should be the guarantor of equity by setting floors on services as a condition for localities obtaining state funding.

5. Greater flexibility in employing existing federal funds, for example through waivers, is desirable, but more resources and absolute terms are needed to adequately serve the chronically mentally ill.

6. Local program directors often do not know how to best utilize the federal entitlements, and the Medicaid system in particular.

7. Though regulation is experienced as distasteful, most people working in state and local agencies prefer regulation to sacrificing equity or cost-containment.

8. On-site mental health services should be more available at places frequented by the elderly, including senior centers and elderly housing.

9. Primary care physicians need better skills in handling common mental health problems of the elderly, such as depression and dementia.

Services Research Priority

Development of outcome measures that permit objective evaluation of a public system's performance. This could bring more objectivity to the discussion of control issues between states, localities, and the federal government, and to arguments about the level of funding necessary to provide adequate care.

Dialogue

A Congressional staff person: Communication from local to state to federal level must be improved.

An economist: Not more paperwork!

A Congressional staff person: No, more understanding. Make sure that people representing your state know what's going on! There is the question, however, of the federal government preempting state policy. Any state that's doing well wants to be exempt from federal standards; the ones doing poorly want to have the federal government raise their standards, particularly if they pay for the improved standards with federal dollars.

A state legislative staff person: Everyone wants a bit of control, so a partnership is an obvious solution. The Medicaid waiver program is a positive example.

A state mental health official: As long as states fund the programs they'll want some control. In our state, the counties go directly to

Washington. And they don't agree about the best way to provide care. So, Washington hears mixed messages.

An economist: How could states coordinate local efforts?

A state mental health official: There are lots of questions. Where should services be provided? When is centralization an advantage? What's the optimum mix of community versus institutional services? For all of these questions, large counties want independence, but small ones want the state to do the job.

An advocate: The federal government can facilitate states' efforts to set priorities. But because the mentally ill are politically disempowered, local communities should not determine the priorities. If localities get more money from the states they must be accountable! If states channel the money, they can set performance criteria. But, to build a local infrastructure, states must relinquish their roles as service providers. Ideally, local communities should deliver local services with constraining structures at other levels of government based on performance criteria.

A state mental health official: States don't run community programs, they monitor them. The states' interest is to reduce the size of the state hospital system, and they can't do that without help from localities. But if states put 50% to 60% of the funding into local programs, they are entitled to a say over priorities. What we don't know, is who is really best served by state hospitals versus community settings?

A state legislator: The state bails out localities when local and federal support is cut back. And as long as they pay, they'd better get a say!

An advocate: But give them the money. Counties won't stop hospitalizing patients unless they can keep some of the cost savings. If you allocated state money to counties to buy hospital care you would change the incentives.

. . . . .

A state legislative staff person: As private providers get interested in providing a service, like home care or long-term care, localities become third-party payers, rather than providers. States and localities serve as *gap fillers, payers,* and *regulators.* If the private sector can handle it, let them do it!

An economist: Should the private sector be offered incentives?

A state mental health official: The private sector has expertise at cost control; business does better at business.

Another state mental health official: What the private sector does is a better job of screening the people out. A few weeks ago there was a strike at a private psychiatric hospital. One day later 50% of their patients were out. They must have been pretty sick! I think the private sector is overrated. . . . They cull out the bad risks. I'd love to see a private sector hospital serve the population we serve. How do you get the private sector into the business?—You force them!

A state legislator: You have to lean on them to take the serious cases. It costs a lot of money to take care of the really sick patients. We like to use the private sector but you need to keep an eye on them.

An economist: Does the public sector do a better job than the private sector for money spent for seriously ill patients?

A state mental health official: Historically, the state hospital is where you put the patients nobody wants. Really sick patients mess up the pristine atmosphere of a private hospital.

A researcher: But you can segment internally and keep stigmatized patients on a special ward. The question is, who is really more efficient?

An advocate: It'll never be profitable to take care of sick patients. The federal government will never pay enough to make it profitable.

. . . . .

A Congressional staff person: I'm not a doctor, but my impression is that it's easier to diagnose and understand cardiovascular problems than to diagnose someone with a little bit of memory loss—is it a disease or just old age?

A researcher: When people are old, what's the return on investment?

A Congressional staff person: Are we going to put a 75-year-old person back to work, even if we found a cure for Alzheimer's disease?

An Alzheimer's disease program official: There are elders out there who do work.

A Congressional staff person: But it's still not the same as with a 35-year-old with so many years of potential employment ahead of him or her.

An economist: Different services go to different people, based on their socioeconomic status. The public/private split makes it easier to do that.

A researcher: No solutions can shift the status quo regarding the sharing of burden between local, state, and federal government. There is a reluctant acceptance of nonegalitarian solutions. There are three values; you can have any two but not all three: deregulation, contained costs, and equity. We are apparently willing to sacrifice equity.

A state mental health official: Reduce federal involvement, except for the dollars! That will help.

A researcher: That is the status quo of state government's position. They want control, but with federal dollars.

A Congressional staff person: People don't like paying federal taxes without federal control.

A researcher: There's a striking contradiction in this meeting. In our earlier discussion of the system, most people seemed willing to accept a status quo that compromises equity. But when our basic values are discussed this isn't so.
. . . . .

A local program official: We need to show elderly people that the public sector delivers quality mental health care.

A state legislative staff person: I wouldn't recommend that to seniors in my state—the system is so overburdened now. The system would have to totally shift gears to properly serve seniors. Plus, we'd be asking those seniors to learn to use a totally new system. Instead, let's build up mental health services in day care, senior centers, etc.

An Alzheimer's program official: Education of primary care providers and case managers makes sense in every state.

An advocate: I think it's better for the general medical care system to take care of these problems (dementia and depression)—that's where the patients are. The *only goal* of the public mental health system should be to treat the severely and chronically mentally ill. Those other patients are more acceptable to the general health system. They would divert attention from the patients who need the state mental health system more.

A researcher: I agree that depressed patients should be mainstreamed.
. . . . .

A state mental health official: The state mental health system is for people who can't be mainstreamed.

Another state mental health official: The state mental system isn't the right place for a depressed senior—he'd be a square peg in a round hole.

A state legislative staff person: There are patients who will need both traditional mental health services and medical services.

Another state mental health official: You can only integrate services if you control them. We used to shuttle patients back and forth between the state psych hospital and the general hospital. Now we just send everyone over 65 to one general purpose geriatric hospital. The diagnosis is interesting, but not always relevant. CMHCs have never picked up the charge of serving the elderly, but they may in the near future. So, elderly and severely, chronically mentally ill people are now in competition for a limited pool of resources.

A researcher: Why does the state need to get involved with the elderly at all?

A state mental health program official: Because the state has money, or can get it thorough Medicare and waivers, and they have control of CMHCs. Not a lot of people want to get into this business of caring for the elderly with mental health problems, and Medicare really doesn't cover it.   . . . . .

A state legislative staff person: Medicare benefits should be more responsive to the needs of the people. A 50% copay on psychiatric services is a deterrent to access.

A researcher: But 50% of Medicare is better than 100% of a totally inadequate Medicaid rate.

An Alzheimer's program official: Any federally supported program for medical education should require that geriatrics and geriatric mental health be taught, as a requirement for federal support. And staff in any senior program should have some training in geriatric mental health.

A Congressional staff person: All the money for all these projects is ultimately coming from the taxpayers. Right now, the public does not perceive that the current system delivers high quality care at a reasonable price—so show the results!

Private Providers

Shared Perceptions of Reality

1. The private sector must answer to its sources of capital, and will not deliver services unless doing so is profitable.
2. Private facilities usually have better access to well-paid experts in new technologies than public facilities.
3. Private providers usually do better than public agencies at tracking and controlling costs, particularly labor costs.
4. The private sector has incentives to skim—to treat less sick patients to make greater profits.
5. The success of private sector health care products depends more on marketing than on scientific proof of their efficacy.
6. The present financing system offers incentives to overutilize inpatient care.

Prevalent Opinions

1. Private sector contracts with government agencies only make sense if they allow adequate margins, and have a long enough term for providers to profit from efficiencies gained through experience.
2. Private providers would welcome greater flexibility and licensing, certification, and reimbursements; this would facilitate their ability to innovate.
3. The private sector is unlikely to assume responsibility for the care of the chronically and severely mentally ill.
4. The private sector's development of new neuropsychiatric services for the elderly probably will begin with high-quality specialty services for affluent elderly.
5. Public-private collaboration will be encouraged by permitting for-profit entities to bid on federal demonstration projects to develop and test new models of care.
6. Some regulation of private providers is necessary to limit skimming of the best-insured and least sick patients.

Services Research Priorities

1. Development of a more equitable system of payment, such as outcome-based reimbursement, that would allow profits to be made caring for sicker and more complex patients.
2. Empirical studies of resource inputs needed for treatment of specific conditions, to enable private providers to cut costs with-

out compromising quality. Cutting inpatient lengths of stay and reducing staff:patient ratios would both be facilitated by empirical support if this could be done without harming patients.

3. Understanding how to influence physicians to utilize hospital resources more efficiently.

Dialogue

An entrepreneur: Can you make money off of government-funded programs? We can't get hospitals to do it if there's no profit in it. Why invest in developing specialty geriatric programs if you can get more profit by putting your resources some place else?

An insurance executive: We have to pay for programs, and have to rate their quality. For example, some head trauma programs are worth $500 a day, but many others are not.

A researcher: The health industry says they can't make money off of the government. Why does the defense industry say they can?

An entrepreneur: The defense industry is now where the health industry was five years ago.
                    . . . . .

An entrepreneur: Private providers will not invest capital in elderly care if they fear they'll lose money, especially if they're likely to make money on, say, adolescent services or a mobile diagnostic unit. With lithotripters, we committed ourselves to buying the manufacturer's entire production of the machines for a year, so that we could get them before the competition. For something technological, we'll commit private capital, but not for developing new services for the elderly.

A physician executive: How will services be developed for the elderly by the private sector? Initially, by developing services for aging yuppies who want to buy high-line services. For example, retirement communities may offer case management as an attractive feature. If these features work out, they'll trickle down, or be seen as indispensable, and then be purchased, in a less luxurious form, by the public sector.

A state mental health official: But who developed case management? The public sector! You're talking about applying CMHC technology for profit! The private sector will borrow what's best from public systems.
                    . . . . .

A researcher: We all agree that there are certain services that should be delivered. There is a need for geriatric psychiatric care in various settings. Our private providers must answer to investors and that constrains them. The nonprofit providers feel freer to pursue values, though the government may constrain them. The payers want evidence of effectiveness, but the evidence is often a matter of packaging. "Centers of excellence," for example, can claim higher fees.

But it's hard to conceive of "centers of excellence" for many areas in geriatric psychiatry. Alzheimer's disease may be an exception—there could be centers that specialize in offering the latest in drug treatment for Alzheimer's disease.

But for many problems, treatment is required on-site, whether at a nursing home or a primary care center. Some of those people are going to turn up in private hospitals. How could the elderly compete as consumers for hospitals' services? Could hospitals start to develop services now, or has the government permanently debased this issue?

A drug company executive: Neither the public nor the private sector can do it alone, especially in long-term care. But be careful! Nursing homes are already stigmatized—nursing homes with psychiatric services will be doubly stigmatized! Demand may not exist, because elderly people don't want to identify themselves as consumers of mental health services.
. . . . .

An advocate: Differences among states in Medicaid eligibility makes it harder. For example, in my state, Medicaid won't fund geropsychiatric inpatient treatment in a psychiatric hospital.
. . . . .

A researcher: Would it help to set up models of excellence in psychogeriatric care—to advance the delivery of services, to reassure certain payers, and to interest the private sector?

An entrepreneur: Look at the auto industry. First, you develop the Mercedes, then General Motors copies it. In nursing homes, look at the payor mix. More government payers usually means lower quality.

A physician executive: But you need four-wheel drive cars as well as Mercedes. Consider day care—there are lots of ways to do it: home care, licensed facilities. . . . Elderly people need more alternatives. Now, you go to a hospital, or you see someone once a week. Where are the partial hospitals? We need a spectrum of care, as well as enthusiasm and high morale.

A researcher: Let's merge the auto industry and centers of excellence metaphors. What do you want in a nursing home . . . amenities? rehabilitation? Excellence can only be defined with respect to given goals. Now, excellence is defined by inputs rather than outcomes.

. . . . .

A nursing home executive: I'd like to offer better psychiatric services to Alzheimer's patients. But Medicaid doesn't pay adequately, so we have to have the right mix of Medicaid and private pay.

What we need desperately is treatment for patients in our nursing homes with chronic psychiatric conditions who develop acute flare-ups. For example, treating acute depression occurring in the nursing home. We can't treat these for two reasons: licensure and reimbursement.

A physician: Why not use consulting psychiatrists?

A nursing home executive: Try to find them. Then try to get them fair reimbursement. Plus, SNFs may not offer acute psychiatric treatment. The only way we could give the services we want is to get Medicare-recognized acute psychiatric beds.

. . . . .

A physician executive: What if a patient is psychotically depressed? A work-up plus a medication trial plus ECT is a money loser. That's why hospitals don't want to do geriatric psychiatry.

Another physician: There's no way to adequately evaluate and treat a psychotic depression in 12 days, or even the 20 that may be allowed under the TEFRA cap. Many patients need six weeks!

An insurance executive: But you've helped me. I might have believed it was *three years.*

A researcher: But you could do some of the evaluation in a lower cost setting. You are saying: How long does it take, and then multiply in the acute hospital rate. What if we specify the amount you had to spend, then if you wanted six weeks you would have it . . . in a less intense and costly setting.

An advocate: If you want us to do that, end the regulations that prevent us from doing it!

A state mental health official: There are lots of alternatives that may be more cost effective, but they're not reimbursed. Only the acute hospital level is reimbursed.

Another advocate: If Medicaid paid for active treatment in nursing homes, when it was needed, fewer patients would wind up in hospitals.

. . . . .

A state mental health official: Not all private care is of high quality, but some private providers have great skills, paradoxically used to take care of less sick patients. We like tapping that talent.

A retirement home executive: Private companies must deal with the bottom line. If there is no profit, they'll sit it out. But, if the field is really big, companies may be willing to experiment to see if there's some profit in it.

A physician executive: Take the example of alcohol rehabilitation. We sold the idea to industry, but it turned out residential treatment centers do it as well, and for about one-third of the cost, as hospitals. So now we're getting out of that business in our hospitals. We limit ourselves to what we do best . . . dual diagnosis patients, and particularly complex patients.
· · · · ·
A nursing home executive: We're really worried about OBRA and their preadmission screening rules. They won't let us consider the availability of other dispositions when we do our screening.

State mental health official: HCFA has the object of cutting benefits to mentally ill elderly. What they'll get is under-diagnosis of mental illness.
· · · · ·
A retirement housing executive: When the defense department needs a new bomb, they put out a contract to develop the technology. HHS could do the same, and private providers should be able to bid.

A state mental health official: Existing HHS contracts go to non-profits. These should be open to for-profits.

An entrepreneur: We have a different problem—with our doctors. We want to get length of stay down to 12 days, but the doctors in Texas think that's malpractice. Develop a good psychiatric product with short lengths of stay, and get the doctors to believe in it, and I've got something I can sell.
· · · · ·
A state mental health official: The public sector doesn't spend enough—that's one thing that distinguishes it from the private sector. Private facilities, if well run, may offer a lower episode cost than public facilities, because their shorter lengths of stay may outweigh a higher daily bed rate.

So much public sector long-term care is bad. More money might help, but some state institutions just aren't flexible enough to make use of more money.

A physician: Why is it expensive *and* bad in some cases?

A state mental health official: Labor costs—expensive union contracts rather than money spent on patient care, and high costs for workers' compensation.

A nursing home executive: Private nursing homes taking patients that used to be in state hospitals, and take care of them for less money. Why? Those state hospitals had poor cost controls. They had an annual lump sum and they spent it.

A physician executive: If inpatient care and outpatient care are options, the hospital industry will promote inpatient care. But as a purchaser, you'd favor the cheaper mode of treatment. We might provide cheap, high-quality care as a loss leader to improve volume—operating an emergency room is a good example. We also provide community services to establish our place in the community.

A nursing home executive: Our Alzheimer's facilities offer free respite care, and this creates a potential customer base for our nursing homes. They find out nursing homes aren't so bad.

A researcher: Let's watch the paeans to private industry. Public systems are accountable to the public in the way that private providers are not. Issues of distribution are important.

A retirement housing executive: The pie is big enough for everybody.

A researcher: Only if you see no limit to the resources you're going to put into care.

A physician executive: Our companies bid on the management of public hospitals. We know how to cut costs, especially labor costs. We can come into a large complex system and bring in excellent management skills.

An entrepreneur: Consider the perils of dealing with the state. A well-known private hospital made contracts and turned around a number of public hospitals—then the state took the contracts away and gave them to Joe's Psych Company, because they offered a lower rate. We need longer contracts for management contracts to make sense.

A physician executive: We can design a hospital building in a day...and get it built in 10 months. The public sector could use those skills.

A retirement housing executive: If we could trust each other.

A researcher: Time for closing thoughts. We've identified some potential areas for collaboration. What do you want me to say tomorrow?

A physician executive: Say nice things about the capabilities of the private sector. Also, emphasize our duties to our sources of capital. We have organizational skills to offer, and less dead wood than the public sector.

A nursing home executive: Access and competence often follow reimbursement.

State mental health official: The private sector should not retreat from the challenge of treating this population. There are areas where the private sector can do a better job than state-operated facilities.

An advocate: Teaching hospitals, whether public or private, can do a better job of educating future providers about the psychiatric problems of the elderly.

An entrepreneur: Development of pilot programs that could be cloned is an acceptable role for private hospitals, and could be sold to a board of directors. But, we hope that the people we deal with would accept the principle that "no margin . . . no mission." A return on capital is a necessary piece of the equation.

Researcher: Let's not blur the for-profit/nonprofit distinction. Let's better define what we want to buy, then we'd communicate better and could haggle over price. But let's buy results, not services!

An insurance executive: For-profit is not bad. The public sector is neither sacrosanct nor totally bureaucratic. Both sectors must work together. But be careful that the privates, in scrambling for market share, don't "skim the cream."

Another researcher: Skimming versus efficiency, that's the $64 question.

Nursing home executive: We need flexibility in licensure, certification, and reimbursement. Without flexibility, we limit families' choices.

Medicare and Medicaid Programs

Shared Perceptions of Reality

1. The government finances health services, but has only indirect influence over their organization and delivery.
2. Medicaid waivers would permit innovative models of care, but the waivers are difficult to use.
3. HCFA, because it must restrain expenditures, does not take an active role in informing the public about its waivers and less familiar benefits.
4. Psychiatric treatment remains stigmatized for many, if not most, older Americans.
5. Elderly patients with psychiatric complications of physical illness do not use the public mental health system.
6. Congress is more responsive to the demands of a broad consensus than to special pleadings by provider groups.
7. Federal health care policy is more responsive to political power than to research findings.

Prevalent Opinions

1. Depression in the medically ill elderly is frequently undiagnosed, misdiagnosed, or improperly treated, despite research evidence that treatment is effective.
2. Impediments to recognition and treatment of depression include providers' knowledge, skills, and attitudes, and patients' fear of stigma.
3. Improving Medicare coverage for the treatment of depression would improve access to care, but would not in itself solve the problem of undertreatment.
4. Access to neuropsychiatric services would be improved by offering them on-site in elderly housing and senior centers.
5. Better education of providers and patients regarding neuropsychiatric disorders is needed; incentives for evaluation could be linked to Medicare support of teaching hospitals.
6. Screening nursing home patients for mental disorders may either improve their care or lead to dumping, depending on whether treatment is actually offered.

Services Research Priorities

1. Better understanding of access to neuropsychiatric care, impediments, and how to promote timely access.

2. Better understanding of how to positively influence provider behavior.

Dialogue

A Congressional staff person: I am rather cool about special pleadings by provider groups and by settings. When they get the ear of the government, incentives are distorted. In some states, a *visit* by a home health service gets more Medicare dollars than a day in a nursing home! My boss feels that nursing home beds would be overutilized if they were covered by Medicare.

Another Congressional staff person: The federal government does not deal explicitly with the organization and delivery of services. It just finances them. . . . We are suspicious of claims of cost offsets. "It'll really be cheaper, trust me!"
     . . . . .

A researcher: I am concerned about splitting services between physical and mental, leaving enormous gaps. There is a convergence between the mentally ill getting physically sick in old age, and physically ill people developing mental illnesses. We've got to separate a difference in labeling from a real difference.

A political scientist: There is a tendency to fragment the community into special interests, shifting costs and shifting patients. Private industry are looking for licenses, and looking for "good patients." It's Calvinistic—"Perdition and redemption preordained by case mix."
     . . . . .

A federal official: People waste my time when they complain the system doesn't work. They should operate the system as if it were to their advantage. Now case management is a nonsense term but nonetheless a valuable idea; Medicaid case management benefits are well-used because intelligence and time are needed to figure out how to use the Medicaid system. It's better to get paid under the case management benefit than under the 50%-reimbursed administrative match. I think there is a lack of attention to what is already available, especially for Medicaid. For example, more could be done with inter-agency agreements, whereunder state Medicaid is supposed to negotiate treaties with other providers of care to Medicaid beneficiaries. Case management is needed both at the state level and at the recipient level. The system is too arcane for people to use without skilled help. . . . Congress acts at the margins, incrementally. Therefore, use the system to the max, find its weaknesses, and then have them fixed, a little bit at a time.
     . . . . .

A psychiatrist: The majority of my visits to the elderly are home visits. A lot of my patients are physically ill as well, and have mobility problems. Providing services on location overcomes stigma. I provided services on-site in a senior citizen building. Before on-site services were available, 2% of the residents used mental health services; now 18% utilize them. I think it would be a good idea to provide a lower copayment under Medicare for on-site mental health services in elderly housing and in nursing homes.

A researcher: This would facilitate access but not necessarily save money. Also, it would be an incentive to patients, but not for providers to go into homes in the first place.

An economist: We need different solutions for different problems. Consider depression: A physician may not recognize depression or may recognize it and not know how to treat it. Better physician education and questions about depression on board examinations might help, but I don't think it would be enough. Could we use the Relative Value Scale somehow to push physicians to recognize depression?

Depression recognition in high-risk conditions such as cancer and stroke should be built into protocols for assuring quality of care. In-hospital consultative follow-up by psychiatrists should be covered.

Also, we have the problem of mental toxicity of prescription drugs—could physicians' training in clinical pharmacology be improved?

A Congressional staff person: Medicare will soon begin paying for drugs, and could then require coordination of drug lists, supplying composite drug lists to primary care physicians.

A government official: HCFA may require that bidders on drug financing contracts be required to screen for adverse drug interactions.

A researcher: But to be effective, the system would have to be real time, and even then, the physicians wouldn't necessarily change their behavior, given the lists of drugs. Thus, how do we educate our providers effectively? Are there financial barriers to provider education?

An advocate: You bet! Medical schools don't educate their students on issues of chronic care, in part because the money isn't in it! If the school and faculty practice are making out well, why change?

A researcher: Education in geriatric care has historically been limited. This needs change!

A Congressional staff person: Negative incentives generally work best—do it or you don't get Medicare dollars.

A hospital chain executive: Hospitals want teaching dollars, so make subsidies for teaching hospitals contingent on adequate geriatric training.

A researcher: For training, a few million here and there make a big difference.

An advocate: Money should be spent to train all physicians, not just specialists, to take better care of the elderly. And, it should be spent early in medical training, even before the bulk of hospital training.

. . . . .

A psychiatrist: Psychiatric services in residential buildings may reduce building-wide anxiety, enabling residents to tolerate deviant behavior, and empower them to deal with neighbors' deviance. I believe there should be tax breaks for office space for mental health providers within housing for the elderly.

A political scientist: Who should have access to this space?

A Congressional staff person: Don't fight over who gets to provide services! That wastes political capital. There are problems, given the boundary between medical and social services, as to whose bailiwick this would be in.

. . . . .

An economist: We have a heterogeneous set of issues. Let's break it up into homogeneous subgroups. Medical patients with psych complications are unlikely to use CMHCs—like patients with post-stroke depressions, post-surgical depressions, and drug toxicity. A second group is the cognitively impaired. A third group is the chronically mentally ill, including alcohol and drug abusers.

. . . . .

A Congressional staff person: Getting nonpsychiatric physicians to recognize mental health problems is crucial. Financial incentives are indirect and inefficient.

A researcher: Financial barriers to access may predominate among traditional users of specialty mental health services, but nonfinancial barriers may predominate among patients seen in medical primary care settings.

An economist: Many patients would be willing to pay for treatment if the problem were recognized. Doctors may hear complaints compatible with a diagnosis of depression and not make the diagnosis.

A researcher: And mental health interventions for secondary depression in the medically ill are effective.

An economist: Granted, but how do you get changes—through the financing mechanism or through education? Physician knowledge and behavior must be addressed.

A hospital chain executive: The relative value scale will pay physicians for cognitive services. Are you saying that physicians don't know how to render these services? Physicians should define screening for psychiatric complications as part of the service they render.

Another researcher: How much time can you expect a primary care physician to devote to a depressed elderly person when he has a waiting room full of sick patients and an average of 11 minutes for each of them? Drug therapy isn't the entire answer—perhaps briefer talking treatments could be developed. RVS will enable physicians to afford to spend more time with patients. But will they spend it with depressed elderly people?

A hospital chain executive: We must raise consciousness, make it clear that mental health assessment is part of cognitive skills.

A third researcher: We must answer the question: Why do providers fail to treat mental disorders they know about? We need research into the reasons for nonintervention.

. . . . .

A Congressional staff person: Perhaps we need education for *patients* to encourage reporting of cognitive and affective symptoms, and how to do it—offer some kind of assertiveness training for patients and families.

A researcher: Who would do that?

A Congressional staff person: The area Administration on Aging, the National Institute on Aging, the Association for the Mentally Ill, the National Institute of Mental Health. There are people who know they have mental symptoms but don't report them.

An advocate: ADRDA has destigmatized Alzheimer's disease, but has identified service gaps. Consumer initiative is important. So educate the general public.

An economist: Depression in the medically ill isn't limited to the elderly. Should indirect education benefits be linked to specific

education on geriatric and mental health issues? Maybe there
should be special RVS codes for medical/psychiatric evaluations,
such as assessment for drug toxicity or a brown bag drug evaluation.

. . . . .

A researcher: The preservation or improvement of function is
going to be a major theme in long-term care legislation. The links
between physical health, mental health, and overall function
need further study.

. . . . .

A researcher: We need a primer of options for funding treatment
under present programs, to increase both provider and beneficiary awareness.

A government official: HCFA is pressured to cut its outlays: you
can't expect them to help people utilize services!

Economist: Why *can't* HCFA provide its own educational publications?

A researcher: And can't Medicaid rates of reimbursement be more
realistic?

Health Insurance Industry

Shared Perceptions of Reality

1. Companies don't choose to take risks they can't accurately estimate, therefore better-defined and more standardized treatments are more likely to be covered.
2. If consumers deny the possibility that they will ever need psychiatric treatment, they will be unwilling to pay more for better
   psychiatric coverage.
3. Escalating medical care costs are forcing companies to emphasize
   utilization review and quality assurance.
4. Executives believe some cost-offset effects of psychiatric care
   might exist, especially for depression, but doubt that the company paying for the treatment will necessarily profit from the
   savings, and worry that increased psychiatric benefits would be
   used by many people for whom there are *no* cost-offsets.
5. Separation of mental health benefits from other medical benefits
   is the rule in the industry, and it persists despite individual
   executives' awareness that physical and mental health may be
   linked in patients.
6. HMOs and other prepaid plans generally retain the tradition of
   separating or "carving out" mental health benefits.

Prevalent Opinions

1. Better utilization review and quality assurance for psychiatric care will make it less costly and more insurable.
2. Capitation carries serious conflict of interest risks.
3. Case management may be useful in very costly or complex cases, but is too expensive to be used routinely.
4. Flexibility in benefit design can save money, as when partial hospital care can be substituted for inpatient care.
5. National standards for coverage would make insurance companies' jobs easier.

Services Research Priorities

1. Better standardization of diagnosis and treatment.
2. Determining which providers and settings deliver particular services most efficiently.
3. Identifying high-risk groups for whom cost-offsetting effects of psychiatric treatment are greatest.
4. Determining patient groups for whom inpatient care can be replaced by less costly alternatives, without compromising outcome or safety.
5. Development of scientifically supported and easily applied protocols for quality assurance for psychiatric care.

Dialogue

A researcher: A major role of private insurance has been Medigap coverage. Should there be products that go beyond just filling the gaps?

An insurance executive: Medigap contributes to the problem of escalating costs by making consumers insensitive to price. We must also ask how well providers are doing in managing themselves, and in dealing with the elderly population.

Another insurance executive: We're not too worried about Medigap driving up costs, but about Medigap becoming obsolete because of the Catastrophic Bill. We are thinking of expanding Medigap to cover long-term care, health promotion, and other new services. But we are driven by the market, and will only offer coverage people want to buy. If a product with better mental health coverage only appealed to the mentally ill, it wouldn't be a good product. Until people want better psychiatric benefits, you'll be at a competitive disadvantage if you offer them. For example, if an indemnity plan has good mental health benefits and an HMO plan does not, the HMO will be able to offer a better deal on other services.

An insurance executive: Employers want to limit total outlays so they will offer flexible plans, and their employees will choose other benefits rather than mental health benefits.

Another insurance executive: You're really looking at a dissolution of the insurance mechanism. People choose to be uncovered for disorders they don't think they'll get, but actually have a substantial chance of getting.

. . . . .

A researcher: Current ideas of long-term care insurance think of long-term care as nursing home care or home help, and they assume that the primary doctor will provide necessary medical services and that Medicare will pay for them. They don't see long-term care insurance as facilitating or paying for specialty mental health services.

Another researcher: The only way I see direct coverage of neuropsychiatric services is as part of a comprehensive capitated plan, like S/HMO.

A third researcher: Should there be a requirement for neuropsychiatric treatment that might prevent the need for higher levels of long-term care services? For example, a required neuropsychiatric assessment every year or two for long-term care insurance customers, to provide early intervention that will both save money and improve quality of life?

An insurance executive: We're not going to right current discriminatory policies on mental health by starting with the elderly. We have to begin breaking discrimination with the general population. We might adopt the strategy of Arkansas, which defined manic-depressive illness as a medical condition. Some of the neuropsychiatric disorders might be pushed over to the medical side of the house...and then you have less of a problem with limits.

An advocate: This idea has been going around the American Psychiatric Association for a while. But if everything is "medical" or "organic," what happens to psychotherapy?

An insurance executive: But most of the mentally impaired elderly need medical management and case management, not psychotherapy.

. . . . . .

An insurance executive: Capitation worries me. Clinicians then take on responsibilities for managing care that directly influence their own incomes. There are other alternatives that hinge on increasing the public's perception of the value of these services. We begin by introducing case management. While not committing to comprehensive neuropsychiatric services for everyone, we employ them on a case-by-case basis. We want to get experience paying selectively for extra benefits to preserve function, not to save money, but to get satisfied customers and good outcomes.

Another insurance executive: Our company is already doing this.

A researcher: It takes a lot of staff to provide comprehensive case management. Is it worth it, particularly for a smaller company?

The second insurance executive: A special program to monitor inpatient psychiatric services used by people covered by our company did save money. Social workers under the direction of a psychiatrist worked out care plans with the attending psychiatrist, and monitored progress every six to eight days.

A utilization review executive: Our firm combines gatekeeping with case management and monitoring, and seeks alternatives to inpatient care before admission. We are seeing increased use of outpatient care and partial hospital care and a slight increase in hospital admissions, accompanied by decrease in total hospital days, and an overall reduction in expense. We did this in California, Michigan, Connecticut, and Ohio.

A third insurance executive: Psychiatric length of stay in managed care systems is about seven days versus fourteen days in an indemnity system. We "flex the benefit" administratively when it looks like the cost of care will be too high if we don't. We can't change benefits generally without approval by employers, employees, and the insurance commission.

A researcher: It works better in states with more flexibility.

The first insurance executive: The elderly offer a unique opportunity, because their long-term care needs are closely related to their neuropsychiatric needs. Even if more comprehensive care adds a point or two to the premium, it will be worth it if the customers are satisfied and their families are satisfied.

An insurance executive: But you can't do that outside of a managed care system. The same party must be at risk for both acute and for long-term care needs. . . . . .

An insurance executive: Especially for the elderly, medical and mental health are intertwined. In most current HMOs, integration is a fiction, because mental health and physical health staffs are separate.

A researcher: Separating medical and psychiatric dollars would defeat our purpose of integrating medical and psychiatric care.

A utilization review executive: Taking off my businessman's hat, I think you're right, for the elderly.

An insurance executive: But most elderly care is not managed care, so you won't get *carte blanche*.

A researcher: Could utilization review be designed to address mental and medical health care utilization simultaneously?

. . . . .

An insurance executive: We want quality standards for mental health services. Perhaps the academic centers can help us.

A utilization review executive: Many of us in the private sector are developing these standards, but we won't share them, because they're proprietary.

A physician: Medical groups will not get excited about quality assurance, because somebody does it for them.

A researcher: Eventually some of these quality assurance methods will make it into the public domain.

A utilization review executive: We don't use fixed algorithms, but we use clinicians to review care according to research-based guidelines. Our clinicians offer a consultation to the service provider. What's the diagnosis? What's the treatment plan? What's the disposition?

A researcher: What can the academic centers do?

Another insurance executive: Help us with risk management. We could use support from the literature when we deny claims for hospitalization.

A third insurance executive: And you could help us with precertification, and selection of the appropriate provider type.

A researcher: With studies of who does what best.

. . . . .

A researcher: How can private insurance help prevent "carve out" of mental health benefits become avoidance of the problem of neuropsychiatric disorders? How about driving all these problems back into the general medical pool?

An insurance executive: We would rather define benefits as mental, so we can limit them. We are, however, responsive to court orders.

Another researcher: It seems no elderly person without a psychiatric disorder wants to buy mental health coverage. But every elderly person knows someone who has suffered from mental illness. What accounts for this discrepancy?

An insurance executive: Denial. There is a sense of potential fatality of physical illnesses, as opposed to mental illnesses.

A second insurance executive: You've got to market and legitimize your services. This generation of elderly is still hung up with stigma.

A third insurance executive: When we lifted limits on outpatient mental health coverage, elderly people didn't use more psychiatric care. Disabled people did.

An advocate: You can frighten people with the prospect of going into a nursing home. If people felt psychiatric treatment would keep them out of nursing homes, they might go for it.
. . . . .

A researcher: If neuropsychiatric disorders are complicators of physical illness, what do we have to show in the way of cost-offsets to get the private sector interested? Twenty-five percent of retirees have primary coverage by private insurance. Even if they're mildly depressed, they see their doctors 2 1/2 times as often as if they weren't. They get barium enemas, colonoscopies. . . . What would be necessary for you to see the relevance of this? What do we have to prove?

A utilization review executive: An employer would be happy to see a 10% cost offset.

A researcher: If we could show you cost-offsets for specific high-risk conditions, would you develop changes in your products? . . . And, should we focus on people who are still working?

An insurance executive: It depends when you get your cost-offsets— months later, or years later.

A state legislator: Many employers have a very short-term focus because of the rapid escalation in premiums.

An advocate: Psychiatric benefits are no longer 7% of total premiums. Some employers are finding they're over 20%. . . .

A researcher: What is most urgent?

Another researcher: Incorporating mental health hypotheses into large demonstration projects.

An insurance executive: Creation of proprietary quality assurance products, with the federal government as a purchaser of privately developed QA products. In these quality measures, mental health dimensions should get more emphasis.

Appendix II

The Organization of the Psychiatric Inpatient Services System

Howard H. Goldman, M.D., Ph.D.
Carl A. Taube, Ph.D.
Stephen F. Jencks, M.D.

Editors' Note: The chapter reprinted here as Appendix II is reproduced with permission from *Medical Care* (Volume 25, Number 9 [Supplement], September 1987, pp. S6-S21). The references cited in the original source were part of an overall bibliography for the supplement and are not reproduced here.

The Organization of the Psychiatric Inpatient Services System

HOWARD H. GOLDMAN, MD, PHD, CARL A. TAUBE, PHD, AND STEPHEN F. JENCKS, MD

This chapter is intended to give the reader an understanding of how psychiatric inpatient facilities differ, why they differ, and how these differences relate to insurance and payment policy. In the following sections, we describe the five kinds of inpatient facilities, review reasons for differences among facilities, describe the magnitude of these differences, examine patterns of change in the system, review differences across states, describe differences in how Medicare and other third parties pay for mental health services and the impact of payment policy on differences among facilities, and summarize the relationship of the structure of the delivery system to the problem of creating a national pricing system.

Kinds of Psychiatric Inpatient Facilities

Psychiatric inpatient facilities are highly differentiated to serve the very diverse needs of the mentally ill. The differences among kinds of facilities, which are much greater than those in most of the general medical system, may be more important for payment policy than, for example, differences between teaching and nonteaching hospitals. In calendar year 1984, Medicare*

paid for 345,898 alcohol, drug abuse, and mental health (ADM) discharges, which resulted in $1,594 million in charges. Five kinds of settings provided this care (Tables 2-1 and 2-2):

General hospital "scatter" beds are general medical and surgical beds used by patients with psychiatric disorders. They are not part of organized psychiatric units and are under PPS. Length of stay for patients in these beds is the shortest of all five groups; frequency of psychotic diagnoses is lowest, and frequency of neurotic and organic diagnoses highest. Most psychiatrists believe that care rendered in these beds is more likely to be delivered on an interim basis and is less likely to provide definitive treatment. Discharges from these scatter beds comprised an estimated 45.7% of Medicare ADM discharges in 1984. For all sources of payment the total number of ADM discharges from scatter beds is probably about equal to the total number of discharges from psychiatric hospitals and units.[5]

Nonexcluded general hospital units are identified beds or wards used exclusively for psychiatric patients, which Medicare pays under PPS. Although nonexcluded units tend to be smaller and to have shorter stays than excluded units, some could have met the exclusion criteria but did not do so, presumably because they decided that inclusion under PPS would be fiscally sound. We estimate that 9.3% of Medicare discharges occurred from such beds. We also estimate that 49% of charges were made for the 55%

---

* In estimating the number of admissions to the five classes of beds, we rely heavily on Taube et al.[4], whose figures include non-alcohol, drug, and mental health (non-ADM) discharges from psychiatric hospitals. In addition, Taube et al. found that 33.1 percent of discharges in hospitals with excluded units occurred from beds which were not part of those units; we assume that the same ratio holds for hospitals without excluded psychiatric units.

TABLE 2-1. Medicare ADM Discharges and Charges by Type of Psychiatric Bed, Fiscal Year 1984

	Scatter Beds[a]	Nonexcluded Units[b]	Excluded Units	Nonpublic Hospitals	Public Hospitals	Total
Percent of Medicare ADM discharges	45.7	9.3	26.5	9.0	9.6	100.0
Percent of Medicare ADM charges	-------------------- 72.7 --------------------			15.2	12.1	100.0
Charge per ADM discharge	-------------------- $4117 --------------------			$7709	$5824	$4607

Source: National Institute of Mental Health, unpublished data.

[a] Scatter-bed discharges is the sum of (1) PPS psychiatric discharges from hospitals with excluded psychiatric units, (2) PPS psychiatric discharges from hospitals without psychiatric units, and

$$(3) \quad \frac{\text{PPS discharges from hospitals with excluded units}}{\text{Total discharges from hospitals with excluded units}} \times \text{Discharges from hospitals with nonexcluded units.}$$

$$[b] \text{ Nonexcluded unit discharges } = \frac{\text{Non-PPS discharges from hospitals with excluded units}}{\text{Total discharges from hospitals with excluded units}} \times \text{Discharges from}$$

hospitals with nonexcluded units.

of discharges that occurred in scatter beds and nonexcluded units, but we cannot separate the charges with confidence.

Excluded general hospital units are distinct psychiatric units, which Medicare pays under TEFRA. Many of these units, especially the larger units and those in urban and public hospitals, closely resemble psychiatric hospitals in patient characteristics and length of stay. There are about 1,272 general hospital units, of which 841 were excluded by the end of 1985. We estimate that excluded units accounted for 26.5% of Medicare discharges in 1984.

Nonpublic psychiatric hospitals are freestanding psychiatric hospitals, owned either by investors or by voluntary boards of trustees, which Medicare pays under TEFRA. These facilities tend to have a very low proportion of patients who are unable to pay and to have lengths of stay that are intermediate between those of general hospital units and public hospitals. Although these hospitals are often spoken of as a group and are represented by a single organization, there are significant differences between voluntary and investor-owned hospitals, one being that almost all facility growth is occurring in the investor-owned group. In 1984, 227 nonpublic psychiatric hospitals had Medicare discharges. Of these, 84 voluntary hospitals accounted for

TABLE 2-2. Diagnostic Category of Medicare Psychiatric Discharges, Percent by Type of Psychiatric Bed

	Hospital Without Unit	Hospital with Excluded Unit		Nonpublic Hospitals	Public Hospitals
		Not from Unit	From Unit		
Percent psychotic	29.0	36.1	70.2	71.7	70.0
Percent organic	33.4	32.4	11.1	12.1	22.1
Percent neurotic depression	18.2	14.4	11.8	10.8	2.3
Other	19.4	17.1	6.9	5.4	5.6
Total	100.0	100.0	100.0	100.0	100.0

Source: National Institute of Mental Health, unpublished data.

3.6% of total Medicare ADM discharges and 6.4% of charges; 143 investor-owned hospitals accounted for 5.4% of discharges and 8.7% of charges. In total, these hospitals accounted for 9.0% of Medicare discharges and 15.2% of charges.

Public psychiatric hospitals are freestanding psychiatric hospitals operated by states or counties, which Medicare pays under TEFRA. These hospitals serve as a safety net for the psychiatric inpatient system; they usually are required by law to accept all patients, and they receive the majority of those who cannot pay, those who are involuntarily committed for care, and those who prove very unresponsive to treatment. They have a higher proportion of disabled and psychotic patients than do other types of hospitals and have the longest average stays. In calendar 1984, 208 public hospitals had Medicare discharges. We estimate public hospitals accounted for 9.6% of Medicare discharges and 12.1% of charges in 1984.

Unfortunately, there are no data allowing comparison of all five classes of facilities. HCFA data on the excluded facilities are only partially analyzed and do not distinguish nonexcluded units from scatter beds. NIMH survey research data on psychiatric hospitalization[6] do not include scatter beds and do not differentiate excluded from nonexcluded units. Sample surveys such as the National Hospital Discharge Survey do not distinguish between discharges from unit and nonunit beds and do not include freestanding hospitals with an average length of stay greater than 28 days. Large data sets such as those compiled by major abstracting services do not indicate which patients are treated in units.

Despite these difficulties with data, the following analysis clearly portrays the five categories of hospitals as a continuum of increasing average length of stay, increasing frequency of patients with psychotic diagnoses, increasing frequency of civil and criminal commitments, and increasing frequency of permanently disabled patients.

Reasons for Differentiation in the Mental Health System

There are several somewhat overlapping reasons why the mental health service system is so much more differentiated than the medical-surgical system.

The Variety of Patient Needs

One reason for the greater degree of differentiation in the mental health system compared with the medical-surgical system is the greater diversity of patient needs. In mental health, needs may be defined clinically in terms of diagnosis, level of impairment/disability, and treatment requirements. This is closely analogous to the medical-surgical system. But in the mental health system, needs are also defined socially in terms of the patient's ability to cope with the social demands of living in sheltered or unsheltered environments and legally in terms of the need of the patient and society to be protected from harm that the patient might cause. Although neurologic and other diseases may cause behavioral problems and impair living skills, these consequences of other diseases are defined as psychiatric problems, given psychiatric diagnoses, and treated in psychiatric settings. The fact that these psychiatric problems can require long-term inpatient intervention creates a need for special capabilities in the service system.

The Variety of Ability to Pay

The need for very long-term services combined with restrictions in insurance coverage means that a substantial population cannot pay for needed services either directly or through public or private insurance. For a variety of reasons, this medically indigent group is far larger for mental health than for medicine and surgery. Table 2-3 shows that psychiatric facilities are highly differentiated with regard to the number of their patients who cannot pay; because inability to pay is so closely related to chronicity of disease (discussed in detail below), this differentiation leads to even more concentration of patients with chronic disease in certain settings than treatment specialization alone would produce.

Variation in Environmental Supports

To a far larger degree than in medical-surgical settings, patients are admitted to psychiatric inpatient settings because society or their living environment can no longer tolerate them rather than because a specific therapeutic objective appears achievable through care that can be provided only in an inpatient setting. This commonly results in a need for medical management and custody functions that are delivered primarily in certain kinds of facilities and that are quite different from the custodial services typically delivered by intermediate care facilities.

Nonresponse to Treatment

To a degree far greater than in medical-surgical care, some hospitals specialize in "treatment failures"—patients who have failed to respond to a moderate period of treatment in another setting. This specialization may be deliberate, as is the case at some voluntary psychiatric hospitals, or may result from inability to refuse to admit treatment failures, as is the case with many state and county hospitals. Sometimes patients who fail to respond before their insurance or other resources are exhausted are defined as treatment failures, resulting in another kind of transfers between settings.

Involuntary Treatment

Involuntary patients are exceedingly uncommon in general medicine and surgery; they are relatively common in psychiatry. These involuntary patients require special treatment facilities, special capabilities, and special treatment approaches. Some facilities simply refuse to accept such patients, whereas others either choose to accept them or are required by law to do so.

TABLE 2-3. Percent Distribution of Expected Principal Source of Payment for Psychiatric Admissions by Type of Facility and Age, 1980

Age/Source of Payment	General Hospitals	Private Hospitals	State/County Hospitals
All Ages			
No payment	3.6	0.9	46.5
Personal resources	6.8	4.1	15.2
Medicare	15.1	15.6	9.6
Other insurance	42.9	62.5	9.5
Medicaid	23.1	6.9	8.3
Other	8.4	10.0	10.9
Under 65			
No payment	4.0	1.0	48.2
Personal resources	7.3	4.3	15.2
Medicare	9.0	7.8	7.9
Other insurance	46.0	68.4	9.9
Medicaid	24.7	7.4	7.5
Other	9.1	11.1	11.3
Over 65			
No payment	—	—	17.1
Personal resources	1.4	1.7	15.3
Medicare	78.1	86.6	39.0
Other insurance	11.6	8.8	2.8
Medicaid	7.0	2.1	21.2
Other	1.9	0.8	4.6

Source: Mental Health, United States, 1985. Rockville, MD: National Institutes of Mental Health, 1985; Table 2.14.

The Magnitude of Service System Differentiation

In discussing service system differentiation and the specialization of individual facilities, we should distinguish specialization in psychiatric disorders (all units and all psychiatric hospitals specialize in psychiatric disorders) from differentiation among psychiatric facilities that specialize in particular kinds of psychiatric care. Specialization in psychiatric disorders presents no problem for a case-payment system because we can determine accurately the average cost of a psychiatric admission. Specialization in particular kinds of psychiatric care creates a major problem if the payment system cannot distinguish among the treatment needs of patients in different kinds of specialized facilities. There are four kinds of evidence of differentiation: differences in the use of different kinds of facilities by Medicare benefi-

TABLE 2-4.   Medicare Status for Psychiatric Admissions by Type of Facility and Age, 1980

	General Hospital Discharges			Private Hospital Admissions			Public Hospital Admissions		
Medicare	<65	65+	Total	<65	65+	Total	<65	65+	Total
Yes	54,379	46,297	100,676	9,991	12,053	22,044	27,599	7,825	35,424
No	552,667	12,957	565,624	117,302	1,863	119,155	321,394	12,231	333,625
Total	607,046	59,254	666,300	127,293	13,916	141,209	348,993	20,056	369,049

Source: Mental Health, United States 1985. Rockville, MD: National Institutes of Mental Health, 1985; Table 2.14.

ciaries, differences in the Medicare benefici- aries who use different kinds of facilities, differences in diagnostic patterns, and dif- ferences in length of stay.

Where Medicare Beneficiaries Receive Treatment

Table 2-1 shows that more than 80% of the episodes for which Medicare pays occur in general hospitals and almost half in scat- ter beds. Table 2-4 suggests that, compared to other patients, Medicare beneficiaries more often receive care in general hospitals' psychiatric units and private psychiatric hospitals rather than in state/county hospi- tals. This appearance may, however, be mis- leading. Tables 2-3 are based on the hospi- tal's expected source of payment, and Medi- care's 190-day lifetime limit on coverage of care in psychiatric hospitals means that hos- pitals know Medicare will not pay for the care of some of its beneficiaries. If Medicare beneficiaries pay for hospitalization with their own money or with other insurance, or if hospitals receive them with no expecta- tion of payment, then they will not appear as Medicare beneficiaries in these tables.

Disabled and Elderly Beneficiaries

An unpublished NIMH analysis of 1984 Medicare data shows that 51.2% of psychi- atric hospitalizations for which Medicare is expected to pay are for individuals less than age 65 (Tables 2-3 and 2-4, which exclude scatter beds, show a higher percentage). These beneficiaries become eligible for So- cial Security Disability Insurance (SSDI) be-

cause of permanent disability incurred after joining the work force and become eligible for Medicare 2 years after they become eligi- ble for SSDI. We can reasonably conjecture that the source of disability is chronic men- tal illness, because the disabled do not dom- inate in other categories of medical-surgical illness, but data to prove this conjecture are not available. Among patients for whom Medicare is expected to pay, the disabled are more often treated in public hospitals and less often in private psychiatric hospi- tals. As noted above, the concentration in public hospitals would probably be even more marked if we had data for Medicare beneficiaries rather than being limited to data about patients for whom Medicare is expected to pay.

Diagnosis

The third edition of the Diagnostic and Statistical Manual of Mental Disorder[7] (DSM-III) is a five-axis system that seeks to describe mental health disorders and prob- lems comprehensively. Three axes (clinical syndromes, personality disorders, and physical disorders) form the basic diagnoses and are recorded in most records; this infor- mation can be supplemented by two addi- tional axes (severity of psychosocial stres- sors and highest level of adaptive function- ing), which appear to have great potential for measuring "severity." Unfortunately, axes IV and V, which might give valuable insights into the reasonableness of differ- ences between components of the psychiat- ric inpatient system, are not systematically

TABLE 2-5. Percent of Principal Diagnoses by Type of Hospital and Medicare Status of Patient

Diagnosis	General[a] Hospital Units		State and County Hospitals		Private Hospitals	
	Medicare	All	Medicare	All	Medicare	All
Mental retardation	0.5	0.4	2.0	1.9	[c]	0.2
Alcohol related	6.4	7.6	13.8	21.71	9.1	9.3
Drug related	1.3	2.9	[c]	4.857	1.1	2.9
Organic disorders	11.2	3.3	10.9	4.2	13.3	3.5
Affective disorders	31.3	31.1	18.4	13.4	43.5	42.9
Schizophrenia	29.4	25.2	46.4	38.0	24.0	21.2
Other psychoses	5.0	4.5	1.3	1.8	2.9	2.5
Acute sit disturb	2.6	3.5	[c]	0.5	2.0	3.4
Personality dis	5.3	4.6	1.5	5.7	1.5	4.8
Other non-psychotic	10.0	13.6	2.1	4.0	1.8	4.8
Other conditions[b]	12.4	3.2	[c]	4.2	0.4	4.6
Total cases	100,676	666,300	35,424	369,049	22,044	141,209

Source: National Institute of Mental Health, derived in part from *Mental Health, United States 1985*, Table 2.16, and in part from unpublished data from 1980–1981 sample surveys.

[a] Nonfederal general hospitals.

[b] "Other conditions" includes preadult conditions, social conditions, no mental disorder, diagnosis deferred, and medical conditions.

[c] Insufficient cases for reliable estimates.

reported in any data system. Further, axis II is not known to be coded reliably, and we are unaware of any studies of reliability in its use. Finally, studies of the effect of concomitant axis I and axis III diagnoses are generally unimpressive. We shall see in the next chapter that, using the standard of effect on length of stay, concurrent physical diagnoses appear to have little predictable impact on the management of a principal diagnosis of psychiatric disorder. Thus, comparison of diagnostic patterns rests on comparison of principal psychiatric diagnosis.

Overall Patterns. Table 2-5 shows the pattern of diagnoses for beneficiaries of Medicare and other insurance plans. Here the frequency of organic mental disorders in the elderly is expected, as is the frequency of schizophrenia among the Medicare beneficiaries. Schizophrenia is presumably concentrated in the disabled because it is less present in the elderly.[6]

Diagnoses in Unit Versus Nonunit General Hospitals. Table 2-6 shows the distribution of diagnoses (classified by DRG) and the corresponding lengths of stay for all alcohol, drug, and mental (ADM) discharges from short-term general hospitals with and without psychiatric units. The data result from linking Commission on Professional and Hospital Activities (CPHA) data on patients, which may not be nationally representative, to American Hospital Association (AHA) data on the presence of units (which does not indicate whether individual patients were treated in units). Thus, the differences are between CPHA hospitals that have units and those that do not, and not between all patients treated in units and all patients not treated in units. We have already pointed out that there are significant numbers of scatter bed discharges in hospitals with units and that patients treated in the two settings differ even in hospitals with units.

Mental disorder diagnoses (MDC 19) account for three quarters of ADM discharges from hospitals with units, whereas these diagnoses account for only half of discharges from hospitals without units. The largest category for unit hospitals was DRG

TABLE 2-6. Diagnosis and Length of Stay for General Hospital Psychiatric Discharges, Hospitals With and Without Units

		Percent of Cases		Average Length of Stay	
DRG	Name	Unit	No Unit	Unit	No Unit
MDC 19					
424	O.R. procs with principal Dx mental disorder	1.8	1.5	28.7	17.3
425	Acute adj react & disturbances of psychosocial funct	5.5	10.4	18.0	4.5
426	Depressive neurosis	16.0	12.9	11.9	7.1
427	Neuroses except depressive	3.9	2.6	11.4	8.0
428	Disorders of personality and impulse control	2.8	1.1	14.7	11.3
429	Organic disturbances and mental retardation	6.1	10.1	14.8	13.1
430	Psychoses	37.5	13.0	16.7	10.3
431	Childhood mental disorder	1.3	0.4	23.9	4.7
432	Other mental disorders	0.4	0.6	9.7	11.3
MDC 20					
433	Substance abuse and substance induced mental dis. left AMA	3.2	3.4	5.5	4.5
434	Drug dependence	2.5	2.8	12.7	16.1
435	Drug use except dependence	1.1	1.0	14.7	14.1
436	Alcohol dependence	3.4	7.9	15.1	13.9
437	Alcohol use except dependence	1.5	2.8	4.8	3.4
438	Alcohol & substance induced	12.9	27.3	10.6	12.1

Souce: Adapted from Taube C, Thompson J, Burns B, et al. Prospective payment and psychiatric discharges from general hospitals with and without psychiatric units. Hosp & Community Psychiatry 1985;36:754–760 (Table 2).

430 (psychoses), with 38% of all ADM discharges; for nonunit hospitals, DRG 438 (alcohol and substance induced organic mental syndromes) was most frequent, with 28% of ADM discharges.[8]

An analysis of Medicare claims from four states showed that although DRG 430 accounted for the largest proportion of unit hospital discharges, DRG 429 (organic disturbances and mental retardation) composed the largest category of discharges for nonunit hospitals.[9]

Diagnoses in State Versus Other Hospitals. A five-state study[10] showed that state hospital Medicare discharges have a different case mix (measured by DRGs) from Medicare discharges in general. For example, less than 30% of Medicare discharges are in DRG 430 (psychosis), compared with 52.9% of state hospital discharges and 73.6% of state hospital residents.

Length of Stay Differences

Differences in length of stay may reflect either differences in treatment programs or differences in patient response to treatment. Although we cannot rigorously distinguish these sources of differences, the fact of differences in length of stay is informative in itself.

General Versus Private Versus Public. Table 2-7 shows that, in 1980–81, the median length of stay in psychiatric units of general hospitals, private hospitals, and state/county hospitals was 12, 19 and 23 days, respectively (mean stays are substantially higher, especially for state/county hospitals). Table 2-7 shows the difference in length of stay between those over and under age 65 across classes of hospitals. Several features of this data are relevant to the problems of creating a psychiatric prospective payment system for Medicare:

TABLE 2-7. Median Length of Stay for Psychiatric Discharges by Setting and Patient Characteristics

	Hospital Type								
	Public			Private			General[a]		
	1970	1975	1980	1970	1975	1980	1971	1975	1980
Condition									
Alcohol-related	33	11	12	9	11	20	5	6	6
Drug-related	17	12	12	17	13	19	5	6	10
Organic disorders	78	63	71	26	18	17	12	14	14
Affective disorders	32	27	22	20	20	20	13	14	14
Schizophrenia	58	41	42	28	23	18	11	13	15
Age									
Under 18	74	66	54	36	36	36	9	17	14
18–24	34	27	17	24	22	16	8	10	10
25–44	37	23	20	18	17	17	10	11	11
45–64	42	21	29	17	18	18	11	14	14
Over 64	61	58	61	24	21	20	17	17	17
All patients	41	25	23	20	20	19	10	12	12

Source: Mental Health, United States 1985. Rockville, MD: National Institute of Mental Health, 1985; Table 2.24.
[a] Nonfederal general hospitals.

1. The downward trend in length of stay in state and county hospitals, which is so dramatic for the overall population, does not occur for those over age 65 in public and general hospitals and is minimal in private hospitals.

2. While lengths of stay are about twice as long in public psychiatric hospitals as in general hospitals, stays are more than three times as long for patients over age 65.

3. Differences between psychiatric hospitals and general hospitals are also smaller for those over age 65 than for those under age 65.

Unit Versus Nonunit Hospitals. Table 2-6 shows large length-of-stay differences between general hospitals with pyschiatric units and those without psychiatric units. In 1982, the mean length of stay for Medicare patients in unit hospitals was 15.9 days, 45% higher than the mean stay of 11.0 days in nonunit hospitals.[8] Unit hospitals have much longer lengths of stay than nonunit hospitals[11] for all mental disorder DRGs except DRG 432 (other diagnoses of mental disorders).[8]

Public Hospitals. Average lengths of stay for even short-term public hospital pa-

tients are substantially longer than those for Medicare discharges in general (e.g., 40.2 days for Medicare DRG 430 [psychosis] discharges in state hospitals vs. 16.4 days for Medicare DRG 430 discharges in general).

Long-Stay Hospitals. A number of psychiatric hospitals are excluded from PPS because they are "long-stay" facilities with an average stay over 25 days. Exact data on the number of psychiatric hospitals so classified are not available, but Morrison[12] found that 17.3% of pre-PPS Medicare discharges were from long-stay hospitals, which is consistent with NIMH survey data. Because the "long-stay" criterion is applied before the psychiatric hospital criterion, these hospitals might remain excluded from PPS even if other psychiatric hospitals were included.

Evidence on Length of Stay. In the past few years, experimental evidence has developed on the effectiveness of long and short hospitalizations. Several investigators and reviewers[5,13–16] found little benefit in extending stays beyond 28 days for the majority of patients. However, these studies excluded important groups of patients, in-

TABLE 2-8. Legal Status of Admissions
by Hospital Type

	General Hospital Units	State and County Hospitals	Private Hospitals
All patients			
Voluntary adms	84.2	41.6	87.4
Involuntary noncriminal	15.1	51.1	12.5
Involuntary criminal	0.7	7.3	0.1
Medicare patients			
Voluntary adms	84.3	36.5	86.0
Involuntary (criminal and noncriminal)	15.7	63.5	14.0

Source: Mental Health, United States 1985. Rockville, MD: National Institute of Mental Health, 1985; Table 2.12.

cluding the suicidal, assaultive, and organically impaired. These exclusions mean that the findings cannot be used directly to determine the appropriateness of long hospital stays for all patients. Thus, research evidence on the effectiveness of long stays is suggestive but not conclusive. Chapter 3 discusses the available evidence as to whether differences in length of stay reflect differences in patient needs or differing treatment philosophies and practice patterns.

Differences in Treatments

Rigorous data on differences in treatment practices across hospital settings are exceedingly difficult to obtain. Although NIMH sample surveys collect such data, the lack of clear definitions makes interpretation difficult. This is especially true because of evolving treatment practices.

Treatment of mental disorders has changed profoundly since World War II, partly because of alterations in the health care financing system and public attitudes toward the mentally ill, but also because of changes in treatment ideology and techniques. A diverse set of psychotherapies has emerged, and psychotherapy has evolved from almost exclusive reliance on psychodynamic models to a diverse set of techniques with diverse theoretical bases. Current treatments include those based on psychoanalytic ideas, as well as treatments based on learning theory, behavioral treatments, and phenomenologic descriptions of behavior.[17,18] A significant consequence of this diversification is that traditional terms such as "milieu therapy" and "intensive psychotherapy" no longer have clear definitions. We must therefore rely largely on widely accepted impressions in saying that public psychiatric hospitals are much less likely to use intensive psychotherapies, such as individual treatment and groups, but that we cannot define whether a patient is more likely to receive these treatments in a private psychiatric hospital or in a general hospital. Although psychiatrists commonly believe that patients in scatter beds receive less intensive treatment than those in organized units, there are no data on this subject.

Voluntary Versus Involuntary. We have good data on one feature of treatment: whether the patient was treated voluntarily.

Table 2-8 shows differences across hospitals in whether patients are treated voluntarily or involuntarily both for Medicare patients and for all patients. Over one half of all state hospital discharges were for involuntarily committed patients, and almost one third of those patients were transfers from general hospitals.[10]

Referrals. Table 2-9 shows differences in the places to which patients are discharged, which also reflect differences in treatment practices. The contrast in such referrals across hospital types also suggests the degree to which state and county hospitals do not have the ability to refer to another facility those patients who do not recover.

Differences in Costs Among Types of Facility

NIMH figures for 1981 show an operating cost per discharge of $3,135 in general hospital psychiatric units, $12,119 in public psychiatric hospitals, and $6,874 in private psychiatric hospitals. These numbers must be treated with great caution because they do not reflect length of stay, case mix, input costs, teaching activities, or urban/rural location. For example, data for public hospitals include very. long-stay, semi-custodial patients; nevertheless, they are the only national cost estimates available. In the first year of prospective payment, charges for Medicare patients were $2,262 in hospitals without excluded units; $3,633 in scatter beds of general hospitals with excluded units; $5,186 in excluded units; $5,186 in public hospitals; and $7,935 in private hospitals. The reader should keep in mind that charges are distantly related to costs in many settings and that the ratio of costs to charges varies across hospitals. Although detailed comparisons on a diagnosis-specific basis are available,[19] they are not particularly meaningful because of the variation in the relationship of costs to charges across settings.

Clearly, the data do suggest a hierarchy of costliness. The lower charges in hospitals without excluded units, even compared to scatter beds in hospitals with excluded units, are consistent with a tendency of excluded units to be located in expensive hospitals.

Transfers

One important indicator of the differentiation of a hospital care system is the frequency of transfers between hospitals. Transfers reflect institutional specialization. In particular, patients are transferred from relatively short-term hospitals and hospitals that require payment to hospitals that specialize in treating patients regarded as treatment failures and patients who cannot pay.

TABLE 2-9. Psychiatric Discharges Referred to Another Inpatient Setting, Percent of Discharges by Setting

	General Hospital Units	Public Hospitals	Private Hospitals
Medicare patients	28.1	14.7	27.8
All patients	16.4	13.8	16.1

Source: Unpublished NIMH analysis of 1980–1981 sample survey.

More than twice as many Medicare patients in the mental health system are discharged to another inpatient facility as in the general health care system: 26% versus 11%. Of Medicare discharges from general hospital psychiatric units, 6.1% are referred to a state mental hospital, 11.5% to a nursing home, and 10.5% to other inpatient settings.† In contrast, only 9% of general hospital discharges for patients over age 65 are to long-term care and only 2% are to other hospitals (unpublished National Institutes of Mental Health Analysis of data from National Institute of Mental Health Sample Surveys and the National Hospital Discharge Survey of the National Center for Health Statistics).

Differentiation complicates designing a prospective payment system because apparently similar patients in different facilities may have arrived at those facilities for reasons as different as treatment failure in one case and acute illness in another. Differentiation makes the hypothesis of random variation in treatment needs, which we discussed briefly in Chapter 1, much more difficult to defend.

---

† In the general health system, 11% of Medicare patients are "discharged" to another inpatient setting, while 27% of Medicare mental health patients are "referred" to another inpatient setting on discharge. The numbers are comparable to the extent that they both indicate the percentage of cases in which the discharging facility identified further patient needs that it believed could be best met at another facility. We do not know how many patients discharged from either type of facility actually enter the hospital to which they are referred.

TABLE 2-10.   Changes in Location of Beds and Inpatient Care Over Time

	Beds			
	1970	1976	1980	1982
Public psych	413,066	222,202	156,482	140,140
Private psych	14,295	16,091	17,157	19,011
General hospital psych units	22,394	28,706	29,384	36,525
Other[a]	75,123	71,964	71,690	51,636
Total	524,878	338,963	274,713	247,312

	Episodes[b]			
	1969	1975	1979	1981
Public psych	767,115	598,993	526,690	499,169
Private psych	102,510	137,025	150,535	176,513
General hospital psych units	535,493	565,696	571,725	676,941
Other[a]	305,254	515,394	530,637	367,769
Total	1,710,372	1,817,108	1,779,587	1,720,392

[a] Includes VA, residential treatment centers for children, and, from 1970 to 1980, federally funded community mental health centers.
[b] Counted as admissions to public hospitals and discharges from others.
Source: Mental Health, United States 1985. Rockville, MD: National Institute of Mental Health, 1985; Tables 2-2 and 2-4.

Changes over Time

We have already mentioned the dramatic changes in psychiatric care that have occurred since World War II. The forces that have changed care have also changed the site of hospitalization, length of stay, and treatments.

Site of Hospitalization

Change in the mental health system is most concretely illustrated by a shift in the settings where mental health treatment has been provided.

Table 2-10 shows the shifts in total beds and total inpatient episodes in the three groups of hospitals. Here the underlying trends of deinstitutionalization of state and county patients are dramatic. The number of general hospital unit beds increased from 22,394 to 36,525 between 1970 and 1982, while the number of state and county hospital beds decreased from 413,066 to 140,140. But total discharges from the private and general beds increased from 638,003 to 833,454 between 1969 and 1981, while episodes in state and county hospitals showed a reciprocal decrease from 767,115 to 499,169.

Deinstitutionalization.   During the 1950s, the population of state and county hospitals began to decline, and psychiatric units in general hospitals began to develop. The movement out of the state and county hospitals (deinstitutionalization) accelerated sharply in the early 1960s, following the 1961 Report of the Joint Commission on Mental Illness and Health and the passage of the Community Mental Health Services Act and at the same time as development of the Medicare and Medicaid programs.

There are indications that deinstitutionalization has not resulted in true community treatment[20–23] and that chronic patients either remain in state inpatient facilities or have been shifted to nursing homes, prisons, and other government-supported settings. Nevertheless, the movement did promote massive development of ambulatory community mental health programs and general hospital units.[6,24] Private clinics and practitioners have increased in number as well.[6,24] Accompanying this growth in community treatment settings has been a tremendous growth in the use of outpatient treatment.

State hospital expenditures in constant dollars decreased from $1.81 billion to $1.76 billion between 1969 and 1981. A 70% reduction in beds in state mental hospital systems over the last 20 years was offset by a dramatic increase in the number of admissions for acute, intensive care. Thus, pressure on state government funds has diminished the capacity of these hospitals to provide acute and long-term care to the public patient even though better staffing ratios and new treatment programs have probably increased the quality of care.

Growth of Private Psychiatric Hospitals and General Hospital Units. General hospital psychiatric unit episodes exceeded those in state mental hospitals in 1977 and are still growing, and private mental hospital episodes have grown since the early 1970s. Table 2-10 shows that an increased number of inpatients is served by private psychiatric hospitals and psychiatric units within general medical hospitals. The number of patients served by Veterans Administration hospitals has also grown, but the relation of these facilities to other parts of the mental health system is exceedingly difficult to define.

Private mental hospitals now represent 8% of available psychiatric beds. The role of these units is still evolving rapidly; in some regions they provide a large part of psychiatric hospitalization and their length of stay is more like that of general hospital units, while in other regions they provide a much smaller portion of overall care and appear to specialize in patients whose needs are beyond the capabilities of general hospital units. Table 2-3 shows that private mental hospitals are either less able or less willing than other hospitals to provide significant amounts of uncompensated care.

General hospitals have experienced increased caseloads of chronic public patients in their emergency rooms and inpatient psychiatric units. Investor-owned general hospitals, like private psychiatric hospitals, generally have been less able and willing to absorb these chronic patients who need intermittent episodes of acute inpatient care, and the burden has fallen more on the public and nonprofit general hospitals. The severity of this problem probably varies with the level of state funding of community care and the restrictiveness of the state mental hospital admission policies.

Trends in Length of Stay in Different Settings

Table 2-7 shows relative lengths of stay and trends in length of stay (in this table, non-Federal general hospitals includes scatter beds as well as units). These changes do create a wider range of mental health treatment options and greater system differentiation, but their importance for our discussion is that they again underline how much the system is changing. Any system that is already in flux tends to be more responsive to incentives than one that is relatively static. To the extent that this is so, the mental health inpatient system may be more responsive to changes in payment incentives than parts of the general medical-surgical system that were less in flux when prospective payment was introduced.

Differences Across States

There are very large differences across states in many of the characteristics we have described, particularly in the rate and extent of deinstitutionalization. Although the metaphor has glaring inaccuracies, it is possible to see states arranged on a continuum from those that have highly traditional public psychiatric hospital systems to those that have tried to phase out the entire system through deinstitutionalization. Likewise, the market penetration of proprietary hospitals varies as does the role of general hospitals and the balance between general hospital units and scatter beds. Further, in states that have expanded nursing home capacity, the long-term resident population of state hospitals has declined; in states that expanded general hospital psychiatric units, especially in public hospitals, acute admissions declined in state hospitals.[25] In designing regional or national per-discharge payment rates, the strong state-to-state variation in the organization of the mental health services system poses special problems.

Evidence

Both the ratio of beds to population and charges per admission vary more across states and regions for psychiatric services than for medical-surgical services. The coefficient of variation for beds per capita at the state level is 4.35 for psychiatric unit beds and 1.80 for general hospital beds. The coefficient of variation for average charges per discharge is 0.84 for private psychiatric hospitals, 0.49 for excluded psychiatric units, and 0.36 for short-stay general hospitals.

The distribution of Medicare ADM discharges across DRGs, average lengths of stay, and average costs vary substantially from state to state.[9,19] A study that compared four selected states with national averages found that the proportion of Medicare discharges with DRG 430 (psychoses) varied sharply. The variance around the length of stay by DRG was greater across states than within states,[9] providing evidence for substantial state or regional variation in lengths of stay. The percentage of Medicare claims from the under-65 population also varies widely across states, implying differences in the percentage of chronically mentally ill Medicare beneficiaries across states.[9,19]

Another kind of evidence for state-to-state variation is the study of mental hospitalization costs by Taube et al.,[26] which was based on the NIMH sample survey. By examining state hospitals, they were able to account for 26% of the variance using patient and hospital characteristics; when they included dummy variables to represent the state in which hospitalization occurred, explained variance rose to 35%. Thus, variation among states appears to account for about 9% of total variation in length of stay. Adding state dummy variables added little to explanation of costs in general hospitals.[27]

Explanations

The resources available for mental health care vary between states and may partly explain why different state patterns appear. The relative availability of state facilities, Medicare certification status of state facilities, state policy regarding voluntary commitment, waiting time to gain nursing home entry, state attitude regarding the enrollment of the chronically mentally ill under SSI, and state Medicaid policy pertaining to psychiatric care have been suggested as reasons why different state patterns appear with respect to Medicare ADM discharges.[10,19]

One solution is to ignore such variation. Medicare does not adjust its per-discharge rates according to the number of nursing home beds in a state even though availability of such beds may influence length of stay and costs. The situation, however, is considerably more complicated because Medicare provides differential benefits across settings and because of idiosyncracies of the cost accounting system.

How Medicare and Other Programs Pay for Psychiatric Services

This section reviews evidence on the diversity of ways in which evolving public policy and the structure of insurance coverage interact to shape the mental health system. Although inferences about the behavior of so highly differentiated a system must be tentative, they are important in understanding the way in which changes in Medicare payments might affect beneficiaries and hospitals.

Medicare Eligibility and Coverage of Mental Health Services

In order to understand how public policy and the structure of insurance coverage affect mental health care, it is necessary for the reader to understand certain features of the Medicare program: who is covered, what is covered, and how much Medicare now pays.

Who Is Covered. Earlier in this chapter, we pointed out the importance of the disabled in use of psychiatric inpatient services by Medicare beneficiaries. Disabled and elderly Medicare beneficiaries have identical coverage for psychiatric services, but the users of psychiatric services, because they are so largely the disabled, are a very atypical sample of Medicare beneficiaries.

While 9.4% of Medicare beneficiaries are eligible because of disability rather than age, 29.7% of all Medicare ADM discharges were disabled individuals. Of Medicare discharges from excluded facilities, 50.1% were disabled, and 56.2% of discharges from psychiatric hospitals were disabled.[4] Thus, in the excluded psychiatric facilities, Medicare is represented primarily by the disabled rather than the elderly.

What Is Covered. Just as the service system for mental health is more complexly differentiated than that for medical-surgical care, so the Medicare benefit structure is different and more limited. There are two other differences of particular significance.

1. There is a 190-day lifetime limit on Medicare coverage of services in psychiatric hospitals; this limit does not apply to services in general hospitals, whether paid under TEFRA or PPS.

2. Medicare payment for outpatient visits that are not hospital services is limited to $250 per year, with an effective copayment of 50%. This amounts to about eight 1-hour visits in a typical state.

TABLE 2-11.   Medicare Expenditures for Psychiatric Services in 1981

Psychiatric hospitals	$190,000,000
General hospitals	$630,000,000
Psychiatrists and psychologists	$115,000,000
Hospital outpatient departments	$45,000,000
Other institutions (e.g., home health, skilled nursing)	$15,000,000
Total	$995,000,000

How Much Is Spent and How.   We have noted that Medicare received charges of $1,593 million for ADM inpatient services rendered in calendar 1984; actual payments will not be available for some time. For a broader picture of ADM expenditures, Table 2-11 shows the most recent complete data.

The $995 million total was 2.4% of Medicare's $41.3 billion total outlays in that year. This 2.4% compares to 7–18% for psychiatric services in other representative insurance programs.[28] Although lower relative outlays for Medicare ADM services may be explained in part by the high general medical costs of the elderly and in part by generally limited provision of ADM services to the elderly, the relative expenditure figure does portray fairly the limited importance of ADM services to the total Medicare budget. Further, these data reflect the greater emphasis on inpatient payments in Medicare ADM services compared to other Medicare services: 16.1% of ADM expenditures were for outpatient services compared to 29.9% of total program expenditures.

Features of Medicare Payment Setting Under TEFRA.   In state and county facilities, acute, chronic, and custodial patients are grouped together in calculating Medicare's per-diem payment for routine care. Since costs are lower for chronic and custodial patients, this would mean that Medicare would pay too much for chronic and custodial patients and too little for acute patients. Medicare, however, does not pay for chronic hospitalization exceeding 190 days or for any form of custodial hospitalization; those costs are paid by local government or by Medicaid. Thus, existence of chronic and custodial state hospital beds actually subsidizes Medicare in two ways—first by providing care to Medicare beneficiaries for whom Medicare no longer pays after their 190-day limit has been exceeded and then by reducing the per-diem cost for those patients who have not exhausted their Medicare benefit.

For these reasons, it is likely that a system that gave general and private hospitals incentives to transfer patients to state and county facilities (as PPS provides incentives for general hospitals to transfer patients to skilled nursing facilities) would actually transfer costs to state and local government rather than simply move patients to a more efficient location of service. Such incentives could not be eliminated by setting payment rates to reflect the percentage of nonacute care delivered in the state system, but rates that did not reflect state characteristics could significantly intensify the incentives to transfer patients to state facilities. An example of a policy that might be studied as an approach to this problem would be one in which payments are adjusted downward for hospitals making significant numbers of transfers and upward for those receiving transfers, an option discussed further in Chapter 5.

Commercial Policies

As in general medicine, reimbursement policies have had a major impact on how and where psychiatric care is provided. Growth of commercial insurance coverage in the 1960s increased general hospital inpatient care and office-based practice of psychiatrists and psychologists. Although commercial insurers generally cover acute general hospital care and are slightly more generous in outpatient benefits (the modal policy allows $1,000 of benefits annually compared with Medicare's $250[29]), they do not have the specific limitations on psychiatric hospitals found in Medicare.

Insurance coverage for mental illness is thus less extensive both in the range of providers covered and in the amount of coverage for mental health when compared to medical-surgical care. In addition, many policies simply exclude mental health services. Of the privately insured United States population under age 65, 82.4% has inpatient and 71.4% outpatient mental illness insurance coverage, compared to 98.0% and 83.3%, respectively, with medical-surgical health insurance.[30]

The Chronically Mentally Ill

The chronically mentally ill present a coverage problem that appears to be different from most chronic medical and surgical conditions. The essential point is that limits on mental health benefits appear to be reached by a far larger portion of the population than reaches limits on general medical benefits, although data on this issue are not available. The number of public psychiatric hospital patients who are over age 65 but for whom Medicare is not expected to pay reflects this problem for the elderly, but we would expect it to be even more intense for the disabled because of their pattern of intensive service use.

Direct Federal-State funding of community-based inpatient and outpatient care through the Community Mental Health Centers Act increased outpatient episodes fourfold between 1965 and 1980; Medicare and Medicaid coverage, although limited, probably contributed to the same trend. Medicaid also enabled a major shift of costs and patients (primarily elderly) from state mental hospitals to nursing homes. This combination of events decreased financial barriers to securing care and ameliorated the impact of economic factors on care received. A major difference, however, is that, in mental health, Medicare did not replace "charity care" to the extent it did in physical health because the mentally disabled (who tend to be impoverished) tend to exhaust their coverage for both inpatient and outpatient coverage.

The degree to which state hospitals serve as the "floor" of the mental health services system is thus partly a result of the structure and extent of insurance coverage. The closest analogy in medical-surgical care is the public general hospital. Public general hospitals, however, account for only 22% of all general hospital beds, for example, whereas state mental hospitals account for 57% of all psychiatric beds. Feder et al. estimated that uncompensated care in community hospitals was 5% of charges in 1982.[31] Table 2-3 indicates that for 17% of admissions to psychiatric inpatient settings, no payment was expected. This ranged from 47% in state mental hospitals to 1.0% in private mental hospitals.

Evidence is unclear on whether these coverage policies affect whether patients are treated or only where they are treated and who pays. For example, when Taube et al.[26] reanalyzed NIMH sample survey data, they found that differences in length of stay among Medicare, Medicaid, and privately insured discharged patients were slight. Frank and Lave's finding[32] that Medicaid payment caps result in increased admissions to public psychiatric hospitals also suggests that the amount of service changes less than the site of service and the payer.

Overview of Relation of Payment System to the Service System

This review of the structure and economics of the mental health inpatient system indicates a number of reasons why the mental health community has responded with such concern to the possible impact of a prospective payment system:

1. Ability to pay already limits access to care in the mental health system even for patients whose insurance provides ready access to care for medical-surgical disorders.

2. The high degree of differentiation in the mental health system is partly a response to payment incentives, so that advocates for that system find it especially easy to see how incentives could result in undesirable system changes.

3. Existing differentiation and a well-developed transfer system provide a ready route by which nonpublic general hospitals and private psychiatric hospitals could direct potentially unprofitable patients to public facilities with even less change in policy than might be needed to achieve the same results for medical and surgical patients.

4. Existing differentiation in the system is sufficient so that it is not inherently likely that variation within a payment category such as a DRG will be the same across hospital types, and this raises serious problems for any payment system based on such categories.

5. Medicare has a far smaller market share in mental health than in general medical-surgical care, and both private psychiatric hospitals and general hospital psychiatric units are experiencing a general growth in demand. For these reasons, many mental health providers may be able to pass up or minimize Medicare business if a payment system emerges that they regard as risky or unfair.

Appendix III

Glossary

ADL (Activities of Daily Living): Basic physical activities essential for daily existence, including feeding, bathing, dressing, walking, and use of the toilet. The best known index of ADLs, developed by Sidney Katz and associates (1963), classifies chronically ill patients according to whether or not they require assistance to carry out specific ADLs. Regardless of medical diagnosis, ADLs tend to be lost in a specific order, with the ability to bathe and dress without help almost always lost earlier in the course of an illness than the ability to feed oneself or remain continent.

ADM (Alcohol, Drug Abuse, and Mental Health Block Grant): Created by the Omnibus Budget Reconciliation Act of 1981 (OBRA), which consolidated federal funding programs into a block grant to each state.

Affect: The outward manifestation of a patient's feelings by facial expression, tone of voice, etc. Affect may be referred to as sad, fearful, angry, etc. Outside of the field of psychiatry and psychology, *mood* and *affect* often are used interchangeably.

Affective disorder: A term used interchangeably with mood disorder.

Assignment (of Medicare benefits): Designation by a Medicare beneficiary that benefits be paid directly to the treating physician. Accepting assignment implies that the physician will regard the Medicare fee as payment in full. The patient remains responsible to the physician for the payment of deductibles and copayments not covered by Medicare.

Alzheimer's disease: A degenerative disease of the brain that is the single most common cause of dementia. Approximately 50% of demented elderly suffer from Alzheimer's disease. Alzheimer's disease refers to a specific neuropathological entity, rather than to a clinical syndrome. Therefore, it is possible for an individual to have Alzheimer's disease pathologically, without being severely enough affected behaviorally to warrant a diagnosis of dementia. The converse, that dementia does not imply Alzheimer's disease, is definitely true. Cerebrovascular disease is the second most common cause of the syndrome of dementia.

Block grant: Funds given to local and state government units by the federal government for a general purpose rather than for a specific contract. While states are required to submit an annual plan explaining how such funds will be used, there is great flexibility in distribution of the grant money as long as the funds are used for acceptable purposes.

Board and Care Home: A non-Medicaid certified residential facility in which three or more persons receive room, board, and some protective oversight. The term comprises a wide variety of facilities and ranges from rooming houses to large, well-organized, and professionally administered group homes.

Capitation: A method of payment of health services in which an individual or institutional provider is paid a fixed, per capita amount for each person served without regard to the actual number or nature of services provided to each person. Capitation is characteristic of health maintenance organizations but unusual for individual physicians.

Case management: Formal management of a patient's access to health care and social services, carried out by a person known as the case manager. Depending on the purpose of case management, the manager's primary emphasis may be on facilitating access to appropriate services, or upon restricting expenditures. Medicaid funding is available for case management services (see Chapter 11).

Catchment area: A geographic area defined and served by a health facility on the basis of such factors as population distribution, natural geographic boundaries, and transportation accessibility. Used in mental health care to identify a geographical area for which a mental health services facility includes or has responsibility.

CCA (Catastrophic Coverage Act):   Legislation passed in 1988 that provides for compulsory insurance for Medicare beneficiaries against catastrophic health care costs. The Act requires that beneficiaries pay an additional premium, the Medicare part C premium, to cover the additional cost of the plan. The CCA does not alter Medicare limits on psychiatric treatment; catastrophic costs of psychiatric illness must still be borne by the patient and family. Another provision of the CCA is that patients covered by Medicare for skilled nursing care may enter skilled nursing facilities without a prior hospitalization. This provision opens the possibility of SNF care being used instead of hospitalization for some acute illnesses.

CCRC (Continuing Care Retirement Community): A residential setting that provides a package of medical, social, supportive, and case management services to enable clients to age in place, with systematic help with intercurrent disabilities and progressive impairments. The target group is affluent; both entry fees and periodic charges are substantial. Restrictions on preexisting conditions may also apply.

CCSE (Cognitive Capacity Screening Examination): An interview-based test designed by Jacobs et al. (1977) to assess patients for moderate-to-severe cognitive impairment. The test is somewhat more sensitive than the MSQ and the PMSQ, and is comparable in sensitivity to MMSE. It does not involve paper-and-pencil items, so may be more convenient in some settings than the MMSE. Like other brief cognitive screening tests, it is relatively insensitive to milder forms of cognitive impairment, and does not test noncognitive aspects of mental status.

Channeling: The National Long-Term Care Demonstration, or channeling demonstration, was a large-scale, multistate demonstration project funded by HHS to test the hypothesis that case management could keep frail elderly persons out of nursing homes, and simultaneously reduce costs. In fact, the demonstration showed that the channeling model did not reduce nursing home care utilization sufficiently to offset the increased expense for community services and case management itself. However, channeling did improve quality of life for clients and caregivers.

CMI (Chronic Mental Illness; Chronically Mentally Ill): A term referring to individuals suffering from severe and chronic mental disorders that cause long-term disability and ongoing needs of treatment. The term comprises individuals with chronic schizophrenia, those with severe and treatment-resistant mood disorders, and some with profound and disabling disorders of personality. Patients with Alzheimer's disease and related dementias are not included in this rubric, even though they may have chronic and disabling mental symptoms.

CMHC (Community Mental Health Center): Public or private nonprofit legal entity through which comprehensive mental health services are provided to residents of a geographic catchment area.

COBRA (Consolidated Omnibus Budget Reconciliation Act): A package of changes enacted in 1985 that, among other things, respond directly to many of the criticisms that have been leveled against the fiscal regulations for home- and community-based services waivers.

Cognitive: An adjective referring to brain functions such as memory, abstract reasoning, planning and judgment, language functions, etc. Cognitive impairment is typical of dementia and delirium, but may also be produced by numerous other neuropsychiatric problems, including prescription drug toxicity and depression. Cognitive mental status refers to that part of mental evaluation that focuses on cognitive function.

Cognitive impairment: A decrease in one or more mental abilities including memory, judgment, abstract reasoning, calculation, language skills, drawing, and visual perception. Cognitive impairment is a very general term that comprises syndromes such as delirium and dementia, as well as stable developmental disabilities and disturbances in thought processes due to psychiatric illnesses such as depression. Cognitive impairment is part of the diagnostic criteria for dementia and delirium. Cognitive impairment of some degree is a virtually universal accompaniment of depression in the elderly.

Cognitive services: A term that refers to medical services that rely heavily upon the knowledge, experience, and judgment of the physician, and are not primarily based upon procedures or the use of high technology. A neurological consultation, an internist's initial diagnostic assessment, and a psychotherapy session are all examples of cognitive services. There is a general consensus that Medicare pays too little for cognitive services, and perhaps too much for procedures. The widespread belief that cognitive services are underpaid was part of the motivation for the Resource-Based Relative Value Scale (see below).

Community Mental Health Centers Act: Federal legislation that authorized federal funding for the creation of comprehensive community-based mental health centers. Such centers were mandated to provide a specific set of services in a geographic catchment area, but could provide other services on a discretionary basis. Federal funding for each center declined over an eight-year time period, and each center eventually was funded mostly through other sources. The act was significantly amended by the Mental Health Systems Act of 1980 and repealed by the Omnibus Budget Reconciliation Act of 1981.

Comorbidity: A medical or psychiatric condition other than the patient's primary diagnosis, that substantially influences the clinical course. For example, depression is a common comorbidity in stroke patients.

Competition: A state of rivalry among sellers, each of whom tries to gain a larger share of the market and greater profits. Under competition, sellers both adapt to existing market conditions (by switching to more profitable items or by operating more efficiently) and attempt to change market conditions (by creating additional demand through product differentiation, combining with other sellers in cartels, or by advertising).

Cost containment: The control of the overall cost of health care services within a health care delivery system. Costs are contained when the value of the resources committed to an activity are not considered excessive. Thus, the determination of adequacy of cost containment is frequently subjective and political, dependent upon the specific population served.

Cost-shifting: See "multiple payers."

CPT (Current Procedural Terminology): A coding system developed and endorsed by the American Medical Association, for describing various physicians' services with numerical codes. HCFA is now committed to providing Medicare reimbursement only if the services are described by appropriate CPT codes. The linkage of coding and reimbursement thus implies a necessity for differential coding if a specialty group is seeking differential reimbursement for particular services.

CPT also incorporates measures of complexity of service, which, if properly applied, may capture the added difficulty of treating elderly patients with multiple interacting diagnoses.

CSP (Community Support Program): A model of community-based services for the chronically mentally ill, established by NIMH in 1977, providing a comprehensive package of services including outreach, clinical mental health services, crisis services, medical and dental care, housing, peer support, family and community support, rehabilitation services, advocacy, and case management. The model, which is rarely fully implemented due to constraints upon funds, describes an ideal system of community-based care for the chronically mentally ill.

Delirium: A relatively acute alteration in mental state due to some organic factor, in which impairment in attention and orientation are prominent, and in which there are multiple symptoms of disturbed cognition, comprising memory, reasoning, and judgment. Further, disturbances of the sleep-wake cycle and of motor function are nearly universal. Delirium is differentiated from dementia because it is acute, because it is usually transient, and because disturbance of attention and orientation predominate over other cognitive signs. Delirium is universal in some conditions, such as extreme fever or dehydration, emergence from anesthesia, and the more severe forms of withdrawal from alcohol and drugs of abuse. Advanced age is a risk factor for delirium, and elderly patients with early or subclinical dementing illnesses are at especially high risk.

Demand-side cost sharing: A relationship between a third-party payer and the patient in which the third party requests additional out-of-pocket payments from the consumer as a disincentive to excessive utilization of care. Mechanisms include additional premiums for high utilizers of services, deductibles, copayments, and annual limits on reimbursement.

Dementia: A persistent and disabling mental disorder, characterized by impairment in memory, judgment, and other cognitive functions, without a disproportionate involvement of attentional processes that would characterize delirium (the acute confusional state). Dementia, by definition, requires that symptoms be persistent, multiple, and functionally disabling. Therefore, an individual in the earliest stages of illness such as Alzheimer's disease does not necessarily warrant a diagnosis of dementia. A dementia is said to be *reversible* if its etiology has a specific treatment, and if the treatment of the etiology can reverse, rather than merely arrest, the symptoms of dementia. A dementia is said to be *treatable* if its etiology can be treated, leading to either arrest or improvement in the symptoms. For dementias such as Alzheimer's disease, which are at present neither reversible nor treatable, treatment may still be available for the symptoms, rather than the etiology, of the illness.

Depression: A word with many meanings. It may refer to a transient mood experienced by a healthy person, or to a disabling mental illness. *Major depression* is the name given to an illness of at least two weeks' duration with multiple symptoms, significant impairment of social and occupational function, and a persistent unpleasant mood. The syndrome of major depression has diverse etiologies, with genetic factors, environmental factors, and physical health status all playing a role. It appears that biologic factors such as genetics, physical health status, and prescription drug use are more potent factors in determining major depression than life circumstances. However, the loss of a spouse is a definite risk factor for major depression in the elderly.

DIS (Diagnostic Interview Schedule): A standardized psychiatric interview for adults designed primarily for population studies of mental disorder. The diagnostic criteria for the conditions included are based on DSM-III; it can also be scored for Research Diagnostic Criteria. This interview can be administered by a lay person and it is computer scored. It was developed for and used in the Epidemiology Catchment Area studies in the early 1980s, and it has since been used in other epidemiological studies in the community and in clinical settings.

DRG (Diagnostic-Related Groups): Method of classifying patients into categories on the basis of diagnosis and treatment. This method is utilized in the prospective payment system employed by the federal government to pay for hospital care of Medicare patients. The classification system was developed by researchers from Yale using large data bases of hospital records from New Jersey, Connecticut, and South Carolina. The major diagnostic categories were derived from the eighth edition of the International Classification of Diseases (ICDA-8). After many trials, 470 DRGs became the standard, and the system was used on a national basis by Medicare to control hospital costs, primarily by encouraging reductions in the length of stay of patients. Empirical studies suggest that the Medicare DRGs for psychiatric disorders are *not* valid predictors of length of stay or of resource consumption.

DSM-III-R (Diagnostic and Statistical Manual of Mental Disorders, Third Edition, Revised): The DSM developed by the American Psychiatric Association is the official manual for classifying mental disorder in the United States. The third edition, published in 1980 and revised in 1987, represents a major shift in psychiatric classification toward quantifying and describing psychiatric symptoms without reference to cause.

Dysphoria: An unpleasant mood state. Depressed patients always have dysphoric mood, but may not label the mood as depressed. Irritability, agitation, and depletion are all descriptions of dysphoria. Persistent dysphoria is necessary for diagnosis of major depression, but is not sufficient, as vegetative disturbance is also necessary to make the major depression diagnosis.

ECA (Epidemiology Catchment Area):   Large-scale studies of mental disorder were conducted under NIMH auspices in five communities and institutions in the early 1980s. The communities are New Haven, Connecticut; St. Louis, Missouri; Baltimore, Maryland; Durham, North Carolina; and Los Angeles, California. Oversamples of populations of special interest, including the elderly, blacks, and Hispanics and rural areas were collected in several sites. The ECA was designed to examine the usual epidemiological concerns such as the prevalence and incidence, etiology and course of illness and also investigated related service use patterns. Thus, it is possible to examine relationships between specific mental disorders and service use in the general health, specialty mental health, and social services sector. With such information, gaps in service use can be identified and planners can, to some extent, predict service use.

Fee-for-service: A method of charging patients for services or treatment whereby a physician or other practitioner bills for each patient encounter, treatment, or service rendered. This remains the most common way of paying physicians in the United States. Fee-for-service contrasts with salary or capitation systems, where physician income does not change with the amount of service rendered. Under fee-for-service, physicians have an incentive to deliver more service.

Functional status: Description of individuals according to what they are able to do, rather than by what diagnoses apply to them. Cognitive function, mobility, social competence, and ability to conduct activities of everyday life are all part of functional status. Numerous formal scales exist for describing functional status, comparing the status of different populations, and measuring changes in individuals over time or with treatment.

Gatekeeping: A feature of prepaid health plans, in which access to specific health services, such as specialists or hospitalization, is controlled by a designated individual, the gatekeeper. The gatekeeper may be the primary care physician or may be a nonmedical health professional hired by the plan with a cost-control mission. Another sense of gatekeeping is the practice by health providers of declining to serve individuals who represent bad financial risks, either because of poor insurance coverage, a poor prognosis, or questionable indications for hospitalization (and therefore a risk of retrospective denial of payment by the third-party payer).

General hospital: An establishment that provides diagnosis and treatment, both surgical and nonsurgical, for patients who have any of a variety of medical conditions. Its components are an organized medical staff, permanent facilities that include inpatient beds, medical services, continuous nursing services, an administrator to whom the governing authority delegates the full-time responsibility for the operation, patients admitted on the medical authority of the medical staff, a medical record maintained for each patient, pharmacy services maintained in or by the institution and supervised by a licensed pharmacist, diagnostic X-ray services, clinical laboratory services, anatomical pathology services, operating room services, and food services.

Geriatrics: A specialty of medical practice concerned with the care of the elderly. Practitioners of geriatrics usually come from the fields of internal medicine, family medicine, and general practice. An internist or family physician wishing to be a *certified* subspecialist in geriatrics must undergo additional fellowship training in geriatric medicine, and pass an examination.

GHQ (General Health Questionnaire): The GHQ is a brief self-report screening questionnaire designed in England by David Goldberg to elicit psychological distress in primary care patients (1972). Primary care patients find this measure easy to complete and acceptable, in part, because somatic symptoms are included. Various versions of the GHQ, based originally on the Cornell Medical Index, have been used widely in this country and many others to identify primary care patients at risk for mental disorder.

HCFA (Health Care Financing Administration): A federal agency under the aegis of the Department of Health and Human Services which focuses on regulations and policies relating to payments for health care, and which administers the Medicare and Medicaid programs.

HIE (Health Insurance Experiment): A well-known study undertaken by the Rand Corporation investigating how insurance coverage influences individuals' utilization of health services and ultimate health status. One finding was that if patient copayments are sufficiently high, individuals will delay seeking treatment for ambulatory medical conditions, including psychiatric disorders.

HMO (Health Maintenance Organization): Organized system for providing health care in a geographic area, which assures the delivery of a set of basic and supplemental health maintenance and treatment services to a voluntarily enrolled group of persons. Services are reimbursed through a predetermined, fixed, periodic prepayment made by or on behalf of each person or family unit enrolled in the HMO without regard to the amounts of actual services provided.

Home- and community-based services waiver: Allows Medicaid dollars to provide a broad range of home and community services to persons who otherwise would require care in an institutional setting.

IADL (Instrumental Activities of Daily Living): Activities beyond the basic ADLs that are part of normal independent existence. These include driving, using public transportation, using the telephone, sending and receiving mail, shopping, and managing household finances. There is less consensus on scales for IADLs than there is for scales of ADLs. IADLs tend to be particularly vulnerable to disruption by mental illness.

ICF (Intermediate Care Facility): An institution licensed under state law to provide health-related care and services to individuals who do not require the degree of care or treatment that a hospital or skilled nursing facility provides. ICF care is not covered by Medicare Part A. Medicaid does cover ICF care, but the rates of payment may be below the market price for ICF services.

IMD (Institution for Mental Diseases): The term given to a nursing home in which half or more of the residents have diagnosed mental illnesses. IMDs must provide some mental health services to their residents, and are reimbursed less favorably by federal Medicaid. Nursing homes have a tendency to underdiagnose mental illness in their residents, so they will not be reclassified as IMDs.

IPA (Independent Practice Association): A group of health service providers who negotiate collectively with health financing organizations concerning reimbursement rates, referral mechanisms, etc.

LCAH (Life Care at Home): A package of services, including medical, nursing, social, and supportive, to enable individuals with functional impairments to remain at home. LCAH is generally funded by private resources, but is less expensive than CCRCs because fees do not include rent. Case management is provided both for access and for cost control purposes.

Long-term care insurance: Policies that provide for various aspects of nonhospital care of functionally impaired elderly. The narrowest form provides for care in a skilled nursing facility. Broader long-term care insurance plans might cover other residential living arrangements, home care, or even physical modifications of the home environment to minimize the effects of a disability.

LTC (long-term care): An expression referring to all forms of continuing services rendered to individuals with chronic illness or handicap. These services include home care, care in a nursing facility, and supportive services such as home-delivered meals that might enable a functionally impaired person to continue residing in the community. On occasion, the term is used as a synonym for care in a nursing home, but this usage is inaccurate.

Managed care: A health care delivery system that attempts to keep costs down by "managing" the care to eliminate unnecessary treatment and reduce expensive hospital care. Management involves both *gatekeeping* (restricting the use of expensive services) and *referral* (the use of appropriate services in time to prevent costly complications). *Precertification* and *recertification* of the need for inpatient care are particularly frequent components of gatekeeping.

Mandated mental health insurance: State laws requiring insurance companies to offer or provide minimum mental health benefits. Mandated insurance may specify a minimum dollar amount of coverage for outpatient care, or a minimum number of days for inpatient care. To date, no mandated mental health plan requires equal coverage for mental and physical illness, or equal coverage for a subset of mental illnesses for which a medical model of treatment is appropriate.

Market segmentation: Division of the market for goods and services into discrete segments, each primarily served by a different vendor type. Segmentation *per se* may be either economically efficient or economically inefficient. If segmentation of a market results from collusion between vendors to support monopoly control over sub-markets, segmentation may be harmful to consumers. On the other hand, if segmentation results from the selection by market forces of the most productive vendor of each type of good or service, the consequences for the consumer may be positive. The segmentation of the health service market by physician and nonphysician providers offers a controversial example.

Medicaid: A federally aided, state-operated and administered program which provides medical benefits for certain low-income persons. The program, authorized by Title XIX of the Social Security Act, is basically for the poor. It does not cover all of the poor, however, but only persons who are members of one of the categories of people who can be covered under the welfare cash payment programs: the aged, the blind, the disabled, and members of families with dependent children where one parent is absent, incapacitated, or unemployed. Under certain circumstances states may provide Medicaid coverage for children under 21 who would not otherwise be eligible. Subject to broad federal guidelines, states determine the benefits covered, program eligibility, rates of payment for providers, and methods of administering the program. Medicaid is considered "assurance," not "insurance," because eligibles receive coverage without paying into the program. It is funded entirely from public sources: about half by federal funds and half by state and local funds. This ratio varies from state to state, with the federal share higher in poorer states. Medicaid eligibles pay no premiums or coinsurance, although some states require a small copayment for prescription drugs and other services.

Medicare: A nationwide health insurance program for people aged 65 and over, for persons eligible for Social Security disability payments for over two years, and for certain workers and their dependents who need kidney transplantation or dialysis. Health insurance protection is available to insured persons without regard to income. Monies from payroll taxes and premiums from beneficiaries are deposited in special trust funds for use in meeting the expenses incurred by the insured. The program was enacted July 30,

1965, as Title XVIII, of the Social Security Act, and became effective on July 1, 1966. It consists of two separate but coordinated programs: hospital insurance (Part A) and supplementary medical insurance (Part B). Catastrophic insurance (Part C) existed briefly between the passage and repeal of the Catastrophic Coverage Act.

Medicare benefits: As outlined in the Social Security Handbook, a person with hospital insurance protection (Part A) may have benefits paid on his behalf or, in certain cases, paid to him or her for covered health care services. The Medical Insurance plan (Part B) adds to the protection provided by the basic hospital insurance plan and covers a substantial part of physicians' services, surgery, and a number of other health items and services. The benefit period includes 90 days of hospital care per episode of illness plus a "lifetime reserve" of 60 days. Medicare Part A is supported by a trust fund that is replenished annually by Social Security payroll taxes paid by both employers and employees. Eligible enrollees pay no premiums for Part A, but are required to pay a significant deductible as well as coinsurance. Approximately 25% of Medicare Part B, which is considered a supplemental insurance program, is funded by enrollee premiums, with the remainder coming from general federal funds. Part B requires a monthly premium and incorporates coinsurance as well as an annual deductible.

Medicare participating physician: A physician who accepts Medicare's fee schedule as payment in full for all Medicare beneficiaries. While physicians are not required by federal law to participate, Medicare payments to participating physicians are slightly higher than payments to nonparticipating physicians, and the total charges of nonparticipating physicians are limited. The current limit is called the Maximum Allowable Actual Charge (MAAC); under the provisions of OBRA 1989, the MAAC will eventually be replaced by 115% of the Medicare payment amount for nonparticipating physicians. Some states, including Rhode Island and Massachusetts, require that physicians charge Medicare beneficiaries no more than the Medicare fee schedule.

Medigap: A private insurance policy designed to augment Medicare coverage, most often by covering copayments and deductibles and thereby reducing the patient's payment liability. In general, Medigap does not expand the scope of covered services. Therefore, while a Medigap policy might reduce the patient's copayment for psychiatric services, it would not change Medicare's restrictions and limits.

Mental health: A euphemism; both a noun and an adjective. As a noun, it generally denotes the absence of significant mental illness. As an adjective, it may designate professionals such as psychiatrists, psychologists, social workers, and psychiatric nurses involved in providing treatment for mental disorders and related conditions. "Mental health problems" may be used as a synonym for "mental illness." When used in this way, the term "mental health" carries a less medical connotation than "mental illness" or "neuropsychiatric disorder."

Mental status: The term has two meanings. It may either refer to the totality of a patient's current mental functioning including cognitive, emotional, and behavioral dimensions, or may refer more narrowly to the cognitive aspects of the patient's mental functioning, specifically memory, orientation, attention, etc. *Mental status examination* refers either to the process of questioning people about their cognition and mental phenomena, or to the formal recording of observations concerning mood, thought, and behavior.

MMSE (Mini Mental State Examination): A cognitive screening test designed by Folstein et al. (1975) that has attained wide acceptance in the medical research community. The test, which involves both verbal questions and some paper-and-pencil items, can be administered in about ten minutes, and screens for moderate-to-severe cognitive impairment. It is somewhat more sensitive to milder cognitive impairment than the MSQ and SPMSQ, but still has a substantial false negative rate. Also, it produces false positives among poorly educated people. It can administered by a lay interviewer. It does not test noncognitive aspects of mental status.

Mood: A person's subjective feeling of happiness, sadness, anxiety, etc. This is distinguished from *affect,* the outward expression of mood. Affect is observed; mood is reported.

Mood disorder: A psychiatric disorder in which a disturbance of mood is primary, and is accompanied by numerous other symptoms. Major depression and manic-depressive illness are examples.

MSQ (Mental Status Questionnaire): A brief questionnaire designed by Kahn et al. (1960) for the detection of moderate-to-severe cognitive impairment. The questionnaire, which relies on simple questions such as stating the date and the current president, is suitable for administration by lay interviewers. The test is not sensitive to more subtle cognitive impairment, and does not evaluate noncognitive aspects of mental status.

Multiple payers: Reverse of the situation where more than one insurance company or public agency has responsibility for paying for an individual's health care. Under these circumstances, there are economic incentives for each payer to shift costs to one of the other payers whenever possible. This is referred to as cost-shifting, or the "problem of multiple pockets." A classic example is when a patient is prematurely discharged from an acute care hospital because of the pressures of the DRG system, and then has a bad outcome creating a need for nursing home care that might be covered by Medicaid. Although the total cost of the patient's care is greater because of the premature discharge from the acute hospital, the acute care hospital has an incentive to push for early discharge because it is not at risk for the long-term consequences of that action.

NAMCS (National Ambulatory Medical Care Survey): A periodic survey of office-based medical practice. This survey, conducted by the National Center for Health Statistics, collects information on reason for visit, diagnosis, procedures, length of visit, etc. An important use of the NAMCS is that service researchers can investigate medical practice patterns in ambulatory settings and by type medical specialty.

Neuropsychiatry: A medical specialty concerned with the diagnosis and treatment of disorders of mood, cognition, and behavior that pays particular attention to disturbances in brain function. The neuropsychiatrist integrates a psychosocial and developmental perspective with a neurological viewpoint. As contrasted with psychiatry, neuropsychiatry gives relatively greater weight to biologic factors in the etiology of mental disturbance, and tends to focus to a greater extent on patients with brain diseases, such as Alzheimer's disease, Parkinson's disease, stroke, epilepsy, or head injury. Neuropsychiatrists are somewhat more likely to use high-technology diagnostic procedures such as brain imaging or clinical neurophysiologic tests in making a diagnosis. Formal training of a neuropsychiatrist may be either as a neurologist, as a psychiatrist, or both.

Neuropsychology: A subspecialty of psychology concerned with the evaluation of the cognitive and behavioral effects of brain injury, and with the systematic characterization of cognitive and perceptual disturbances due to medical, neurological, and psychiatric illness. Neuropsychologists work in the neurological, psychiatric, and neuropsychiatric settings. Their usual role is in diagnostic evaluation, treatment planning, and in objective follow-up of longitudinal course or effects of treatment.

NF (Nursing Facility): The new term for ICF (intermediate care facility) introduced by OBRA 1987.

NIMH (National Institute of Mental Health): A federal agency, part of the Alcohol Drug Abuse and Mental Health Administration (ADAMHA), which is itself a subdivision of the Public Health Service. The primary mission of the NIMH is research on mental disorders, which is conducted both intramurally and extramurally through grants and contracts. To a lesser extent, the NIMH participates in, and funds, education and training of mental health care providers and participates in providing information to the public.

Nursing home: Institutions other than hospitals, that provide various levels of maintenance, personal, and nursing care to people who are unable to care for themselves. These include freestanding institutions and identifiable components of other health facilities which provide nursing care and related services. Nursing homes include skilled nursing facilities, intermediate care facilities, and extended care facilities but not board and care homes.

OBRA 1987 (Omnibus Budget Reconciliation Act of 1987): In the discussion of mental health policy, this refers to the provisions of OBRA 1987 related to the mental health of the elderly. These included an increase in the annual ceiling for outpatient Medicare psychiatric treatment, and several nursing home reform provisions, including a requirement for preadmission screening and annual resident review for mental illness and mental retardation. See PASARR.

OBRA 1989 (Omnibus Budget Reconciliation Act of 1989): In the discussion of mental health policy, this refers to the provisions of OBRA 1989 related to the mental health of the elderly. These included the elimination of the annual ceiling for outpatient Medicare mental health treatment, the addition of psychologists and clinical social workers to the list of providers reimbursable by Medicare, and specific amendments to the nursing home reform provisions of OBRA 1987. The latter included a deadline for HHS to develop final requirements on preadmission screening of nursing home residents for mental illness (see PASARR), a delay in screening requirements for private-pay nursing home residents, and an exemption from screening for nursing home residents readmitted to a nursing facility after a hospital stay.

Partial hospitalization: A general term that encompasses a variety of outpatient psychiatric programs that are more encompassing than a traditional office visit, and usually involve the services of several different disciplines. Partial hospital programs include day hospital and day treatment programs, as well as day care and night care centers. Partial hospital services *per se* are not covered by Medicare, but components of them may be under the outpatient hospital benefit. When they are, the institutional (nonphysician) component is not subject to the annual outpatient limit. Medicaid plans may cover partial hospitalization; policies vary from state to state.

PASARR (Pre-Admission Screening and Annual Resident Review): This provision of OBRA 1987 requires that nursing homes that receive Medicare and Medicaid payments screen all prospective residents for mental illness and mental retardation, and that they rescreen long-term residents annually for these disorders. If mental illness or mental retardation is present and the resident requires active treatment for them, a determination is made whether the resident requires nursing home care because of physical disability, mental illness, or functional impairment. Residents who need active treatment for mental illness and do not otherwise require nursing home care must be discharged. Residents who require nursing home care but also need active treatment for mental illness must be provided with that treatment, at other than federal expense.

PPO (Preferred Provider Organization): A group of health care providers that contracts with a health care financing organization to provide services to its beneficiaries. Clients of a health plan that contracts with a PPO must obtain treatment from members of the PPO, if they are to enjoy their full benefits. Usually, members of the PPO are paid less than a market rate for their services, in exchange for a larger volume of patient referrals. In theory, however, the PPO system can also be used as a method of quality assurance for the care received by clients of a health plan. Discounts and utilization review are primary sources of support.

PPRC (Physician Payment Reform Commission): An agency set up by Congress in 1986 to investigate alternatives for reforming physician payment by Medicare and to make recommendations to Congress and HHS concerning a new physician payment schedule. The PPRC was specifically directed to focus on eliminating excessive payments for invasive procedures and to promote more equitable payment for primary care services.

PPS (Prospective Payment System): A system for reimbursing medical care prospectively, according to a patient classification system, rather than retrospectively according to the actual costs of the patient's treatment. In theory, this creates incentives for the provider of services to render services most efficiently and economically. In practice, it may encourage manipulation of case mix to emphasize treatment of patients on whom the institution can make a profit, while excluding those who require costly treatment and have an uncertain prognosis. Diagnosis-related groups (DRGs) are one system of prospective payment. However, other models of prospective payment could take into account factors other than a patient's diagnosis, such as age and functional status. To date, no method of classification of psychiatric patients has proved sufficiently predictive of resource utilization to form a rational basis for a PPS for mental illness.

Prepayment: The payment for health care services in advance. Insurance companies, PPOs, HMOs, or related health care organizations are paid a set fee for health care services to be provided if needed during the period of coverage.

QA (Quality Assurance): A generic term for activities designed to monitor and hopefully improve the quality of medical care. QA efforts may be *process-based*, focusing on the completeness of charts, the use of laboratory tests according to protocol, etc., or may be *outcome-based*, targeting specific rates of improvement, mortality, complications, etc. A third kind of QA is *structural* QA, focusing on the adequacy of physical facilities and equipment.

RBRVS (Resource-Based Relative Value Scale): A system for reforming physician payment by Medicare, and possibly eventually by other third parties. The scale, developed by Hsiao et al. (1989) under a federal contract, assigns a relative value to various physicians' services, based on the time involved, the specialized knowledge needed, the risk assumed, and other resources necessary to deliver the service. The concept of an RBRVS has been endorsed by the American Medical Association. However, many physicians and subspecialty groups, including the American Psychiatric Association, have challenged the provisional assignment of relative values for specific services, questioning the methodology upon which the relative values were assigned.

RCT (Randomized Controlled Trial):   A type of clinical research in which a group of patients with a given condition is randomly divided into two groups, one that will receive the treatment of interest and the other that will receive a control or placebo treatment. The RCT is the "gold standard" of treatment trials, as it is relatively free from biases encountered in before-and-after investigations or in naturalistic comparisons between treated and untreated groups. RCTs are widely performed to test the effects of medications and surgical procedures; they are increasingly being used to test alternative forms of service delivery.

Respite care: Temporary placement of an ill person in institutional care to provide relief for family caretakers. Respite care is distinguished from other forms of long-term care by its temporary nature and by the intended beneficiary being the caretaker, rather than primarily the patient himself. Respite care can be provided by nursing homes, by other institutions, or by specially trained volunteer families, who function as foster relatives.

RUGS (Resource Utilization Groups):   A method of classifying nursing home patients by diagnosis enacted in New York State, in an effort to predict the resource inputs required to care for them properly. This could form a basis of a prospective payment system for nursing home care.

S/HMO (Social/Health Maintenance Organization):   A prepaid health plan for the elderly that combines medical services with social and supportive services in a single package. As with the HMO, the S/HMO strives to recruit relatively healthy elderly to average down the service utilization of the more impaired elderly. The S/HMO uses case management as a cost control mechanism (see Chapter 10).

SNF (Skilled Nursing Facility):   An institution that has a transfer agreement with one or more participating hospitals, and is primarily engaged in providing to inpatients skilled nursing care and rehabilitative services; meets specific regulatory certification requirements. SNF care is partially covered by Medicare Part A.

Somatization: A tendency to express emotional distress as physical symptoms. Somatization *disorder* refers to a lifelong pattern of multiple somatic complaints without a physical basis. Other causes of somatization apart from somatization disorder include depression and anxiety disorders.

SPMSQ (Short Portable Mental Status Questionnaire): A brief instrument (Omer 1983) for screening patients for moderate-to-severe cognitive impairment. Like the MSQ, it can be administered by lay interviewers. It is not sensitive to milder forms of cognitive impairment, and does not test noncognitive aspects of mental status.

SSA (Social Security Administration): An agency of the Department of Health and Human Services which manages the Social Security program.

SSDI (Social Security Disability Insurance): Disability insurance provided under the Social Security Act to individuals who have paid into the Social Security system for at least five years prior to becoming totally and permanently disabled. Compared with SSI, SSDI benefits are substantially greater, and Medicare coverage is included regardless of the patient's age.

SSI (Supplementary Security Income): A program of income support for low-income aged, blind, and disabled persons, established by Title XVI of the Social Security Act. SSI replaced state welfare programs for the aged, blind, and disabled. This federally administered program pays a monthly basic benefit; states may supplement this basic benefit amount. Receipt of a federal SSI benefit or a state supplement under the program is often used to establish Medicaid eligibility.

Supply-side cost sharing: A relationship between a third-party payer and a provider of health services that places the provider at risk if the cost of services rendered exceeds a predetermined guideline. Prospective payment systems are one form of supply-side cost sharing.

TEFRA (Tax Equity and Fiscal Responsibility Act of 1982): Developed in the U.S. Senate and passed by Congress in response to the mandate of the First Concurrent Budget Resolution to increase government revenues by approximately $100 billion for the first three fiscal years. TEFRA's four principal objectives include: 1) to raise revenues to narrow anticipated budget deficits; 2) to insure that both individual and business taxpayers pay their fair share of the total tax burden; 3) to reduce distortions in economic behavior resulting from the present tax system; 4) to charge groups benefiting from specific government programs with the costs of those programs. Under TEFRA, a prospective payment system by DRGs was instituted for hospitals receiving funds from HCFA. Psychiatric units and rehabilitation units were exempted, but per-discharge limits were placed on the total reimbursement paid by HCFA to exempt psychiatric and rehabilitation units. These limits, the "TEFRA limits," are usually substantially less than the actual expenditures incurred for taking care of the most ill psychiatric patients. For example, TEFRA limits often provide for less than 20 days of inpatient hospitalization, while a severely depressed elderly person requiring electroconvulsive therapy may require four weeks or more.

UR (Utilization Review): A process for evaluating whether medical care services, particularly hospitalization, are being used appropriately and efficiently. UR can be either prospective, concurrent, or retrospective, and may or may not be linked to third-party reimbursement decisions.

Vegetative signs: Disturbances in eating, sleeping, and energy that accompany mood disorder. Vegetative signs are required for the diagnosis of major depression.

Veterans Administration Hospital: A health care facility where medical, mental health, and dental services are rendered to veterans. Preference is given to patients with service-connected disabilities. The Veterans Administration reimburses VA hospitals for mental health services on a capitation basis. Therefore, VA hospitals are encouraged to develop community services, partial hospitalization, etc. if the effect of these services is to reduce inpatient lengths of stay.

Waiver: Permission, granted by HCFA for a specific project, to use Medicare or Medicaid funds to provide services not ordinarily covered by those programs. Waivers may involve predetermined caps on the total amount spent, or may involve restricting clients' access to HCFA-funded services not included in the program. Most innovative service delivery programs for the elderly, such as On Lok, rely upon waivers to provide their funding and allow case managers control over services used.

Sources

Ammer C, Ammer DS: Dictionary of Business and Economics. New York, NY, The Free Press, 1984

Craig RT, Wright B: Mental Health Financing and Programming: A Legislator's Guide. National Conference of State Legislatures, May 1988

Folstein MF, Folstein SE, McHugh PR: Mini-Mental State. J Psychiatric Research 12:189-198, 1975

Furino A: Glossary of Terms Used in the Economics of Health Care and Medical Practice (unpublished document). San Antonio, The University of Texas Health Science Center at San Antonio, 1987

Goldberg DP: The Detection of Psychiatric Illness by Questionnaire. Maudsley Monograph No. 21. London, Oxford University Press, 1972

Hsaio WC, Braun P, Becker E, et al: A National Study of Resource-Based Relative Value Scales for Physician Services: Final Report. Boston, Harvard School of Public Health, 1988

Jacobs JW, Bernhard MR, Delgado A, et al: Screening for Organic Mental Syndromes in the Medically Ill. Ann Intern Med 86:40-46, 1977

Kahn RL, Goldfarb AI, Polack M, et al: Brief objective measures for the determination of mental status in the aged. Am J Psychiatry 117:325-328, 1960

Katz S, Ford AB, Moskowitz RW, et al: Studies of illness in the aged. The index of ADL: a standardized measure of biological and psychosocial function. JAMA 185:914-919, 1963

Omer H, Foldes J, Toby M, et al: Screening for cognitive deficits in a sample of hospitalized geriatric patients: a reevaluation of a brief mental status questionnaire. J Am Geriatr Soc 31:266-268, 1983

Spiegel AD, Kavaler F: Cost Containment and DRGs: A Guide to Prospective Payment. Owings Mills, MD, National Health Publishing, 1986

Stoline A, Weiner JP: The New Medical Marketplace. Baltimore, MD, The Johns Hopkins University Press, 1988

Timmreck TC: Dictionary of Health Services Management, 2nd ed. Owings Mills, MD, National Health Publishing, 1987

Appendix IV

Conference Participants

The following individuals participated in the National Conference on Access and Financing for Neuropsychiatric Care for the Elderly (October 1988)

Participant	Institution Represented
Linda Aiken, R.N., Ph.D.	University of Pennsylvania
Senator Louis Bertonazzi	Massachusetts State Senate
Daniel P. Bourque	Voluntary Hospitals of America
Kenneth Bowler	House Ways and Means Committee (Staff Director)
J. Gregory Boyer	The Upjohn Company
Steven Brody, J.D., M.S.W.	University of Pennsylvania
Barbara Burns, Ph.D.	University of Maryland
Nancy Cannon, Ph.D.	John Hancock Insurance Company
Alfredo Cardillo	Office of New York State Senator Tarky Lombardi
Gene Cohen, M.D., Ph.D.	National Institute on Aging (Deputy Director)
Richard Connard, M.D.	Southmark Foundation
Clement Delahunt	The Upjohn Company
Golda Edinburgh, M.S.W.	National Association of Social Workers
Mary Jane England, M.D.	The Prudential Insurance Company
David Espino, M.D.	University of Texas Health Science Center, San Antonio
Sam Fager, M.D.	Aetna Insurance Company
Christine Ferguson	Office of U.S. Senator John Chafee (Legislative Director)
Barry S. Fogel, M.D.	Brown University
Ann Ford, R.N., Ph.D.	Department of Health and Rehabilitative Services, State of Florida
Antonio Furino, Ph.D.	University of Texas Health Science Center, San Antonio

Gwen Gampell	Subcommittee on Health, House Ways and Means Committee (Professional Staff)
Lori Gibson	Office of U.S. Representative Claudine Schneider
Howard Goldman, M.D., Ph.D.	University of Maryland
John Gorman	Blue Cross and Blue Shield of Rhode Island
Gary Gottlieb, M.D., M.B.A.	University of Pennsylvania
Lois Grau, R.N., Ph.D.	American Nurses' Association
David Greer, M.D.	Brown University
Lee Grindheim, Ph.D.	American Psychiatric Association
Lauren Gross	Office of U.S. Senator Claiborne Pell
Barry Gurland, M.D.	Columbia University
Barbara Herzog, Ph.D.	American Association of Retired Persons
Peter Hollman, M.D.	Zambarano Memorial Hospital
Thomas Hoyer	Health Care Financing Administration
Beth Jackson, Ph.D.	Brown University
Robert Kane, M.D.	University of Minnesota
Rosalie Kane, Ph.D.	University of Minnesota
Judith Lave, Ph.D.	University of Pittsburgh
Senator Tarky Lombardi	New York State Senate
Hal Mark, Ph.D.	University of Connecticut
Danna Mauch	Department of Mental Health, State of Rhode Island
James Morone, Ph.D.	Brown University
Joseph Munley	The Upjohn Company
Nancy Orr, M.S.G.	Hillhaven Corporation
Harold Parrish	Department of Mental Health, State of Texas
Susan Pettey, M.P.A., J.D.	American Association of Homes for the Aging
Anne Powell, M.S.W.	Office of California Assemblyman Bruce Bronzan (Principal Consultant)
Joseph Raso	Blue Cross and Blue Shield of Rhode Island
Russell Ricci, M.D.	Voluntary Hospitals of America
Gail Robinson, Ph.D.	Mental Health Policy Resource Center
Thomas Romeo	Department of Mental Health, Retardation and Hospitals, State of Rhode Island
Mark Schlesinger	Harvard University
Steven Sharfstein, M.D.	Sheppard and Enoch Pratt Hospital
Michael Smyer, Ph.D.	American Psychological Association
Martin Stein, M.D.	Hospital Corporation of America

David Strachan	Blue Cross and Blue Shield Association
Major Loree Sutton, M.D.	American Psychiatric Association
William Waters, Ph.D.	Department of Health, State of Rhode Island
Anne Weiss	Senate Finance Committee (Professional Staff)
Terrie Wetle, Ph.D.	Braceland Center for Mental Health and Aging
Stephen White, Ph.D.	Preferred Health Care, Ltd.
Peter Whitehouse, M.D., Ph.D.	Alzheimer's Disease and Related Disorders Association
Paul Widem	National Institute of Mental Health
Cora Yamamoto	Office of U.S. Senator Spark Matsunaga

Index

Academic institutions, role in
    regional planning, 275, 276
"Active treatment," 261
Activities of daily living (ADL), 184
    definition of, 323
    effect of neuropsychiatric
        disorders on, 37
    in determining program
        eligibility, 185
    measurement of, 192
    methodological concerns in
        assessing, 185
Acute confusional state. See
    Delirium
ADL. See Activities of daily living
Administration on Aging, 297
ADRDA. See Alzheimer's Disease
    and Related Disorders
    Association
Adverse selection, 99, 100
Affect, definition of, 323
Affective disorder, definition of,
    323
Affordable long-term institutional
    care, Medicare coverage of,
    33
Agitation, 40, 50
    in dementia, 52–54
Akathisia, 53
Alcohol, drug abuse, and mental
    health (ADM) block grant,
    323

Alcoholism
    consequences of, 12
    dementia associated with, 12
    funding of treatment, 12, 13
    prevalence of, 12
    treatment of, 12
Alcohol rehabilitation, 290
Almshouses, 85
Alprazolam, 46
Alzheimer's disease, 4, 38, 240
    and family caretakers, 4
    case management for, 214, 216
        policy recommendations,
        217
    definition of, 323
    Medicare benefits for, 103
    psychiatric services for, in
        nursing homes, 289
    specialized centers for, 288
Alzheimer's Disease and Related
    Disorders Association
    (ADRDA), 216, 272, 297
American Association for Geriatric
    Psychiatry (AAGP), 139
American Association of Pastoral
    Counseling, 140
American Board of Psychiatry and
    Neurology, 138
American Psychiatric Association,
    300
American Psychological
    Association, 138

AMI. *See* Association for the
    Mentally Ill
Amitriptyline, 44, 46
Anticholinergic effects, 44
Antidepressants
    side effects of, 44
Antipsychotic drugs. *See*
    neuroleptics
Anxiety disorders, prevalence of,
    13
Area Agencies on Aging, 72
Arkansas policy on
    manic-depressive illness, 300
ASPA/CCH Survey, 30
Assessment, 39
    as component of case
        management, 202
    in long-term care services, 167,
        184–186
Assistance to long-term care
    clients, 186, 187
    need for, 28
Association for the Mentally Ill
    (AMI), 297
Autonomy, tradeoffs with safety,
    187

Behavioral and emotional
    consequences of brain
    disease, 7–11
    paranoia, 7
Behavioral problems and nursing
    care costs, 41
Benefit coordination, 229, 230
Benzodiazepines, 46
    for agitation, 52
    in dementia, 52
Bereavement, 1, 2
    depression in, 13
Beta blockers
    for agitation, 52
    in dementia, 52
Block grant, definition of, 324
Blue Cross/Blue Shield
    coverage of inpatient
        psychiatry, 98
    "dental/mental trade-off," 100
    High Option, adverse selection
        in, 100
    payment for inpatient
        psychiatry, 99
Board and care homes

case management needs, 217
    definition of, 324
Brokerage model, 162

Capitated mental health system
    in Rhode Island, 250
    in Rochester, N.Y., 250
Capitation
    definition of, 324
    effect on mental health service
        use by elderly, 132
    for care of chronically mentally
        ill, 250
    in On Lok model, 169
    Medicaid, 251
    problems with, 299, 301
Care coordination. *See* Case
    management
Care management
    distinction from "case
        management," 273–275
    requirements for patient
        participation, 274
Care planning, 194, 195
    as component of case
        management, 202
    for nursing home residents,
        policy recommendations,
        217
Caregiver
    stress, 40
    support groups, 187
"Carve out," 259, 267, 298
    problems for psychiatric
        services to elderly, 228
Case coordination. *See* Case
    management
Case management, 201–220,
        273–275
    aggressive, 227
    "brokerage" model, 203
    components of, 202
    controlled studies of, 207
    costs of, 299
    definition of, 202, 324
    for chemically dependent
        persons, 210
    for chronic schizophrenics, 210
    for elderly neuropsychiatric
        patients, 214–216
    populations served, 214
    funding by Medicaid, 88

history of, 203
in community support
programs, 162
in developmental disability, 206
in long-term care, 206–209
in long-term care insurance
plans, 209
in mental health
controlled studies of, 211,
212
critique, 211
in S/HMOs, 209
mental health versus long-term
care, 211
policy recommendations,
216–218
population-based, 205
rationale for, 201
rehabilitative model, 211
risk-based, 230
selection of, 301
standards for, 208
supportive model, 211
synonyms for, 202
variation in models, 212–214
Case mix, 294
measures for long-term care,
193
Casefinding, as component of case
management, 202
Catastrophic Coverage Act (CCA),
89, 233, 259–260, 299
definition of, 324
Catchment areas
as basis of Community Mental
Health Center
organization 249
definition of, 324
CCA. *See* Catastrophic Coverage
Act
CCRC. *See* Continuing care
retirement communities
CHAMPUS, 225
Channeling Demonstration,
163–166
analysis of results, 207
characterization of clients, 165
definition of, 163, 325
eligibility, screening questions
for mental disorder, 164
evaluation of, 165
financing of, 165

lack of cost savings from, 165
Chemical dependence, case
management in treatment
of, 210
Chemical restraint, 54
Child welfare system as case
management model, 205,
206
Chronic mental illness (CMI),
definition of, 240, 325
Chronic schizophrenia
case management for, 210
Chronically mentally ill
and housing needs, 244, 252
and PASARR, 261
and Social Security disability,
252
care of, 243–245
case management in care of,
244
community care of, 244
in nursing homes, 244
inpatient care of, 244
insurance coverage of, 320, 321
models for long-term care for,
174
state responsibility for, 246
Clinical social workers
Medicare reimbursement of,
262–264
CMHC. *See* Community Mental
Health Centers
CMI. *See* Chronic mental illness
Codes for medical/psychiatric
evaluation, 298
Cognitive mental status, 43
definition of, 320
impairment, definition of, 326
measurement of, 185
"Cognitive services," 109, 123, 264
definition of, 326
Commercial health insurance,
psychiatric benefits of, 320
Commission on Professional and
Hospital Activities (CPHA),
311
Commonwealth Fund, 208
Community mental health centers
(CMHC), 99, 160, 210, 216
as locus of treatment for
schizophrenia, 7
case management in, 287

definition of, 326
lack of use by medical patients,
    296
linkages to nursing homes and
    senior centers, 159
need for central authority over,
    249
underfinancing of, proposed
    remedies for, 249
underservice of elderly by, 214,
    215
Community Mental Health
    Centers Act, 320
definition of, 327
requirement for services to
    elderly, 159
Community support program
    (CSP), 92
case management in, 215
components of, 161
definition of, 328
Comorbidity, 110, 118, 122
definition of, 327
relation to longer hospital
    lengths of stay, 129
Competition, 144, 145
definition of, 327
Complexity of services and
    relative value, 121–123
Concurrent review, 226
Confusional states, 1, 2
    See also Delirium
Consolidated model of care
    management, 162, 163
Constraints on service programs,
    192, 193
Consultants, management
    function in choice of, 274
Continuing care retirement
    communities (CCRC)
clients served in, 170, 171
definition of, 170, 325
Continuum of care, 72
Contracts, 93
between government agencies
    and private providers, 286
optimal duration of, 291
Control groups for outcome
    studies, 195
Copayments, 258
in Medicare, 285
Cost containment, 259, 280, 284

definition of, 327
Cost sharing
demand side, 100, 328
supply side, 100, 342
Cost shifting, 196, 229, 232, 233,
    243, 258, 259, 280, 320
definition of, 327
Cost-offset effect, 125–134, 257,
    269, 294
analysis of, 130
and methodological flaws of
    studies, 128
definition, 125
evidence for, 126
industry skepticism regarding,
    298
methodology studying, 131
reasons for, 128–130
relation to age, 128
research priorities, 131, 132
Counseling. *See* Psychotherapy
"Counselors and therapists," 140
CPT. *See* Current Procedural
    Terminology
"Creative dining," 54
CSP. *See* Community support
    program
Cuing
importance in ADL
    measurement, 192, 193
in ADL assessment, 185
Current Procedural Terminology
    (CPT) 104–106, 111–117
APA recommendations for
    changes in, 105, 111
AMA response, 106
definition of, 327
modifiers for severity, 118
psychiatric medical
    management code, 111

DAT. *See* Dementia of the
    Alzheimer's type
Death rates, 240
Decision analysis, 149
Defensive medicine, 190, 191
definition of, 323
Degenerative dementia
goals of treatment for, 180
Deinstitutionalization, 86, 91, 99,
    243

and interinstitutional transfers,
316
public criticism of, 248
role of local government, 248
shift of patients to nursing
homes, 160
Delirium
and PASARR, 261
consequences of, 8
definition of, 328
funding of treatment of, 8, 9
medical treatment of, 8, 9
prevalence of
after hip fracture, 8
after open heart surgery, 8
in hospitalized elderly, 8
Delusions, 41
Demand-side cost sharing, 100
definition of, 328
Dementia, 67
agitation in, 50
behavioral symptoms in, 50–53
treatment of, 50–52
caregiver needs in, 182, 183
coexisting with depression, 38
cost effectiveness of evaluation
of, 182
cost of nursing home care in, 29
definition of, 328
delusions in, 50
depression in, 50
early identification of, 198
effects of early diagnosis of, 183
effects of treatment on, 197,
198
effects on course of physical
illness, 183
evaluation of, 49
funding of treatment for, 5
hallucinations in, 50
medical intervention in, 5
multi-infarct, 4
prevalence, 38
in community, 4
in nursing homes, 4
of reversible cases, 181
psychosis in, 50
role of CT scan in evaluation
of, 181, 182
treatable causes of, 49
treatment of, 38, 49–51, 54–55
nonphysicians' role in, 54

physicians' role in, 54
service delivery, 54
See also Alzheimer's disease;
Degenerative dementia
Dementia of the Alzheimer's type
(DAT). *See* Alzheimer's
disease
Demography, 24, 25
Demonstration projects, 150
effects of time on, 195, 196
Departments of elderly affairs, 272
Dependency ratio, 26
Depression, 1, 2
and bereavement, 13
and disability, 38, 129
and frequency of physician
visits, 38
and major medical illness, 13
and motivation, 39
and PASARR, 261
and retirement, 23
as drug side effect, 42, 43
attitudes of primary care
physicians toward, 271
case management for, 214
coexisting with dementia, 38
cognitive impairment in, 42
definition of, 329
diagnosis of, 42
effects on course of physical
illness, 183
family intervention in, 43
funding of treatment of, 6
hospitalization for, 48
in dementia, 4
medical causes of, 42
misdiagnosis of, 102, 293
premature discontinuation of
treatment, 48, 273
prevalence of, 37, 38
in ambulatory medical care,
5
in nursing homes, 6
in the community, 5
rationale for case finding, 198
treatment of, 6, 37, 41, 44, 47,
48, 55
efficacy of, 297
goals of, 180
in general health sector, 258
physician role, 198, 199
service delivery issues, 48

service providers, 48
site of, 199
"treatment resistant," 50
underdiagnosis of, 293, 296,
    297
Depressive symptoms in dementia,
    39
Deregulation, 280, 284
Desipramine, 44, 46
Developmental disability, 206
Developmental Disability Act, 206
Diagnostic and Statistical Manual of
    Mental Disorders, Third
    Edition (DSM-III), and
    Revised (DSM-III-R), 65
    definition of, 329
    multiaxial system, 310, 311
    problems with coding of Axes
        II, IV, and V, 310, 311
Diagnostic Interview Schedule
    (DIS), 65
    definition of, 329
Diagnostic-related groups (DRGs)
    100, 102, 312, 429, 430, 438
    definition of, 329
    differentiation and validity of,
        321
    inappropriateness for
        psychiatric services, 103,
        104, 225
Diazepam, 52
Differentiation of inpatient
    facilities
    magnitude of, 309–315
    reasons for
        variation in ability to pay,
            308
        variation in environmental
            supports, 309
        variation in involuntary
            treatment, 309
        variation in patient needs,
            308
        variation in treatment
            response, 309
    relation to payment incentives,
        321
DIS. *See* Diagnostic Interview
    Schedule
DIS/DSM, 66
Disability, 28
    attribution of, 32

depression and, 32
in chronic mental illness, 247
Dorothea Dix, 98
Doxepin, low dose, 44
DRGs. *See* Diagnostic-related
    groups
Drug prescriptions, monitoring
    of, 80
DSM-III and DSM-III-R. *See*
    Diagnostic and Statistical
    Manual, Third Edition,
    Revised
Dysphoria
    definition of, 330
    in dementia, 39

ECA. *See* Epidemiologic
    Catchment Area
Economic growth rates
    implications of, for
        neuropsychiatric care,
        33, 34
Economic outcome measures,
    258, 259
Economic productivity, 257
ECT. *See* Electroconvulsive therapy
Education
    incentives for, 296
    of patients, 293, 297
    of providers, 293
Effectiveness
    definition of, 148
    measurement of, 193
Efficacy of interventions for
        depression and dementia,
        37–61
    definition of, 148
    distinction from effectiveness,
        148
Electroconvulsive therapy (ECT),
    42, 48
    and memory loss, 47
    efficacy for depression, 47
    side effects, 47
Eligibility for service programs,
    192
Epidemiologic Catchment Area
    (ECA) study, 65, 240, 242
    definition of, 330
Epilepsy
    depression in, 10
    drug interactions in, 10

prevalence of, 10
treatment of, 10
EPO. *See* Exclusive provider
    organization
Equity, 280, 284
Ethnic minorities, implications for
    regions, 26, 27
Evaluation and management
    (EM) services, 110
Excluded units, 1981
    per-discharge costs in, 315
Exclusive provider organization
    (EPO), 230–232, 234
    demonstration for elderly
        mentally ill, 232
    "locking in" of beneficiaries,
        231
    risk of underservice by, 231, 232
Expectations, role of in assessment
    design, 185, 186

Falls, 44
    relation to agitation, 40
Family, 54
    educational intervention, 54
    intervention in dementia, 54
    payment of caregivers, 191
    service needs of, 5
    therapy for elderly, lack of, 215
    understanding of
        neuropsychiatric
        disorders, 271
FASB. *See* Financial Accounting
    Standards Board
Federal Employees Health
    Benefits Program (FEHBP),
    100
Federal HMO Act, 222, 223
Feedback programs for changing
    provider behavior, 149
Fee-for-service, 146, 147, 223
    definition of, 330
FEHBP. *See* Federal Employees
    Health Benefits Program
Financial Accounting Standards
    Board (FASB), and retiree
    health benefits, 229
Fluoxetine, 46
Functional assessment, 184
    definition of, 330
    in standards for entitlements,
        268

GAO. *See* General Accounting
    Office
Gatekeeping, 301
    definition of, 331
General Accounting Office
    (GAO), 158
General health care providers, 63,
    258
    relationship with mental health
        specialists, 72
    role in treating dementia and
        depression, 284
    treatment of mental disorders
        by, 139
    use by elderly for mental
        health care, 242
    use of psychotropic drugs by, 77
General Health Questionnaire
    (GHQ), 66
    definition of, 331
General hospital inpatient
    psychiatric units
    discharges to nursing homes,
        315
    excluded, 307
    growth in, 317
    increases in numbers and use,
        316
    nonexcluded, 306
General hospitals
    and chronically mentally ill, 317
    definition of, 331
    unit versus nonunit psychiatric
        services, 311
Geriatric assessment, 196
Geriatric medicine
    psychiatry training for
        specialists in, 140
Geriatric mental health specialists
    maldistribution of, 270
    shortage of, 258, 270
Geriatric psychiatrists, 139
    and physician payment reform,
        266
    assumption of risk by, 266
    Medicare disincentives for, 289
    shortage of, 258
Geriatrics
    definition of, 331
    goals
        of dementia care, 193, 194
        of service systems, 179–184

GHQ. *See* General Health
    Questionnaire

Halfway houses, 247
Hallucinations, 41
Harvard Relative Value Study. *See*
    Resource-Based Relative
    Value Scale
HCFA. *See* Health Care Financing
    Administration
Head trauma programs, 287
Health Care Financing
    Administration (HCFA)
    261, 262, 290, 293, 295
    definition of, 331
    lack of assistance to providers,
        298
Health Insurance Experiment
    (HIE), 147
    definition of, 332
Health insurance industry, debate
    on role of, 298–304
Health maintenance organization
    (HMO), 100, 298–299
    and chronically mentally ill, 250
    basis for cost savings, 223, 224
    case management in, 223, 224
    common features of, 222, 223
    comparison with fee-for-service
        plans, 147
    definition of, 332
    mental health services in, 224
    models of, 222, 223
    open-end, 227
    specialized, for mental health
        services, 146
    staff model, appropriateness
        for elderly mentally ill,
        227, 228
Health promotion programs, 30
HIE. *See* Health Insurance
    Experiment
Hip fracture, 127
HMO. *See* Health maintenance
    organization
Home care, 79, 295
    Medicare coverage of, 33, 294
Home- and Community-Based
    Waivers
    and OBRA 1986, 251
    definition of, 332
Homelessness, 99

and mentally ill, 243, 252
    relation to failures of SSI, 248
Hospice, 79
Hospitalization for depression, 48
    expense of, 29
    See also Inpatient care
Housing, 252, 253
    and chronically mentally ill, 252
    integration with mental health
        services, 253
Housing and Urban Development
    (HUD), 252
HR 1325, 267
HR 2470. *See* Catastrophic
    Coverage Act
HUD. *See* Housing and Urban
    Development
Hypothyroidism
    cognitive impairment in, 10
    depression in, 10
    prevalence of, 10
    treatment of, 11

IADLs. *See* Instrumental activities
    of daily living
ICFs. *See* Intermediate care
    facilities
IMD. *See* Institution for Mental
    Diseases
Imipramine, 44, 46
    in depressed demented
        patients, 50
Incentives
    effect on families, 191
    for underservice, 235
    in long-term care, 187
    outcome-based, 188–192
Income, 27
Incomes of Older Americans, 239
Independent practice association
    (IPA), 223
    as managed care providers, 225
    definition of, 333
    insolvent, 231
    open-end, 227
Indigent Insane Act of 1854, 98
Indirect grants, 93
Informal care, 28
    givers of, 186
Innovation
    legal barriers to, 192, 258, 259
    regulatory barriers to, 258, 259

Innovative training, 148, 149
Inpatient psychiatric care
    alternatives to, 299
    changes over time
        due to deinstitutionaliza-
            tion, 316
        in site of hospitalization, 316
    incentives for overutilization,
        286
    See also Hospitalization
Inpatient psychiatric units
    differences in costs among, 315
    use by elderly, 87
Inpatient psychiatric units,
    306–321
    in general hospital, 78
    types of, 306–308
    use by elderly, 242
"Inside limits," 99
Institute of Medicine Study, 188
Institution for Mental Diseases
    (IMD), 247
    definition of, 332
Institutionalization, 40
    prevention by psychiatric
        treatment, 129
Instrumental activities of daily
    living (IADLs), 184
    definition of, 332
    in determining program
        eligibility, 185
    methodological concerns in
        assessing, 185
Intergenerational wealth transfers,
    26, 31, 32
Intermediate care facilities (ICFs)
    cost of care in, 29
    definition of, 332
Involuntary treatment, 314
IPA. *See* Independent practice
    association

Kennedy, Senator Edward, 268

Labor costs
    control by private sector, 291
    in public sector facilities, 291
LCAH. *See* Life care at home
LCCs. *See* Life care communities
Length of stay, 287
    and treatment efficacy, 312–314
    difference by payer, 321

differences among inpatient
    settings
    general versus private versus
        public, 312, 313
    in long-stay hospitals, 313
    unit versus nonunit
        hospitals, 313
    in general hospital inpatient
        psychiatric units 306, 307
    in managed care system, 301
    in psychiatric hospitals, 307, 308
    in "scatter" beds, 306
    relation to psychiatric
        comorbidity, 129
    trends in, 317
    variation across states, 318
Licensing and certification of
    nursing homes, 276
Life care at home (LCAH), 170,
    171
    definition of, 171, 333
    services provided by, 171
    target population of, 171
Life care communities (LCCs),
    163, 170–173
    definition of, 170
    nursing home care in, 171
    options for mental health care,
        171, 172
Lithium and augmentation of
    antidepressants, 46
Litigation, fear of, 190, 191
Locked-door units, 54
Long-stay hospital, 313
Long-term care
    approach of aging field, 157
    approach of mental health
        field, 157
    case management in, 173,
        206–209
    community-based, 208
    cost containment in, 173
    definition of, 333
    federal legislation, 268, 269
        role of neuropsychiatric
            assessment in, 268, 269
    financing of, 88
    in public sector, 290
    incentives in, 1987
    limitations for mental health
        care, 173

linkage to neuropsychiatric
care needs, 301
measurement of quality in,
187, 188
need for psychiatric
components of, 172
regulation of, 187, 188
services, assessment in, 184–185
shortfalls in coverage for, 106
treatment in, 186
Long-term care insurance
and mental health services, 300
case management in, 209
definition of, 333
home health benefits, 89
regulation of, 266
Long-term care models,
psychiatric component of,
157–177

Maladaptive emotional
consequences to predictable
crises
consequences of, 13, 14
funding of treatment, 14
treatment of, 14
Managed care, 69, 221–237
and the elderly mentally ill, 225
definition of, 333
potential for decreased
hospitalization, 250
problems specific to elderly
populations, 228, 229
untested assumptions, 234
Managed care systems, 274
access to mental health services
in, 259
Management function of medical
care. See Care management
MAOIs. See Monoamine oxidase
inhibitors
Market segmentation, 135–155
definition of, 334
research recommendations
regarding, 147–150
Market share
of Medicare in mental health
services, 321
of various mental health
providers, 136
Mayo Clinic, 226
Medicaid, 2, 5, 6, 25, 29
and chronically mentally ill, 243
and cost-shifting, 245, 320, 321
and general hospital
psychiatric are, 249, 250
and transfer from state
hospitals to nursing
homes 320, 321
as payer of last resort, 90
capitation in, 251
coverage of mental health
services, 79
coverage of partial
hospitalization, 79
debate on role of, 293–298
definition of, 334
effects on states' responsibility,
86
eligibility of mentally ill for, 247
differences among states,
288
funding of case management
by, 88, 251, 294
funding of mental health
services, 246, 247
in nursing homes, 262
funding of nursing home care,
158, 260
limitation of reimbursement to
CMHCs, 159
perverse incentives in, 247
policy on organic mental
disorders, 103
"Spend down," 88
Medicaid waivers, 192, 206–208,
276, 281
coverage of case management
under, 207
difficulties in using, 293
Medical education, geriatrics in,
285
Medical evaluation for elderly
persons with behavioral
disorder, 264, 265
Medical management
amount of, 104
benefits for, 102
distinction from
psychotherapy, 103, 105
risks of, 104
Medicare, 29, 32, 93
and access to hospital care, 239
and chronically mentally ill, 243

and funding of home health
care, 232
as "earned entitlement," 90
"at risk" contracts with HMOs,
146
benefits, definition of, 335
capitated payments to HMOs,
223
claims
variation across states, 318
for nonaged beneficiaries,
318
copayments and caps, 87, 88,
285
coverage of mental health
services, 318–321
190-day lifetime limit, 319
and TEFRA, 319
and PPS, 319
and prospective payment
system, 319
limits abolished by OBRA
1989, 319
debate on role of, 293–298
definition of, 334
effects on states' responsibility,
86
eligibility, disability and, 319
expenditures for psychiatric
services, 319, 320
funding of mental health
services, 109
limits on coverage, 126
funding of psychiatric-medical
units, 79
incentives for inpatient
psychiatric treatment, 199
"medical management"
benefit, 102
participating physician,
definition of, 335
patients, interfacility transfers
of, 315
payment for cognitive services,
78
payment for psychologists' and
social workers' services,
262–264
payment setting under TEFRA,
319, 320
payments to nonparticipating
physicians, 110

program priorities, 33
prospective payment system,
245
scope of coverage, 5, 6
of psychiatric treatment, 98,
246
of treatment for depression,
293
shortfalls of, 101
use of psychiatric inpatient
services by beneficiaries,
310
use by nonaged disabled,
310
Medicare waivers, 206, 207, 276
and caregivers, 192
and community care, 192
coverage of case management
under, 207
Medigap
definition of, 335
possible expansions of, 299
psychiatric benefits of, 87
Mental disorders
disability from, 66
in the elderly, 257
prevalence in nursing homes,
160
problems with diagnosis of, 283
producing physical illness, 129
relation to general health care
service use, 125
underdiagnosis of, 257
undertreatment of, 257
See also Psychiatric disorders;
Neuropsychiatric
disorders; Mental illness
Mental health, definition of, 336
Mental health benefits
as proportion of total
insurance costs, 304
in prepaid plans, 224, 225
Mental health HMO, 250
Mental health measures in
demonstration projects, 258
Mental health professionals
differences among, 141
in general health settings, 80
direct versus indirect
services by, 92–94
training needs of, 258

Mental health services
  at senior centers, 284
  availability in elderly housing,
      281
  by general health care
      providers, 77, 78
  recommendations, 77, 78
  differences across states in,
      317, 318
  federal role in funding of, 90
  in day care, 284
  integration with housing, 253
  options for change in, 77
  provision by generalists, 69
  provision by specialists, 73
  research recommendations, 80
  state role in, 91
  use in community, 73–76
  use in institutions, 76
  use of current system, 72, 73
Mental health services for elderly,
    financing of, 222–224
Mental Health Systems Act of
    1980, 92
Mental illness, 2
Mental status, definition of, 336
Mental Status Questionnaire
    (MSQ), 167
  definition of, 336
Mental symptoms of physical
    illness, 64
Methylphenidate, 45
Mianserin, 46
Milieu therapy, definitional
    problems, 314
Mitchell, Senator, 268
Models of excellence, 288
Monitoring, as component of case
    management, 202
Monoamine oxidase inhibitors
    (MAOIs)
  efficacy for depression, 45
  in depressed demented
      patients, 45
  orthostatic hypotension, 45
  side effects, 44, 45
Mood
  definition of, 336
  measurement of, 185
Mood disorder, definition of, 336
Moral hazard, 99, 100

MSQ. See Mental Status
    Questionnaire
Multi-infarct dementia, 49
Multiple payers, 85–108
  definition of, 337

National Association of
    Insurance Commissioners
    (NAIC), model long-term
    care insurance regulation,
    266, 267
National Conference on Access
    and Financing for
    Neuropsychiatric Care for
    the Elderly, 279
National Hospital Discharge
    Survey, 308
National Institute of Mental
    Health (NIMH), 297
  definition of, 338
National Institute on Aging
    (NIA), 297
National Long-Term Care
    Demonstration. See
    Channeling Demonstration
National Nursing Home Survey,
    157, 160
National Register of Health
    Service Providers in
    Psychology 138
Near-poverty, 239
Need for mental health services,
    63–66
Neuroleptics, 53
  in dementia, 51
  relation to deinstitutionaliza-
      tion, 243
Neuropsychiatric assessment,
    14–16
  examination in, 14, 15
  functional assessment in, 15
  history in, 14
  importance of timely access to,
      32
  laboratory tests in, 15
  linkage to long-term care
      insurance, 300
  table of components of, 16
  work-site based, 31
Neuropsychiatric needs, linkage
    to long-term care needs, 301

Neuropsychiatric problems
  cost implications of, 40
  recognition of, 269–273
  treatment of, 16
Neuropsychiatry, 3
  definition of, 337
Neuropsychology, 138
  definition of, 337
NIA. *See* National Institute on
  Aging
NIMH. *See* National Institute of
  Mental Health
Nomenclature, 2
  "emotional problems," 3
Nortriptyline, 44, 45
Nursing
  case management elements in,
    203, 204
  diagnosis in, 204
  geriatric nurse practitioners,
    137
Nursing facility
  definition of, 338
  See also Nursing homes
Nursing Home Reform Act,
  260–262
  See also Omnibus Budget
    Reconciliation Act of
    1987
Nursing homes, 2, 79
  and chronically mentally ill
    residents of, 245
    medical comorbidity in, 245
    services available for, 245
  and stigma, 288
  case mix in, 245
  consultation to, 258
  costs of, comparison with home
    care, 207, 208
  coverage of services
    in S/HMO plans, 167
    in Life Care Communities,
      171
  definition of, 338
  effects of screening patients for
    mental disorders in, 293
  estimates for use by elderly,
    157, 158
  lack of mental health
    professionals in, 245
  licensing and certification of,
    276

  management function in
    choice of, 274
  Medicaid funding of, 158
  placement in, role of
    nonpsychiatric factors,
    132
  prevalence of mental disorders
    in, 160
  psychogeriatric units in, 80
  reform, implications for, and
    mentally ill elderly, 253,
    254
  residents of
    case management for, 214
    disincentives to service by
      private psychiatrists, 159
    underdiagnosis of mental
      problems in, 159
    undertreatment of mental
      problems in, 159
    underrecognition of mental
      disorders in, 215

O<small>BRA</small> 1981, 208
OBRA 1986, 251
OBRA 1987. *See* Omnibus Budget
  Reconciliation Act of 1987
OBRA 1989. *See* Omnibus Budget
  Reconciliation Act of 1989
Office of Technology Assessment,
  216
Ohio program for SSI
  determinations for mentally
  ill, 252
Older Americans Act, 135, 215
Older workers, 29, 32
  labor force participation rate,
    30
Omnibus Budget Reconciliation
  Act (OBRA) of 1987, 79,
  103, 104, 188, 253, 290
  definition of, 338
  mandate for uniform data set
    in, 262
  nursing home reform
    provisions of (Nursing
    Home Reform Act),
    260–262
  and assessment, 261
  and psychotropic drug
    therapy, 261
  and social services, 261

psychosocial outcome
measures in, 261
preadmission screening, 89
Omnibus Budget Reconciliation
Act of 1989, 110, 121
definition of, 338
elimination of Medicare
outpatient cap, 262–264
Medicare reimbursement of
psychologists and social
workers, 262–264
On Lok, 146, 163, 168–170, 173,
233, 253
adaptation of model for
chronically mentally ill,
174
characterization of clients, 169
definition of, 168
eligibility for, 169
evaluation of, 170
financing of, 169
history of, 168, 169
service components in, 169
On-site services, 293
Medicare payments for, 295
subsidies for, 296
Organic delusional disorder, 41
Organic hallucinosis, 41
Organic mental disorders
in Medicare beneficiaries, 311
Outcome-based quality measures,
188, 189
Outcome-based reimbursement,
286
barriers to, 190
Outcomes
of long-term care, 188, 189
linkage to goals, 194
Outpatient commitment, 227
Outpatient treatment, increases in
use of, 317
Over-the-counter drugs, risks of, 11
Oxazepam, 52

Paranoia, 7
Paraphrenia, 7
Parkinson's disease
cognitive impairment in, 9
confusional states in, 9
dementia in, 9, 49
depression in, 9
prevalence of, 9

psychosis in, 9
treatment of, 9
Partial hospitalization, 288, 299,
301
definition of, 339
PASARR. *See* Pre-Admission
Screening and Annual
Resident Review
Pastoral counselors, 140
lack of geriatric training for,
141
Pew Memorial Trust, 208
Phenelzine, 45
Physical restraint, 54
Physician payment reform,
109–124, 264–266
Physician Payment Reform
Commission (PPRC), 109,
122
definition of, 340
Placement. *See* Institutionalization
Polypharmacy, 11
Poorhouses, 85
Postural hypotension, 44
Poverty, 27, 239
PPO. *See* Preferred provider
organization
PPRC. *See* Physician Payment
Reform Commission
PPS. *See* Prospective payment
system
Pre-Admission Screening and
Annual Resident Review
(PASARR) 290
and chronically mentally ill, 261
and delirium, 261
and depression, 261
and stress reactions, 261
cost shifting function of, 260
definition of "active
treatment," 261
definition of, 339
Preadmission screening
disincentives for use of
community services, 158
GAO 1979 recommendations
for, 158
Preadmission screening and
Annual Resident Review. *See*
PASARR
Precertification, 226

Preferred provider organization
(PPO), 100
appropriateness for elderly
mentally ill, 227, 228
as managed care providers, 225
definition of, 339
Prepaid plans
mental health benefits and
utilization in, 224, 225
Prepayment, 100, 147, 210, 223
definition of, 340
Prescription drug abuse, 1, 13
Prescription drug psychotoxicity,
1, 272, 295
treatment by general health
care providers, 258
President's Commission on
Mental Health, 240
Prevalence of mental disorders in
elderly, 63–65
in institutions, 67–69
in nursing homes, 67–69
Primary care physicians
attitudes toward depression,
271
education of, 272, 273
efforts to modify detection of
mental disorders by, 140
limitations of, 40
mental health skills of, 281
misdiagnosis of neuropsychiatric problems by, 270
training in mental health of, 78
training needs of, 258
underrecognition of
psychiatric disorders by,
122
"Primary nurses," 78, 204
Private medical insurance
exclusion of psychiatric care by,
98
mental illness coverage by, 229
benefit limits of, 229
copayments for, 229
Private providers
cost control by, 286
debate on role of, 286–292
increase in, 317
lack of interest in chronically
mentally ill by, 286
"skimming" by, 286, 292

Private psychiatric hospitals, 283,
307, 308
1981 per-discharge costs in, 315
growth in, 317
investor-owned, 308
role in regional planning, 275,
276
use by elderly, 87
voluntary, 307
Private psychiatrists
in nursing homes, 159
treatment of elderly by, 138, 139
Productivity, 23, 29
Program evaluation, 258
costs of, 196, 197
Prospective payment system
(PPS), 13, 93, 163, 199, 131,
225, 245
definition of, 340
Protriptyline, 44
Provider disciplines
effects of, 143
relative roles of, 2, 3
Psychiatric complications of
physical illness, 64
Psychiatric consultation, 79, 258
under-utilization for aged
patients, 127
Psychiatric emergency services
as point of access to care, 250
Psychiatric liaison services, 131
effect on acute care costs, 127,
128
effect on post-discharge
dispositions, 127
Psychiatric-medical units, 79
Psychiatrists
effects of competition on fees
of, 144
geriatric training of, 139
licensure and certification, 138
training for work in primary
care settings, 78
Psychologists
Medicare reimbursement of,
262–264
OBRA 1989 requirement to
consult with attending
physicians, 263
specialization in aging, 138
training and licensure, 138

Psychoses
  in dementia, 4, 52
  prevalence in elderly, 241
Psychostimulants, 45
Psychotherapy
  changes in practice since WW
    II, 314
  determinants of practice
    patterns, 142
  for depression, 47
  in general health sector, 80
  standards for, 142
Psychotherapy, intensive
  definitional problems, 314
Psychotoxicity of prescription
    drugs
  anxiety, 11
  common causes of, 11
  delirium, 11
  depression, 11
  incidence of, 11
  insomnia, 11
  memory loss, 11
  treatment of, 12
Psychotropic drugs, 76, 79, 80
  in nursing homes, 54
Psychotropic medications. See
    Psychotropic drugs
Psy.D. degree, 138
Public hospitals
  1981 per-discharge costs in, 315
  treatment of disabled in, 310
  uncompensated care in, 321
Public mental health system, and
    chronically mentally ill, 280,
    284
Public psychiatric hospitals
  length of stay in, 308
  public sector role in treatment
    of, 230
  types of patients in, 308
Public-private collaboration, 286

Quality assessment, 188
Quality assurance (QA)
  definition of, 340
  proprietary products for, 304
  role in cost containment, 299
Quality of care, 148

Randomized controlled trial
  (RCT), 148

  definition of, 341
RBRVS. See Resource-Based
  Relative Value Scale
RCT. See Randomized controlled
  trial
Referrals
  between inpatient settings, 314
  to mental health professionals,
    77, 78
Regional differences, 275, 276, 280
  in Medicaid, 275
  in psychiatrist supply, 275
  in state mental health systems,
    275
Regulation, 281
Rehabilitation, 197
Relative value scale, 295, 109–124
  effect on diagnosis of
    depression, 297
  See also Resource-Based Relative
    Value Scale
Residential treatment, 247
Resource coordination. See Case
    management
Resource utilization groups
    (RUGS), 193
  definition of, 341
Resource-Based Relative Value
    Scale, 104–106, 109–124
  adjustment for time, 123
  definition of, 340
  Harvard study, 110, 117–119,
    264
    criticisms of, 105
    cross-links between
      specialties, 119, 120
    limitations of psychiatric
      vignettes, 118
    medicine services, 117, 118
    relative values for
      psychiatric versus internal
  research priorities, 119, 122,
    123
  risks of inappropriate relative
    values, 121
  special considerations for
    elderly psychiatric
    patients 264
Respite care, 79, 186, 187
  as "loss leader" for private
    nursing homes, 291
  definition of, 341

lack of coverage by Medicaid,
88
outcomes of, 193, 194
Restraints, 40
Retiree health benefits, FASB
standards, 229
Retirement, 13, 29, 30
and depression, 23
Retirement age, 26
Rhode Island
capitated mental health system
in, 250
Risk management, 259
Robert Wood Johnson
Foundation, 208
program for chronically
mentally ill, 91, 210
Rochester, N.Y., capitated mental
health system in, 250
RUGS. *See* Resource utilization
groups

Scatter beds, 78, 306, 311
1981 per-discharge costs in, 315
Schizophrenia, 1, 2, 67
funding of treatment for, 7
in Medicare beneficiaries, 311
increase in prevalence in
blacks, 241
long-term course, 241, 242
prevalence, 6, 7
prevalence in elderly, 241
Screening tools, 78
Senile dementia. *See* Alzheimer's
disease
Senile dementia of the
Alzheimer's type (DAT). *See*
Alzheimer's disease
Senile dementia of the Alzheimer
type (SDAT). *See*
Alzheimer's disease
Senility, 85
Service needs, 80
S/HMO. *See* Social/health
maintenance organizations
Short Portable Mental Status
Questionnaire (SPMSQ),
164
definition of, 342
Skilled nursing facilities (SNF)
cost of care, 29
definition of, 341

elderly mentally ill in, 229
Social/health maintenance
organization (S/HMO) 163,
166–168, 224, 234, 300
case management in, 209
characterization of clients of,
166
definition of, 166, 341
eligibility for, 166
evaluation of, 168
financing of, 168
mental health treatment in, 168
low utilization, 168
shortage of psychiatrists, 168
shortcomings of, related to
mental health, 168
Social Security, 31
Social Security Administration
(SSA)
definition of, 342
Social Security Disability, and
chronically mentally ill, 252
Social Security Disability
Insurance (SSDI)
and chronically mentally ill, 243
definition of, 342
Social skills training, 80
Social work, 137
"auxiliary function model," 204
case management elements in,
203, 204
Somatization, 129
definition of, 342
SNF. *See* Skilled nursing facilities
Specialty mental health inpatient
settings. *See* Inpatient
psychiatric units
Specialty mental health sector
profiles of providers, 136–139
See also Mental health
professionals
SPMSQ. *See* Short Portable Mental
Status Questionnaire
SSA. *See* Social Security
Administration
SSDI. *See* Social Security Disability
Insurance
SSI. *See* Supplemental Security
Income
Staff:patient ratios, 287
Standardization
of care, 149, 150

of diagnosis and treatment, 299
Stark, Congressman Fortney ("Pete"), 267, 268
State and county mental hospitals
use by elderly, 87
See also Public hospitals
State and local agencies
debate on role of, 280–285
private sector relations with, 282, 283
State Care Acts, 85, 86, 98
State governments
responsibility for chronically mentally ill, 258
role in funding community care, 249
State hospitals, 86, 283
as locus of treatment for schizophrenia, 7
case mix of Medicare discharges, 312
expenditures by, 317
State mental health systems
collaboration with nursing homes, 262
inappropriateness of for acute depression, 285
uncompensated care in, 321
States
relationship to local agencies, 282
role in regional planning, 276
Stigma, 2, 32, 101, 102, 126, 263, 265, 268, 270, 271, 293
and nursing homes, 288
Stroke
depression in, 9
treatment of, 9
prevalence of, 9
Suicide, 38
as consequence of depression, 6
Supplemental Security Income (SSI)
and chronically mentally ill, 243, 247
definition of, 342
eligibility for, 247
Supplier-induced demand, 143
Supply-side cost sharing, 100
definition of, 342

Tax Equity and Fiscal Responsibility Act of 1982 (TEFRA)
and copayment to psychiatric hospitals, 307, 308
and Medicare payments to HMOs, 223
cap on reimbursement of inpatient care, 289
definition of, 342
"TEFRA Cap," 289
TEFRA. *See* Tax Equity and Fiscal Responsibility Act of 1982
Third-party payments, 93
Tort reform, 276
Transfers between hospitals
cost-shifting effects of, 320, 321
Trazodone
for agitation, 52
in dementia, 52
in depressed demented patients, 46
lack of anticholinergic effect, 46
Tricyclic antidepressants, 42–44
low dose, 44
Trimipramine, 44

Uncertainty, in medical practice, 136
Underrecognition of mental disorders, 126
Underservice
of elderly mentally ill, 242
Undertreatment of mental disorders, 126
Underutilization, need for research on causes of, 273
Uniform Data Set, 262
Unmet need
estimates of, 222
in community, 76
in institutions, 76
UR. *See* Utilization review
Use of mental health services by elderly, 125, 126
Utilization review (UR)
definition of, 343
effects on care, 226
role in cost containment, 299

Values
    relevance to outcome
        assessment, 189
Variations among regions. *See*
    Regional differences
Vegetative signs, definition of, 343
Veterans Administration Hospitals
    as locus of treatment for
        schizophrenia, 7
    definition of, 343
    use by elderly, 87
Violence, 40
Vitamin B$_{12}$ deficiency
    cognitive impairment in, 11
    confusion in, 11
    depression in, 11
    prevalence of, 11

treatment of, 11
Vocational rehabilitation
    counselors, 205

Waiver
    definition of, 343
    See also Medicare waivers;
        Medicaid waivers
Wandering, 53, 54
    nondrug treatment of, 53
Waxman, Congressman Henry, 268
Women, economic issues
    concerning, 26
"Woodwork effect," 234
Workers' compensation, 291

Yuppies, aging, 287